Endorsements for *The Tribes of the Person-Centred Nation (3rd edition): An introduction to the world of person-centred therapies*

This landmark third edition of *Tribes* offers a cornucopia of person-centred concepts, protocols and practices. Here we have a rich array of contemporary approaches to person-centred therapy that will be valued by practitioners, trainers, supervisors, as well as trainees seeking to understand more about the multiple ways that person-centred therapy has been envisioned and practised. This book is not to be missed. It will become a classic for those seeking to access valuable narratives on the contemporary person-centred therapy landscape. Mick Cooper is an excellent editorial lead, stepping into the shoes of the much-missed Pete Sanders to foster this enormously engaging, multidimensional collection of narratives on traditional and contemporary approaches to person-centred work. As Mick notes in the concluding chapter, each of the tribes has much to contribute to the rich kaleidoscope of person-centred theories and practices.
Lynne Gabriel OBE, Professor of Counselling & Mental Health, York St John University

This text is one of a kind in bringing together for comparison and clarification the vibrant range of developments within the person-centred nation. It provides clear, expert descriptions of each 'tribe', up to date in theory and research, and brings to life the practice in each tribe with engaging case vignettes that highlight both the differences and the commonalities across these vibrant and evolving approaches. It represents a unique, must-read text for all students on professional trainings, as well as for experienced therapists across orientations.
Peter Pearce, Director of Clinical Training, Metanoia Institute

Carl Rogers' influence on the development of psychotherapy was wide-ranging. In this much-awaited third edition, Mick Cooper has brought together a remarkable range of authors and proponents of the different therapies that have roots in Rogers' work. Cooper challenges us to consider the boundaries of person-centredness and the commonalities and differences of these approaches. It is essential reading for students and anyone interested in the wider legacy of Rogers and the health of humanistic therapies today.
Professor Stephen Joseph, University of Nottingham, and author of *Think Like a Therapist*

This is a magnificent book presenting a range of distinctive work and important developments within the person-centred nation. Mick Cooper has done a magnificent job in bringing together this stimulating, rich resource that is both scholarly and accessible, with its theoretical insights, case examples of therapist key skills, suggested reading and further sources for exploration. It will be of enormous value to those in training and seasoned person-centred therapists alike. I also recommend it to therapists of all orientations as it is full of inspiration for contemporary therapeutic practice.
Divine Charura, Professor of Counselling Psychology, York St John University

A number of branches have grown from the roots of person-centred hypotheses and philosophy. In this accessible text, each chapter author lays out a rationale for why their 'tribe' belongs in the person-centred family. For students seeking clarity and for practitioners looking to locate themselves within the branches, this is essential reading.
Janet Tolan, counselling, supervisor and co-editor of *People Not Pathology*

Cooper's new edition of Sanders' work wonderfully elucidates the theoretical/clinical clusters we gravitate to as practitioners. It beautifully highlights the historical and contemporary developments within our vibrant kaleidoscope of practice groupings. It is significant reading for both students and qualified therapists alike.
Christine Brown, Founding partner, LC&CTA

This book is an important resource for readers keen to understand, explore and debate the similarities, tensions and differences that exist in the various branches of the person-centred nation. It is a potent demonstration of Margaret Warner's assertion that 'Person-centred therapy should not be considered a single form of psychotherapy, but rather a cluster of therapies sharing some broad values'.
Colin Lago, independent therapist and writer, inspired by person-centred thinking and practice for more than 50 years

3RD EDITION

The Tribes of the Person-Centred Nation

AN INTRODUCTION TO THE WORLD OF PERSON-CENTRED THERAPIES

EDITED BY MICK COOPER

PCCS BOOKS

First edition published 2004
Second edition published 2012
Third edition published 2024
Product code – 012026700

PCCS Books Ltd, Wyastone Business Park, Wyastone Leys, Monmouth NP25 3SR
admin@pccs-books.co.uk
www.pccs-books.co.uk

The Tribes of the Person-Centred Nation (3rd edition): An introduction to the world of person-centred therapies

British Library Cataloguing in Publication data: a catalogue record for this book is available from the British Library.

ISBNs
paperback – 978 1 915220 47 9
epub – 978 1 915220 48 6

Cover design Jason Anscomb
Cover image: AureliasDreams / Alamy Stock Photo

Typeset in-house by PCCS Books
Printed in the UK by Bell & Bain Ltd, Glasgow

Contents

Dedication

To Pete Sanders, with all our love

Acknowledgements

With particular gratitude to all the authors in the first and second editions. Your work laid the foundations for and flows into what appears here, and has inspired and nourished several generations of practitioners over the past decade.

Special thanks to Catherine Jackson and the team at PCCS Books, who have worked tirelessly to bring out a new edition of this text.

About the editor

Mick Cooper is Professor of Counselling Psychology at the University of Roehampton and a practising counselling psychologist. Mick is author and editor of a range of texts on person-centred, existential, and relational approaches to therapy, including *Working at Relational Depth in Counselling and Psychotherapy* (2nd ed., Sage, 2018, with Dave Mearns), *Pluralistic Counselling and Psychotherapy* (Sage, 2011, with John McLeod), and *Integrating Counselling and Psychotherapy: Directionality, synergy, and social change* (Sage, 2019). Mick has led a series of research studies – both qualitative and quantitative – exploring the processes and outcomes of person-centred counselling with young people, and has published in a range of leading international psychotherapy journals.

Mick is a Fellow of the British Association for Counselling and Psychotherapy and the Academy of Social Sciences. Mick's latest book, *Psychology at the Heart of Social Change: Towards a progressive vision for society* (Bristol University, 2023), explores the contribution that therapeutic theory and practice can make to wider social progress and justice.

He is the father of four children and lives in Brighton, on the south coast of England.

Introduction

Mick Cooper[1]

Something a lot of people didn't know about Pete Sanders was that he was great at table tennis. I didn't know that either, until he came to the house where my family and I were then living, in Glasgow, and was zipping around our table like lightning, slapping the ball at me and all full of tricks and techniques – wow! Like many of us across the person-centred, counselling and radical psychiatry communities, I miss Pete enormously. He was an extraordinary figure: vivacious, warm, passionate, fiercely intelligent. Being brilliant at table tennis was just the start of his superpowers.

It was a great honour to be invited by PCCS Books to edit the third edition of this book, and a testament to Pete's work, creativity and vision that it has already achieved such a standing in the person-centred field. *The Tribes of the Person-Centred Nation*, with a first edition in 2004 and a second in 2012 (both edited by Pete), was the first text to comprehensively, accessibly introduce the principal schools of thought and practice that had evolved from the work of American psychologist Carl Rogers. I remember Pete's excitement and enthusiasm for the book when he first described it to me, back in the early 2000s. Pete loved the person-centred field; he loved its values and its commitment to individual and social empowerment. I think the book was a way for Pete to share his love for the person-centred approach: to show – not just to those starting out in the field but also to those already in it and those outside of it – its richness, depth and complexity, and to help trainees find their way around this multifaceted and, at times, seemingly contradictory field.

I also think Pete, as a loving and community-oriented man, wanted to bring the person-centred nation closer together. As he wrote in his Introduction to the second edition (Sanders,

1. Sections of this Introduction are taken or adapted from the introductions to the first and second editions, written by Pete Sanders. I am, in this respect, not the sole author of this Introduction. But, of course, Pete is no longer with us; I take full responsibility, therefore – but not full credit – for what is written here.

2012a): 'Our mission is to bring the UK person-centred community into a more intimate relationship with its natural "family" – some of the other tribes of our nation' (p.xi).

What is a tribe of the person-centred nation?

Tribes of the person-centred nation can be defined as approaches to therapy that are grounded, substantially or wholly, in the teachings of Carl Rogers. These are approaches that emphasise in particular the therapist-provided conditions of empathy, acceptance and congruence, and a high degree of client self-direction. The term comes from Margaret Warner's (2000) paper, 'Person-centered psychotherapy: One nation, many tribes', published in the *Person-Centered Journal*. In that paper she writes: 'Person-centered therapy should not be considered a single form of psychotherapy, but rather a cluster of therapies sharing some broad values' (p.28). That is, person-centred therapy is not one thing but a collection of approaches emanating from a shared source. Warner goes on to state that we should celebrate and debate our diversity, 'while remembering that we are, at core, "one nation" whose commonalities far outweigh our differences' (pp.37–38).

Warner's call to celebrate difference and diversity across the person-centred tribes has not always been heeded. I remember an almost stand-up fight between two eminent advocates of different person-centred approaches at the first world person-centred conference I ever attended, in Egmond aan Zee (Netherlands) in 2003 – hardly a demonstration of unconditional positive regard! Readers of this book may have only a patchy knowledge of what is sometimes referred to as the 'turf wars' in the field of person-centred therapies. These are the tensions that occur when any new strand of theory and practice emerges in any area of human endeavour. These tensions are to do with ownership of the ideas; the tendency to wonder whether they are correct, and what happens when and if they are amended, superseded or added to as a result of new thinking or new evidence. The history of psychotherapy is a history of big ideas, developments, disagreements and splits. The world of person-centred therapy is no different. Carl Rogers (1957, 1959) had a big idea in the shape of his 'if… then' hypothesis regarding the six 'necessary and sufficient' conditions, which threw down the gauntlet at the feet of his establishment peers. Since that time, there have been developments, vigorous disagreements and a following of different paths in the person-centred field. Indeed, Pete and I came to develop quite different views of the person-centred approach: his always more classical (see Chapter 2, this volume); mine moving increasingly in a pluralistic direction (see Chapter 9, this volume). However, the vast majority of person-centred practitioners worldwide are dedicated to working together, uncomfortable though that might sometimes be, to further refine their understanding and practice in the service of clients. This is the spirit in which this book has evolved.

But what makes a 'tribe' a tribe? Is, for instance, the 'person-centred cognitive behaviour therapy' developed by Canadian psychologists Josefowitz and Myran (2005) a 'tribe' of the person-centred approach? What about Natalie Rogers' (1993) person-centred expressive arts therapy? The answer to this question is somewhat arbitrary, in that there is no definitive set of criteria 'out there' against which such a decision can be made. Different people have different views, and they are highly dependent on how the term 'person-centred' itself is defined. For the purposes of this book, I am following Pete in defining 'person-centred' as approaches to therapy grounded, substantially or wholly, in the teachings of Carl Rogers. However, a definition of 'person-centred' that is based, for instance, on the six 'necessary and sufficient conditions' (Rogers, 1957, 1959) could lead to a very different conceptualisation of the tribes. Any answer is also likely to be parochial, in the sense that what qualifies as a tribe in one region of the world may not be identified as such in another.

For the purposes of this book, my selection is based around the following criteria:

- There must be a coherent and distinctive theoretical base for the approach, with clear and explicit links to the work of Rogers.
- There must be literature available in the UK that lays out these basic elements of the approach.
- There must be training opportunities available in the UK, either as a specialist training or as a significant proportion of existing person-centred trainings.

In these respects, a 'tribe' is not simply a new idea, however elegant or however it might revolutionise our practice. Mearns and Thorne's (2000) 'configurations of self' or Warner's (2013) 'fragile processes', for instance, are important ideas for the person-centred field, but they have not, in themselves, spawned new schools of theory or practice that have developed their own identity. Having said that, so difficult is this brief that not all of these criteria have been fully met by all the tribes represented in this book. It seemed reasonable to bend the rules a little, since part of this book's mission is to encourage and give support to fledgling practitioners in the UK and to issue a call for training and literature in approaches that in mainland Europe are taken for granted. For example, there is no UK training exclusively devoted to existentially informed person-centred therapy, yet these ideas are given substantial coverage in a range of courses.

A gathering of the tribes

My aim in this third edition, like Pete's in the first and second, is to provide an opportunity for readers interested in person-centred approaches to counselling and psychotherapy to find out more about the history of these ideas and practices and how they developed into stand-alone approaches. My hope, again shared with Pete, is that this will not only enrich your current understanding but also better inform your choices of further training and ways of working. The authors of the various chapters have covered the value-base, philosophical roots, theory, practice and relevant research relating to each approach to help readers explore where they stand. They are not presenting a cast-iron definition of each tribe –indeed, most would assert that the definitions are constantly adapting. Each chapter is the author's (or authors') own interpretation of the approach they represent, although in all instances they are founders or key representatives of that approach. Readers will find overlap and disagreement. This is as it should be, since we are swimming in muddy waters. If tolerating discomfort while struggling for meaning and clarity is not to your taste, then you may find the reading difficult.

The tribes identified for this third edition of the book are as follows:

- Classical person-centred therapy (Chapter 2) – the 'original' approach, the starting point of it all, as described in Carl Rogers' early writings, but still pervasive today.
- The relational approach to person-centred therapy (Chapter 3) – a contemporary modification of the classical approach, emphasising a two-person, dialogical encounter.
- Focusing-oriented therapy (FOT, Chapter 4) – evolving from the work of Eugene Gendlin, Carl Rogers' close colleague.
- Emotion-focused therapy (EFT, Chapter 5) – integrates active therapeutic methods from Gestalt and other humanistic therapies within the frame of a person-centred relationship.
- Person-centred experiential counselling for depression (PCE-CfD, Chapter 6) – combines classical and emotion-focused approaches for implementation in England's NHS.
- Motivational interviewing (MI, Chapter 7) – initially developed for problem drinkers, uses a range of active methods to draw out the client's own motivation for change.
- Existentially-informed person-centred therapy (Chapter 8) – draws existential philosophical insights, such as the inherent freedom of human being, into a person-centred, relational practice.
- Pluralistic person-centred therapy (Chapter 9) – emphasises flexibility, integration and collaboration to personalise therapy to the unique, individual client.
- Person-centred creative arts therapies (Chapter 10) – uses a wide variety of arts media, including visual art, movement and music, to facilitate creativity and growth.
- Pre-therapy (Chapter 11) – empathic and closely reflective methods that aim to re-establish 'contact' with those experiencing severe psychological disconnection.
- Child-centred play therapy (CCPT, Chapter 12) – extends and develops non-directive principles to working with children.

As with any great thinker, Carl Rogers' work was manifold, and different tribes can be seen as actualising different elements of his teachings. For example, the classical person-centred approach tends to take forward Rogers' emphasis on non-directivity; EFT, his focus on emotions; and person-centred creative arts therapies, his beliefs in the power of creativity. In this way, multiple approaches can be 'Rogerian' without necessarily all saying the same thing. Like a tree, one trunk can branch off in many directions.

The book begins with a historical introduction to Carl Rogers and the person-centred approach in Chapter 1 and concludes with reflecting thoughts on difference, integration and development across the tribes.

No doubt, some will take issue with this selection of tribes, and different taxonomies have been proposed (see, for instance, Tudor, 2022). It has been argued, for example, that pluralism is incompatible with a person-centred understanding of human beings (see, for instance, Ong et al., 2020), or that emotion-focused therapy and motivational interviewing are too directive to be 'truly' person-centred. Whether or not such criticisms are 'correct', you, the reader, will now at least be better able to judge. In the spirit of the person-centred approach, my hope, echoing Pete's, is that the chapters will stimulate reflection, dialogue and debate. Indeed, it might be argued that this very willingness to engage with other positions and perspectives from a standpoint of openness, listening and respect is, ultimately, what it means to be person-centred.

Format of the chapters

Following Pete's format, for each chapter, I asked authors to cover:

- the basic theoretical underpinnings of the approach, including how it develops from Rogers' work
- key practices
- examples of practice, with at least one case study and one client–therapist dialogue
- key research evidence on the approach
- resources – key books and websites.

I also asked our authors to keep the 'spirit of Pete' and write in a way that is informal, accessible and engaging. Pete wanted, as do I, the book to be lively and interesting and to stimulate its readers with a diversity of ideas and practices.

The readership

The book is primarily aimed at students of the person-centred approach: those who, perhaps, have an initial basic understanding of person-centred therapy and skills but would like to know more about its development and the different forms it can take. If nothing else, we hope the book will help you, in your assignments, to say which form of person-centred therapy you are writing about, rather than using the more imprecise and general 'the person-centred approach'. Of course, the book in itself is not a training in these different tribes (or in person-centred skills, more generally), but there is enough here to help you decide which you may want to follow up and signpost you to key further resources, including training pathways. We also hope that qualified practitioners will find much of interest and value here: new ideas, new practices and new possibilities to help you develop, grow and diversify in your professional career.

Changes in the third edition

In the first edition of this book, there were five tribes; in the second edition, there were six and four 'new developments'. In this third edition, I have included 11 tribes. I discussed these changes with PCCS Books and we agreed we needed to simplify the structure, and that the previous distinction between 'tribes' and 'new developments' was a bit too arbitrary. We also wanted to explore some of these 'new developments' in more depth. Hence, four of the second edition's 'new developments' are now included here as fully fleshed out tribes: the relational/dialogical approach (Chapter 3), person-centred and experiential counselling for depression (Chapter 6), creative therapies (Chapter 10), and pre-therapy (Chapter 11). In addition, we have brought in chapters on motivational interviewing (Chapter 7) and child-centred play therapy (Chapter 12). Two other significant changes are that, in this edition, the chapter on integration focuses more specifically on pluralistic person-centred therapy (Chapter 9), and we have dropped our chapter on experiential person-centred therapy, given the coverage of experiential work in our focusing, EFT and existential chapters (4, 5 and 8, respectively). Readers may, however, find much of great value in those chapters on experiential and integrative person-centred approaches in the second edition (Baker, 2012; Worsley, 2012). Similarly, while we've replaced Pete's final chapter in the second edition – 'Mapping person-centred approaches to counselling and psychotherapy' (Sanders, 2012b) – with a briefer conclusion, Pete's 'position statement' from the second edition remains an important read for those interested in conceptualising and defining the person-centred field.

With respect to the authors, Sheila Haugh, one of the most experienced and respected figures in the person-centred world, has come in to update Pete's chapter on the history of Rogers and the person-centred approach (Chapter 1) and Tony Merry's chapter on the classical person-centred approach (formerly titled 'Classical client-centred therapy', Chapter 2). In addition, we have a slew of new contributors – all of them leading national and international figures, including Gina Di Malta, Steve Cox, Richard Doyle, David Murphy, Bill Miller, Siebrecht Vanhooren, Nicola Blunden, Ani de la Prida, Dion Van Werde and Dee Ray.

There are also some changes to the formatting of the book that, I have to confess, I do not think Pete would have liked. Pete did not like having to go 'off-page' to find the references for in-text citations, and introduced an additional side column so he could place them, and any necessary footnotes, right beside the text to which they referred. Pete also loved footnotes. In this edition, we have returned to a more standard format, with references at the end of chapters and minimal use of footnotes. We felt that a simpler structure provided a cleaner, easier read and one that could support more complexity in the text. In addition, and probably even worse in Pete's eyes, we've used the standardised American Psychological Association (APA) formatting for the references, in line with PCCS Books' current house style. I don't think I ever saw Pete more impassioned than when he was berating APA reference formatting for its cultural imperialism… along with its excessive use of full stops. But we feel it's a consistent system that everyone can stick to and it's helpful for students to know how they should be referencing their academic work if they are required to use APA. So, sorry, Pete!

Finally, an important note on terminology. We decided to use the term 'classical person-centred therapy' throughout the book, rather than 'classical client-centred therapy'. As Sheila Haugh explains more fully in her update to Chapter 1, this has long been the preferred and more familiar, terminology in the UK. We also use UK spelling over US spelling ('centred' rather than 'centered') other than in direct quotes and published titles.

And what stayed the same

There are a couple of important things that we didn't meddle with, along with the general style, structure and aims of the book.

The first is that we decided to keep the use of the term 'tribes', even though some have expressed preferences for alternative terms, such as 'branches', 'strands' or 'schools'. The term 'tribes', for some, evokes notions of warring factions, arguably with nationalistic and colonialist connotations. Nevertheless, for others, the term 'tribes' brings up positive connotations of identity and belonging. Given how well known – nationally and internationally – this book has become, we also felt that changing its title to something like 'The branches of the person-centred tree' might disorientate potential new readers and erroneously suggest a lack of continuity. Moreover, as I explained at the start of this introduction, it is a quote from Margaret Warner's work (2000) – an author for whom many of us in the person-centred field have enormous respect.

Second, in our title and across much of the book, we decided to retain the term 'person-centred', rather than 'person-centred and experiential' (PCE), to describe the extended family of Rogerian and post-Rogerian approaches. The latter term is widely used in the literature – for instance, in the title of the principal journal for the field, *Person-Centered & Experiential Psychotherapies* – and in the name of one of the talking therapies currently offered in NHS primary care services, 'person-centred experiential counselling for depression' (Chapter 6). 'Experiential' refers to those post-Rogerian approaches such as focusing and EFT that tend to focus on clients' emotions and experiences, in contrast to approaches that adopt a more non-directive stance. In this respect, the term 'person-centred and experiential' may be seen as making a more explicit divide between classical and 'process-directive' post-Rogerian approaches, with only the former identified as 'person-centred'. This goes back, then, to the question of how 'person-centred' is defined. Our decision to retain the term 'person-centred' in a relatively broad sense is based on a number of factors. First, it maintains consistency with previous editions of the book; second, it feels more concise; third, we are aware that, in many regions of the world (for instance, Ukraine and Belgium), 'person-centred' is used in this broad and comprehensive way; fourth, at a personal level, it feels most inclusive – most in the spirit of Rogers' desire to welcome and affirm different ways of being. But I accept, very much, that this may be a reflection of my own 'pluralistic' tendencies – towards valuing and embracing otherness. To others, a distinction between 'person-centred' and 'experiential' may feel more precise or, indeed, more respectful of the differences between them.

Conclusion

This book is dedicated to Pete, in the names of all the people who loved and learnt from him. Our aim is to continue his work – to build a vibrant, diverse, welcoming person-centred community that can flourish and grow across multiple perspectives and practices. More than that, we seek – through encouraging reflection and learning, dialogue and debate – to build a community that knows itself and can robustly meet the challenges from the wider field, standing up for a client-directed, non-pathologising and empowering approach to mental wellbeing work. We hope that you find much in these chapters to stimulate and engage you, to make you think, and to encourage you to take forward the person-centred vision in its multiple forms.

References

Baker, N. (2012). Experiential person-centred therapy. In P. Sanders (Ed.), *The tribes of the person-centred nation: An introduction to the schools of therapy related to the person-centred approach* (2nd ed.) (pp.71–102). PCCS Books.

Josefowitz, N. & Myran, D. (2005). Towards a person-centred cognitive behaviour therapy. *Counselling Psychology Quarterly, 18*(4), 329–336.

Mearns, D. & Thorne, B. (2000). *Person-centred therapy today: New frontiers in theory and practice.* Sage.

Ong, W.T., Murphy, D. & Joseph, S. (2020). Unnecessary and incompatible: A critical response to Cooper and McLeod's conceptualization of a pluralistic framework for person-centered therapy. *Person-Centered & Experiential Psychotherapies, 19*(2), 168–182. https://doi.org/10.1080/14779757.2020.1717987

Rogers, C.R. (1957). The necessary and sufficient conditions of therapeutic personality change. *Journal of Consulting Psychology, 21*(2), 95–103.

Rogers, C.R. (1959). A theory of therapy, personality, and interpersonal relationships as developed in the client-centred framework. In S. Koch, (Ed.), *Psychology: A study of a science. Vol. 3: Formulations of the person and the social context* (pp.184–256). McGraw-Hill.

Rogers, N. (1993). *The creative connection: Expressive arts as healing.* Science and Behavior Books.

Sanders, P. (2012a). Introduction – read this first. In P. Sanders (Ed.), *The tribes of the person-centred nation: An introduction to the schools of therapy related to the person-centred approach* (2nd ed.) (pp.vii-xvii). PCCS Books.

Sanders, P. (2012b). Appendix: Mapping person-centred approaches to counselling and psychotherapy. In P. Sanders (Ed.), *The tribes of the person-centred nation: An introduction to the schools of therapy related to the person-centred approach* (2nd ed.) (pp.233–246). PCCS Books.

Tudor, K. (2022). There and back again: Re-envisioning 'relationship therapy' as the center of a contemporary, cultural, and contextual person-centered therapy. *Person-Centered & Experiential Psychotherapies, 21*(2), 188–206. https://doi.org/10.1080/14779757.2022.2066562

Warner, M.S. (2000). Person-centered psychotherapy: One nation, many tribes. *Person-Centered Journal, 7*(1), 28–39.

Warner, M.S. (2013). Difficult client process. In M. Cooper, P.F. Schmid, M. O'Hara & G. Wyatt (Eds.), *The handbook of person-centred psychotherapy and counselling* (2nd ed.) (pp.343–358). Palgrave.

Worsley, R. (2012). Integrating with integrity. In P. Sanders (Ed.), *The tribes of the person-centred nation: An introduction to the schools of therapy related to the person-centred approach* (2nd ed.) (pp.125–147). PCCS Books.

1. Carl Rogers and person-centred therapy: A historical overview

Pete Sanders and Sheila Haugh

Introduction

The first national conference organised by the British Association for the Person-Centred Approach (BAPCA), held in Durham in September 2002, was titled 'Dialogues' and featured dialogues between 'classical' person-centred therapy, Gendlin's 'focusing', and existential therapies. Those of you embarking on training in person-centred therapy (PCT) might wonder what it was all about. You may think everyone knows that there is one unitary (if fairly broad) 'school' of person-centred therapy. It is more complicated than that. We hope you will find this quick tour of the history of events and ideas in the tradition of PCT will not only bring you up to date with the strands of thinking in the approach – the identities of the 'tribes' of the person-centred 'nation' (see Warner, 2000) – but also help you understand person-centred theory in general. It may also help you identify the subtle variations of person-centred theory and practice taught in your own training and help you decide which tribe(s) you identify with (if any). An ongoing debate about the range of approaches claiming to be 'person-centred' has been bubbling away for many years in books, journals, unpublished papers, seminars, cafés and hotel bars at international conferences. In this chapter, we will try to outline the debate as a backdrop to, or even the raison d'être of, this book.

Client-centred or person-centred?

First, we need to understand a little about the different names given to the therapy described by Rogers, at least in the UK. It was only in the very late 1970s that Rogers started using the term 'person-centred' to describe his work. Previously he had used the term 'client-centered'. In the UK we are accustomed to using the terms 'person-centred counselling', 'person-centred therapy' or 'person-centred psychotherapy', and 'the person-centred approach', or PCA. Also, given the central place of the PCA in the development of counselling outside of medical settings in the UK, the term 'person-centred' was quickly preferred to the term 'client-centred' to indicate the egalitarian, non-expert nature of the helping relationship. This then encouraged only a weak distinction between the notions of the therapeutic and non-therapeutic applications of Rogers' work in terms of nomenclature. It was during his time in California that Rogers started using the term 'person-centred', but he used it almost exclusively to describe the application of his ideas to fields other than therapy. Thus, in his final book, *A Way of Being* (Rogers, 1980), Chapter 6 was titled 'The Foundations of a Person-Centered Approach'. Rogers wrote in the introduction:

> [T]he old concept of 'client-centered therapy' has been transformed into the 'person-centered approach'. In other words, I am no longer talking simply about psychotherapy, but about a point of view, a philosophy, an approach to life, a way of being which fits any situation where growth – of a person, a group or a community – is part of the goal. (p. ix)

Rogers was careful to use the terms to delineate between the therapeutic aspects of his approach ('client-centred therapy') and the broader non-therapeutic (but still obviously change-oriented) philosophy and applications (the PCA, including encounter groups, education, peace project and so forth). In all his later publications, including his biographies, he consistently calls his approach to one-to-one therapy 'client-centered'. For example, in the months before he died, in interviews with David Russell (Rogers & Russell, 2002), he uses the term 'client-centered' in this context.

It is not altogether clear why, in the UK, the majority of counsellors evidently preferred to use the term 'person-centred' to refer to the therapeutic practice, rather than to the wider applications of Rogers' ideas. But UK practitioners had, to all intents and purposes, stopped using the term 'client-centred therapy' (in its UK spelling) by the 1990s. For this reason, in the present edition of this book, we primarily use the term 'person-centred' where Rogers and his contemporaries, and also our US colleagues today, would have used 'client-centered'. In this chapter, with its historical focus, we retain 'client-centered'.

With regard to the vexed issue of counselling, therapy and psychotherapy, we have used these terms interchangeably, since most therapists following Rogers' general approach see no difference between the processes of counselling and psychotherapy.

Those of you finishing a certificate in counselling or just starting a diploma might think that the history of person-centred therapy and the person-centred approach is fairly straightforward, and that it might go something like this: Carl Rogers thought up the basic idea in the 1940s, calling it 'client-centered' to shift the emphasis of psychotherapy from an expert therapist-based affair to an enterprise in which the patient (Rogers, importantly, called this person the 'client') and their needs were put at the centre. His ideas culminated in his 'necessary and sufficient conditions' writings in 1957 and 1959. Then, after moving to California in the 1960s, he introduced the term 'person-centred' to further de-emphasise the formal medical/clinical nature of the proceedings and restore more qualities of equality and personhood to the helping relationship. Rogers then went on to invent encounter groups and work towards world peace, until his death in the mid-1980s.

There is of course much more to this truncated story. At the personal level in Rogers' life, the gaps can be filled by reading a decent biography of Rogers (such as Kirschenbaum, 2007, and Thorne, 2012). For the wider social and political context of Rogers' development, Barrett-Lennard's *Carl Rogers' Helping System: Journey and substance* (1998) is the book to read. In this present chapter, our aim is to dash through the history of the development of the ideas – which requires a little digging around to winkle the information out of other texts. This is a tall order, given the space available, but we hope it will provide a good foundation for your understanding of the diverse ways the person-centred approach to therapy has differentiated and diverged – for us, it's rather like a piece of string: first woven together from, then fraying back into, different strands.

Non-directive therapy

In 1928, aged 26, Rogers joined the Child Study Department of the Rochester Society for the Prevention of Cruelty to Children. During his time there, he moved away from the psychometric measuring approach of professional psychology and became more interested in the practical approach to helping children and parents practised by social workers. Here he was particularly influenced by the developments emanating from the Pennsylvania School of Social Work and Philadelphia Child Guidance Clinic, including the work of Otto Rank (a psychoanalyst) and his student, Jessie Taft.

Rogers published his first book in 1939 – *The Clinical Treatment of the Problem Child*. Even in this early book, the seeds of his later work are clearly evident. He realised that a good relationship with the parents of the 'problem child' was one of the keys to success, and he listed the factors that he found to be important:

- It only works with parents who want to be helped.
- The relationship between the helper and the parent is the 'essential feature… The worker endeavours to provide an atmosphere in which the parent can come freely to experience and realise his own attitudes' (p.197).
- The effect on the parent is to help clarify their feelings and bring about self-acceptance.
- It relies on the parents themselves to independently arrive at their own parenting solutions.
- Its essence is one of non-interference.
- It relies on the 'individual's own tendency toward growth' (p.200).

In 1939, Rogers moved to Ohio State University as a full professor. In the following year, he gave a talk at the University of Minnesota titled 'Newer Concepts in Psychotherapy'. This presentation, given on 11 December 1940, is seen by some as the birth of client-centered therapy. Rogers' second book, *Counseling and Psychotherapy: Newer concepts in practice,* was published in 1942. In it he presented, for the first time ever, the verbatim transcripts of real therapy sessions. The book included a transcript of an entire eight-session case – the case of Herbert Bryan – complete with notes and analysis. This was nothing short of a revolution in the study and understanding of the previously mysterious world of psychotherapy.

In addition to his revolutionary use of the new technology of wax-disc recordings, Rogers continued to draw together further elements of the framework of what he was soon to call 'non-directive therapy'. The name emphasised the key feature that distinguished it from other therapeutic approaches: namely, the reliance on the client's own, self-directed growth processes rather than the expertise of the therapist. The client was their own expert.

It is important to appreciate that these ideas did not descend on Rogers out of the blue. He was renowned as an integrator of ideas, taking influences from many leading-edge theorists and practitioners. For example, as well as Otto Rank and Jessica Taft, Rogers also referenced Karen Horney, a post-Freudian feminist psychoanalyst. Her theory on the needs of children to be accepted and loved suggests Rogers' theory of conditions of worth (see Chapter 2, this volume) (Horney, 1937). He was also influenced by the work of his early graduate students, such as Richard Hogan's unpublished PhD thesis on threat and defence (Hogan, 1952), and most notably, Stanley Standal's exploration (1954) of the notion of unconditional positive regard (UPR).[1]

Client-centered therapy – University of Chicago

Rogers moved to the University of Chicago in 1945, where he set up the influential Counseling Center. He gathered around him a group of staff who all became extremely influential, either in association with Rogers or in their own right. This group included Godfrey Barrett-Lennard, Eugene Gendlin, Thomas Gordon, Nathaniel Raskin, Julius Seeman, John Shlien and Fred Zimring. It also included Virginia Axline, who would go on to found the field of child-centred play therapy (Chapter 12, this volume). Later generations of Counseling Center staff included Barbara Brodley and Ned Gaylin.

In 1948, Nat Raskin described the University of Chicago Counseling Center approach under Rogers as 'The development of nondirective therapy', but within a couple of years Rogers had changed the name to 'client-centered therapy'. The approach was announced and explained in his comprehensive, impressive 1951 volume, *Client-Centered Therapy: Its current practice, implications and theory*. It was very well received at the time and is still considered by many to be the best starting point for understanding this approach. The language of 1950s academia can be challenging, requiring patient and dedicated reading from some of us. Nevertheless, it was, and remains, a formidable and revolutionary text.

Chapter 11 of *Client-Centered Therapy* includes Rogers' 19 propositions, which represent the first systematic outline of his theory of personality, motivation and change. Whether Rogers was influenced by phenomenology as a philosophy at this stage in his theorising remains a moot point, but he made repeated references to the 'phenomenal field' in his writings. Phenomenology is a philosophical approach in which understanding of the world is rooted in the immediate experience of the individual (vs an understanding of the

---

1. You can follow these ideas further in Barrett-Lennard (1998) and Moon et al. (2001).

world based on religious doctrine or scientific analysis). Edmund Husserl (1859–1938) is credited with developing contemporary phenomenology. Each individual perceives events and gives them meaning, so in order to understand the behaviour of another, we need to understand the meanings they give to events. Hence Rogers proposed empathy as a core factor in effective therapy (vs behaviourists' search for meaning in external, objective events, and psychoanalysts' search for meaning in Freud's symbols to allow expert analysis by the therapist). The first of Rogers' 19 propositions, 'Every individual exists in a continually changing world of experience of which he is the center' (1951, p.483), leaves little doubt that a phenomenological attitude was at the forefront of his thinking.

It was not until the late 1950s and early 1960s that Rogers more formally acknowledged phenomenology, and also existentialism, as influencing his work (see Chapter 8, this volume). During the 1950s, the University of Chicago was definitely the place to be. Rogers developed the first-ever research programme to investigate the effectiveness of psychotherapy. He and his team attracted large grants, and a huge amount of research was done, not least in the area of trying to develop appropriate methods of study, since no one had attempted to evaluate psychotherapy in such a systematic way before. The team published their results widely (see, for example, Raskin, 1949; Seeman & Raskin, 1953; Rogers & Dymond, 1954), and the first body of empirical research into psychotherapy was, as a consequence, almost entirely client-centered. This first flush of research was, for the most part, received enthusiastically by the therapeutic community.

Howard Kirschenbaum (2007) notes:

> When Rogers first entertained the idea of undertaking research in psychotherapy, there were no precedents for him to follow… Recording or transcribing actual interviews was unheard of. One had only the psychotherapist's word as to whether a particular method was effective or not… It was, indeed, to use Rogers' phrase, 'an art which made a pretense of being a science'. (p.198)

Another feature of the Chicago team was that Rogers deliberately made it as egalitarian as possible, with a flat management structure. John Shlien, in a private conversation, recalled his astonishment when, arriving at his first faculty meeting, he found Carl Rogers writing the entire staff's salaries (with his own at the top) on the chalkboard and asking his assembled colleagues if everyone was happy with the rates of pay and the differentials between each grade. Organising the faculty in such a way had a profound – indeed, life-long – impact on many of the members of staff. New ideas in theory and research were circulated as University of Chicago Counseling Center Discussion Papers in a system formalised by Jack Butler. Many of the theory developments and key research projects that advanced 'client-centered therapy' can be found as germs of ideas in these discussion papers. The academic environment was vibrant, and everyone was encouraged to share, co-operate and support each other.

While at Chicago, Rogers 'not only read but really studied' (Kirschenbaum, 2007, p.224) the work of psychologists, Karl Marx and, of particular interest here, the existential philosophers Kierkegaard and Sartre. Of Kierkegaard, he wrote (1961): 'Though Kierkegaard lived one hundred years ago, I cannot help but think of him as a sensitive and highly perceptive friend. I think this paper shows my indebtedness to him' (pp.199–200).

In the late 1950s, Rogers began using Kierkegaard's phrase 'to be the self one truly is'. In *On Becoming a Person* (1961), he adopted Kierkegaard's 'This is true for me, but I realise it may not be true for a lot of other people' (Rogers & Russell, 2002, p.170) style of writing. It seems that, during this time, Rogers' reading 'caught up' with his earlier ideas. His theorising up to this point had had distinct touches of existentialism and phenomenology (see Chapter 8, this volume), but now he was more systematically integrating some strands of these traditions.

The work of Rogers and the team at Chicago culminated in his seminal 'necessary and sufficient conditions' hypothesis, which he was invited to write up for publication as a chapter for the prestigious collection *Psychology: A study of a science* (1959) by its editor, Sigmund Koch. Rogers considered this chapter to be the best, most complete and comprehensive formulation of his theory, subject to possible revision in the light of experience or research. However, he never did revise the theory to any notable extent.[2] He might have extended it or elaborated it in the sense of considering some areas in more detail, but there were no changes to these basic tenets:

1. That two persons are in contact.
2. That the first person, whom we shall term the client, is in a state of incongruence, being vulnerable, or anxious.
3. That the second person, whom we shall term the therapist, is congruent in the relationship.
4. That the therapist is experiencing unconditional positive regard toward the client.
5. That the therapist is experiencing an empathic understanding of the client's internal frame of reference.
6. That the client perceives, at least to a minimal degree, conditions 4 and 5, the unconditional positive regard of the therapist for him, and the empathic understanding of the therapist. (Rogers, 1959)

No other conditions are necessary for Rogers (1959). If these six conditions exist, and continue over a period of time, this is sufficient: the process of constructive personality change will follow.

This statement was one of the pivotal writings in psychotherapy generally in the second half of the 20th century. Rogers deliberately set about demystifying, decoding and operationalising those aspects of a human relationship that might facilitate constructive personality change. It was nothing less than revolutionary, for a number of reasons:

---

2. Rogers' 1957 paper, 'The necessary and sufficient conditions of therapeutic personality change' in the *Journal of Consulting Psychology* seems to have become better known than the 1959 chapter. However, the 1957 paper is a statement concerning the conditions for therapeutic personality change generally, whereas the 1959 chapter is specifically dedicated to therapeutic personality change within a 'client-centered' *framework*.

- It uncovered the previously arcane world of therapy, exposing it to public scrutiny.
- It made the relationship between therapist and client the agent for change.
- It presented the factors required for change as an 'if–then' predictive hypothesis: i.e. if such and such is present, then such and such will happen.
- It made the whole area of psychotherapy amenable (for the first time) to research based on experimental science (although some thought this to be a mistake on Rogers' part).
- It declared that no other conditions are necessary. This was, and continues to be, a direct challenge to approaches based on the theoretical knowledge or expertise of the therapist, or those predicated on the diagnosis of specific symptoms and the application of targeted techniques.
- It was, and still is, deeply counter-cultural, as in the pseudo-medical-scientific world of psychotherapy of that time it was (and still is) seen as imperative to mimic medical science, and the knowledge, expertise and scientific application of skilled techniques are regarded as the hallmarks of 'quality'.

When combined with Rogers' previous statements on non-directivity and motivation (the healing potential of the actualising tendency), and personality (the idea that incongruence between the self-concept and experience causes psychological tension), within the world of psychotherapy, the revolution was complete. The 1959 chapter (and 1957 paper) remains as radical today as it was then. Rogers made the client clearly the locus of the healing process, including the nature and direction of change. The client was at the centre of a self-directed process facilitated by another (the therapist), and experts were effectively written out.

This did not go down too well in most circles in the psychological therapies. Its challenge to psychological therapies was all the more threatening because the team at Chicago was producing work at a prodigious rate. Research was continuing on many fronts and the Counseling Center attracted funding and had recruited specialists such as Jules Seeman to help develop and validate new methodologies for the emerging discipline of psychotherapy research.

Then, at the height of the Chicago Counseling Center's success, in 1957, Rogers left to take up a new challenge at the University of Wisconsin. He was 'head-hunted' by the university to a professorship, uniquely, in both psychology and psychiatry, and he soon attracted substantial funding for research. Once in post, he invited some of the Chicago Counseling Center team to join him and, along with Charles Truax and others, embarked on a study at the Mendota State Hospital (this research is often referred to as the 'Wisconsin Project'). Rogers wanted this research to silence those who criticised the Chicago research for being too small in scale and using clients whose symptoms were not 'severe'. In his own words (Rogers & Russell, 2002) it was to be 'the research to end all research'.

In brief, the aim of the Wisconsin Project was to evaluate the hypothesis that the conditions proposed by Rogers would determine the outcome of therapy with people diagnosed with schizophrenia and receiving treatment in a state mental hospital. Simply put, the suggestion was that, if therapists provided high levels of the six conditions, the patients should improve more than if the therapists provided low levels of the conditions.

However, in order to anticipate predicted criticisms of the methodology and make it as perfect as possible, Rogers and his team elaborated the design to the point of being practically unmanageable. Even though 'there were no precedents for him to follow' (Kirschenbaum, 1979, p.205), the Wisconsin Project is considered by some to be a heroic failure – over-ambitious and flawed in its design and inconclusive in its results. Others thought that the whole effort was both ground-breaking and disappointing. The positive points of the project included the development of counsellor rating scales by Truax; the use of Barrett-Lennard's Relationship Inventory to measure the client's perception of the relationship, and a greater focus on the therapeutic role of congruence. Whatever your position on the Wisconsin Project (see Rogers et al., 1967), it is universally seen as a great opportunity lost and a professional disaster. It was a fraught time for the research team. The Wisconsin method and results were eventually written up, mainly by Rogers (Rogers et al., 1967) after he left Wisconsin for California.

It was during this time at Wisconsin, however, that Rogers worked most closely with Eugene Gendlin. Gendlin had been a student of Rogers and a staff member at Chicago, and Rogers had invited him to join the Wisconsin team. This continued association influenced the development of client-centered therapy in important ways. Gendlin was developing his theory of experiencing (see Chapter 4, this volume), and Rogers was giving much thought to the process within the client during therapy. Although there are differing versions of history, Gendlin and Rogers appeared to develop a simultaneous interest in the internal experience of the client during therapy. To begin with, it appears that Gendlin's ideas took a lead and there then followed a short phase in which each influenced the other.

Rogers presented his ideas in his address to the American Psychological Association in 1956, when he received the Distinguished Scientific Contribution Award. What he called at the time his emerging 'process conception of psychotherapy' later surfaced as Chapter 7 in *On Becoming a Person* (Rogers, 1961). He presented a seven-stage process of change within the client along a series of loose dimensions, such as openness to experience, positive self-regard, flexibility of personal ideas about oneself (personal constructs), and greater emotional expressiveness. In summary, the client moves from separateness to integration in structure and from rigidity to flexibility in internal process.

The Wisconsin Project design required the measurement of movement in the client as well as the counsellor-provided conditions. Gendlin, as research director and author, or co-author, of eight of the 21 chapters on method and results (Rogers et al., 1967), had therefore turned his attention to client process and its measurement. This represented only one strand of Gendlin's prodigious thinking on experiencing, which included being the theoretical driving force behind the developments of the experiencing scale. He went on to develop an entire theory of human experiencing and how this intersects with therapeutic change. This was the first genuine new thinking from one of the client-centered therapy group that grew up around Rogers in Chicago and after. Springing from a shared interest in what was happening in the experience of the client during the change process, Gendlin elaborated his theory of experiencing into a formal description of a) the moments of change that occurred as the client contacted their present experiencing, and b) the resulting change (Gendlin, 1962, 1974). This is the process he called 'focusing' (see below and Chapter 4, this volume).

This work on how the client touches their inner stream of experience in the present moment released the proverbial genie. There was no getting it back in the bottle. There were now two tribes (focusing and client-centered therapy), and soon there would be three when 'experiential' therapy was born, along with the debates and disagreements that exercise the person-centred nation to this day. Over the space of a few years, from around 1958 to 1964, the original client-centered river had divided into three streams, each of which would become a river in its own right, travelling in parallel yet still linked to, and fed by, the same source.

The source continued to be refined by Rogers, but he added little new theory after the early 1960s. There was an increase in the influence of existential philosophy, and Rogers continued to extend the application of the basic concepts to areas other than one-to-one psychotherapy, and there were changes in emphasis along the way, but no substantial new theory.

Some of Rogers' students and colleagues from Chicago contributed to the refinement and subtle adaptation of the original client-centered theory. These included Jules Seeman (on personality integration and psychological health (1983)), Fred Zimring (on the application of cognitive theory to person-centred practice (1974)), and John Shlien (on the existential edge of internal congruence and consistency (2003)). Others developed wider applications of the ideas, most notably Thomas Gordon (parent effectiveness training and teacher effectiveness training).

Focusing and focusing-oriented therapy

During and after the Wisconsin Project, Eugene Gendlin continued to set his own course with focusing, the practical application of his theory of experiencing. Gendlin was responsible for a piece of clear, original thinking when he unpacked the therapeutic process in the experience of the client. He looked at the course that successful therapy took and tried to describe the process. He believed that the same process happened in all cases where therapy was successful, even though it would be uniquely experienced and expressed by each client and uniquely facilitated by each therapist. His attempt to write down the process as a formula or series of steps divided the client-centered community (1978). The objections to focusing included:

- Gendlin's description of this process in terms of six 'steps' was seen by the classical client-centered therapists as a crucial move away from the non-directive dictum at the core of the approach, since it seemed that Gendlin was advocating instructing the client in the focusing steps and directing their progress through the steps.
- Making a description of a possible process into a general rule by saying that the steps were followed in all cases, albeit uniquely, was also deeply unpopular with some in the classical client-centered community. This was because, in principle, it irons out the change process into a 'one size fits all', even if we all do it differently. The classical client-centered therapists believed that individual clients' processes would be unique both in the 'steps' of the process, if indeed there were any, and in the expression of the process.

As Gendlin's ideas developed, 'focusing' became the term applied to a general process of change, irrespective of the setting. In therapeutic settings, where the client and therapist's shared goal was therapeutic change requested by the client, the term 'focusing-oriented psychotherapy' emerged as the preferred title. The 'six steps' are a suggested protocol for a personal change process that can be practised alone or with a friend or helper, regardless of the setting. This was the formal activity of 'focusing'.

Part of the mission of this book is to disentangle the varied positions that have been taken up over the years. What is focusing-oriented psychotherapy really, and what is its real relation to classical person-centred therapy? Chapters 2 and 4 will help us answer those questions.

Emotion-focused therapy

For some, Gendlin's descriptions of the process of experience opened a door to new possibilities. Rather than follow Gendlin and focusing, they took the idea of contacting the internal flow of experience and looked for interventions that might assist the client in accessing it. This was a much broader palette than focusing and soon became a river of its own – neither focusing nor client-centered. Experiential psychotherapy springs from Gendlin's experiential work, yet is rooted in the egalitarian, non-interpretative tradition of classical client-centered therapy, with the client and their actualising tendency at the centre of the therapeutic process (see Chapter 5, this volume). The approach also sought to integrate ideas and methods that aim to put the client in contact with their flow of experience in the present. Experiential psychotherapy distinguishes between directing the content of the client's world and assisting, guiding or directing the client's process in a collaborative manner. In 1984, Leslie Greenberg and his associates in North America made their mark with *Patterns of Change* (Rice & Greenberg, 1984). In Europe, Germain Lietaer has been advocating and developing experiential therapy for more than 40 years. Several of his writing are available in English – for example, *The Client-Centred Approach after the Wisconsin Project* (1990) and *The United Colors of Person-Centered and Experiential Psychotherapies* (2002).

As Leslie Greenberg and his associates, Laura North Rice and Robert Elliott, developed their ideas and practice, they also developed the terminology to describe their therapeutic approach. 'Process experiential', 'process directive' and 'process guiding' are among their attempts to describe the nuances within it. The most recent functional title of their work, and so far the most durable, is 'emotion-focused therapy' (see Chapter 5, this volume).

Things fall apart in Wisconsin

Meanwhile, Rogers' most popular and influential book, *On Becoming a Person: A therapist's view of psychotherapy*, was compiled and published while he was at Wisconsin in 1961. It was a collection of more than 20 papers that he drew together, edited and linked to present as a complete book. In it, Rogers hit just the right note: a balance between the personal and the professional/theoretical. The book was well received and proved tremendously popular among a very wide range of readers. There was plenty of theory and, indeed, philosophy of both human nature and science, but what came through in the relaxed style of writing was Rogers' personal involvement in the material. True to the title, Rogers the person was there. It was – uncharacteristically for psychology texts at the time – personally reflective and revealing.

But Rogers was not happy at Wisconsin University, which he found too rigid and wedded to a view of academic credibility based almost entirely on passing exams and failing those who did not make the grade. Rogers preferred to encourage individual creative thinking in a much more relaxed environment. He did not favour relaxing the academic standards but began to believe that the narrow academic tramlines within which the graduate students were expected to stay strangled original thought and creative learning. He sent memos to the academic hierarchy and the exchanges became increasingly ill-tempered as Rogers wrote papers on his views on the best conditions for graduate education. He resigned from the university to take up a position at the Western Behavioral Sciences Institute in California (which he had earlier had a hand in founding) to work with his old friend and former student from Chicago, Richard Farson.

Alongside Rogers' personal problems with the institution, the Wisconsin project research was not going well either. Rogers' keenness to test out his ideas away from the middle-class world of academia at the University of Chicago, while admirable, was not enough to maintain the project in all its necessary thoroughness against the myriad other pressures. These were, most notably, the decision of the project team to give up much of their control over which patients were to be involved in the interviews, and the disappearance of crucial data. It would seem that some patients were not able to give consent to being a part of the research and not all the therapists were if fact client-centered. On top of this, the researchers, who included Gendlin, were not able to function effectively as a team, and relationships soon became fractured as the project lost steam and direction when Rogers moved out to the Californian coast. Rogers believed that the problems arose because he 'failed to take the time and care needed to allow the Psychotherapy Research Group to become a truly group-centered, self-directing group' (Kirschenbaum, 1979, p.281). Others in the group thought the basic problem was Rogers' lack of leadership – indeed, by the time of the writing-up phase of the project, Rogers had already left Wisconsin University. The tensions reached their final messy and tragic conclusions after Rogers had left for California in 1964.

And get back together again in California

Rogers moved to La Jolla, a small coastal town in the northern outskirts of San Diego, and stayed there until his death in 1987. In biographies and notes on Rogers' life, accounts of these years often use the term 'freedom' to describe this period in personal and professional terms. Rogers had freed himself from the strictures of academic life and was able to pursue his interests with little or no hindrance.

Some see this move as the beginning of the end for client-centered therapy as a mainstream school of thought in American universities, and assert that Rogers was running away from the difficulties at Wisconsin, both at the university itself and at the research project. Others believed that he was so deeply affected by the professional disappointment at the university and disaster at the research project that he initially simply retreated to reconsider his options. He was 61 years old and in what many at that age would consider to be the twilight of an illustrious career. Peaceful retirement beckoned; there was no real need for him to break new ground and tread new paths in the application of humanistic psychology. But that is exactly what he did.

Once settled in California, Rogers carried the development of the applications of client-centred therapy into new areas. He was encouraged to do this as a result of several influences:

- His discontent with the rather rigid, narrow approach to graduate education in Wisconsin encouraged him to develop his ideas on education, resulting in the 1969 publication of *Freedom to Learn*.
- Meeting Michael Polanyi at Stanford University, where Rogers had spent a year while at Wisconsin, stimulated his interest in the philosophy of science and human nature. He increasingly included thoughts on science and humankind in his publications and a dialogue with Polanyi appeared in *Man and the Science of Man*, which Rogers jointly edited with William Coulson and published in 1968.
- Shortly after arriving in California, Rogers acted as consultant to a group of world-renowned physicists at California Institute of Technology, including Murray Gellman and Nobel Prize-winner Richard P. Feynman. This experience no doubt helped him regain confidence after his experiences at Wisconsin.
- Whether Rogers was disenchanted with individual therapy is debatable, but he turned his attention to the application of client-centered therapy principles in groups. He was not interested so much in formal group therapy as in unstructured, non-directive groups that encouraged congruent, empathic exchanges between participants. These came to be called encounter groups, and Rogers authored the definitive book on the topic, *Carl Rogers on Encounter Groups*, which was published in 1970.
- Rogers was able to turn his attention to one of his long-term dreams: using client-centered therapy principles to help reduce international tensions. He had been interested in conflict resolution in social settings for a very long time, and now he became interested in using the approach to foster world peace. The Peace Project – co-ordinated from the Center for Studies of the Person by its director, Gay Swenson (Barfield) – involved large group meetings in, among other places, Central America, Europe, South Africa and the USSR.

Carl Rogers 1902–1987

When Carl Rogers died in 1987, client-centered therapy and the person-centred approach had been established throughout the world. In some countries, he was best known for his work as a psychotherapist, in others for his work in conflict resolution, cross-cultural work and international peace efforts.

During his time in California, Rogers turned his attention almost exclusively to applications other than individual therapy: namely, encounter groups, education, politics and peace. Since this book is concerned with therapeutic applications of 'client-centred' therapy, with individuals, families and groups, you can now see why, in this 'history' of events and ideas, we have concentrated mainly on the period before he went to California. To all intents and purposes, Carl Rogers stopped working as a therapist when he left Wisconsin. Some readers may have seen films or videotapes of him working with individual clients. He (along with Albert Ellis and Fritz Perls) is known by many students of psychology, psychotherapy and counselling for the first *Three Approaches to Psychotherapy* series (Shostrom, 1965), featuring the client 'Gloria', which was filmed in 1961 and released in 1965. This was followed by a second series (Shostrom, 1977), featuring another client, 'Kathy', with Carl Rogers, Arnold Lazarus and the director, Everett Shostrom, himself.

The 'Gloria films' attracted wide publicity at the time of their release and have been used in training continuously since the mid-1960s. The films were remarkable because, first, they were the first to show real therapy, rather than dramatised therapy or role play. Second, they showed three therapists – founders of their respective approaches – demonstrating real therapy (effectively an advertisement for their particular approach) with a real client. This enabled comparison between the approaches. The films consequently attracted much comment from both inside and outside the helping professions – indeed, at various times, for a variety of reasons, it would not be an exaggeration to say that the films were infamous.

John Shlien, in an unpublished interview, expressed his view that making the 'Gloria' films re-awakened Rogers' interest in one-to-one therapy, which had dwindled in the aftermath of the Wisconsin Project. According to Shlien, Rogers was very nervous before the filming, uncomfortable under the hot lights and worried that he might not be able to give a good demonstration of how he worked. Rogers telephoned Shlien immediately on his return from the filming, saying that he felt he had done a good job and that his confidence – which had taken a bit of a hammering at Wisconsin – was restored. Rogers and 'Gloria' continued to correspond after the recording (see Thorne, 2012, p.52), and there is also an account of the aftermath of the films by 'Gloria's' daughter, Pamela Burry (Burry, 2008). In addition, Rogers continued to do 'demonstration' interviews at workshops where the 'clients' were workshop participants or staff. However, arguably, these occasional, one-off single sessions cannot be considered to be work as a therapist.

One of the consequences of Rogers turning his attention away from one-to-one therapy is that, for those who looked only to him for innovation, client-centered therapy theory effectively stood still for more than 20 years between the mid-1960s and the late 1980s. Rogers published brief, occasional essays related to therapy in this time, but none presented new theory. Similarly, his books *Carl Rogers on Personal Power* (1977) and *A Way of Being* (1980) were both overwhelmingly concerned with other applications of his ideas. Some believe the chapter on empathy in *A Way of Being* presented no new theory and was, rather, an attempt to 'rescue' the beleaguered concept of empathy after it had been so often ridiculed by other psychologists as wooden parroting – a criticism that can still be heard today in some circles. Rogers himself had turned away from empathy as a result of this criticism. Nick Baker (2012), among others, took a different view. He argued strongly that Rogers' 'Empathic: An unappreciated way of being' (reprinted as Chapter 7 in *A Way of Being*) and Rogers' work with Jim Brown did indeed present new theory. Specifically, Baker suggested (2012) that this theory of empathy (originally published in 1975) was 'marinated in the experiential approach' of Gendlin (p.80). Rogers returned to empathy as a key concept in therapeutic relationships at the very end of his life.

'Presence'

As Carl Rogers gave his attention to these extensions and applications of person-centred principles, most would agree that he did not advance the theory in the sense of adding new elements or changing existing ones. There is one possible exception to this when, in 1986, he referred to a particular quality of some relationships:

> When I am at my best, as a group facilitator or a therapist… when I am closest to my inner intuitive self, when I am somehow in touch with the unknown in me, when perhaps I am in a slightly altered state of consciousness in the relationship, then whatever I seem to do seems full of healing. Then simply my presence is releasing and helpful. There is nothing I can do to force this experience, but when I can relax and be close to the transcendental core of me… at those moments it seems that my inner spirit has reached out and touched the inner spirit of the other. (pp.198–199)

This has come to be what must be one of the most frequently quoted passages from Rogers' work. It seems that, again, Rogers' sharing of his personal experiences in therapy struck a chord with many people. It can certainly be taken many ways (and has been). There are two main interpretations. First, it was read by many as the latest evidence in Rogers' writing that he was, in his later years, acknowledging a transpersonal or spiritual dimension to human existence. This view is probably best elaborated in the work of Brian Thorne (1991, 1998, 2002). In terms of the development of person-centred therapy and the PCA, Rogers had given voice to an unspoken dimension of the lives of many therapists as person-centred therapy embraced the spiritual.

Second, it has caused some speculation as to whether Rogers was suggesting a further condition – that of 'presence'. Some argue that presence is a transitory, somewhat enhanced type of interpersonal contact between people that happens in 'mature' relationships. It seems to happen in therapeutic relationships characterised by a depth of relating facilitated by high levels of trust, therapist congruence and ability to stay with processing in the present. Another view is that presence is another condition of successful therapy but may not be necessary.

The person-centred approach finds its heart

Others take Rogers' quote to emphasise the point, central to person-centred therapy, that it is the relationship that is the key, not the skills or abilities of the therapist, and furthermore that this relationship is co-created by the therapist and client. And this latter view draws attention to a 'maturing' of person-centred therapy during Rogers' time in California.

Theory and practice were not advanced, but the person-centred approach more generally deepened, consolidated and, as Mearns and Thorne (2000) have it, 'genuinely found its "heart"' (p.89). This grew into a greater, more sharply defined notion of the relational nature of PCT itself. The emphasis became:

- the human qualities of the therapist, rather than the skilled 'doing' of therapy
- the idea of therapist congruence as the 'being' of the whole self of the therapist in the relationship, rather than 'using' congruence as a 'technique'
- therapy as a co-created relationship, rather than the application of therapist-provided conditions.

These ideas, increasingly evident in Rogers' writing, shifted the leading-edge emphasis slowly but surely towards other themes and elements that would continue to develop after his death.

After Rogers

For some years after Rogers died, development of the person-centred approach seemed to stagnate. The conferences of what was then known as the International Conference for Client-Centered and Experiential Psychotherapy (ICCCEP) more often contained re-iterations of Rogers' work or numerous discussions on what Rogers once said at a dinner party, rather than anything new, theoretically or in practice. Nevertheless, slowly but surely, new shoots could be discerned. Around 1993, Maggie Taylor-Sanders and Pete Sanders set up PCCS books at their kitchen table (literally and figuratively), with the intention to publish person-centred writings. In 1997, the World Association for Person-Centered and Experiential Psychotherapy and Counselling (WAPCEPC) officially came into being. By that time, a number of person-centred training programmes had been developed in the UK, some accredited by the British Association for Counselling (BAC) (later to become the British Association for Counselling and Psychotherapy (BACP)). While none of these events could be described as a definitive moment in the 're-awakening' of person-centred theory and practice in the UK (or more widely), they were indicative of a renewed energy and interest in the approach.

As the tribes of the person-centred nation have developed their identities, genuine new theory and applications have been advanced. For some it has been facilitated by the cross-fertilisation of ideas between the tribes; for others, by taking ideas from psychology, theology or philosophy. Agreeing with Rogers' values and ideas, some have brought activities other than therapy under its umbrella. It is clearly beyond the brief of this historical introduction to detail all these developments; most diploma-level trainings should have a sufficiently good library to take your reading further. These topics should be considered 'leading-edge' ideas, but not in the sense that they are tentative or undeveloped. Most have passed their period of gestation and have now been absorbed into the best contemporary person-centred literature. They are leading edge in the sense that, in terms of understanding theory, they should be tackled after the basics have been thoroughly understood.

Trends in ideas

Spirituality and the PCA

For many years, practitioners and writers struggled to establish human spiritual experience as valid territory for psychotherapy, regardless of therapeutic orientation. In the PCA tradition, Brian Thorne was a pioneer in encouraging practitioners to include spiritual experience and practice in their repertoire of therapeutic possibilities. Collections of his essays and chapters (Thorne, 1991, 1998, 2002) continue to be sources of inspiration for practitioners, not least because of the challenging nature of Thorne's message.

Person-centred therapy as a fundamentally ethical activity

Related to his writing on person-centred therapy as a dialogical approach, Austrian scholar Peter Schmid positioned person-centred therapy as an ethical activity at the heart of ancient European philosophy. He described person-centred therapy as a fundamentally ethical way of conducting oneself as a human being, rather than a set of qualities limited to specifically therapeutic relationships (Schmid, 2001a, 2001b, 2001c, 2002, 2013). Across the Atlantic, American psychologist Barry Grant published what has become, for some, a seminal paper on the understanding of the ethical base of 'principled non-directive' person-centred therapy (Grant, 1990). His paper outlined the difference between using non-directivity (and, indeed, other person-centred therapy 'conditions') as instruments or tools rather than holding them as qualities and values as a person. This strand of thinking has developed in the work of some North American practitioners (Grant, 2003) to become an 'ethics-only' approach to therapy.

A dialogical, relational approach

A dialogical approach is concerned with the 'between'. It is an approach to therapy that emphasises, or even rests completely on, dialogue – that is, the co-created relationship between the helper and person helped (see Chapter 3, this volume). This is different from the 'traditional' phenomenological approach of PCA, wherein we look at the experiences of the therapist and client separately, as though unconnected. We have to be careful here to understand that 'dialogue' does not necessarily mean only talking or a conversation, although that can help most relationships to some extent. One of the most prolific writers on a dialogical approach from within the person-centred tradition was (again) Peter Schmid (2001a, 2001b, 2001c, 2002). He saw human beings *as* dialogue rather than *having* dialogues (2013). Dave Mearns' work reflected this emerging dialogical influence. In the mid-1990s, Mearns (1996) began writing about the profound nature of moments he encountered in his work as a person-centred therapist. This work directly challenged the popular, if ill-informed, notion that person-centred therapy could only work at superficial levels; that person-centred therapy was only fine for the beginning of therapeutic work. He started to use the term 'relational depth' to describe these moments of intense contact between therapist and client that have the potential to shift gears in the change process. He developed the idea with Mick Cooper (Mearns & Cooper, 2018), and it became a stimulus for both theory development and evidence gathering (see Knox et al., 2013). The descriptions of relational depth captured, in practice, the notion of humans as dialogical creatures.

Difficult processes

Historically, and particularly in the UK, person-centred theory had little to say about working with people with traditional psychiatric diagnoses. Continental colleagues addressed some of these areas – for example 'schizophrenia' (van Blaricom, 2006) and 'borderline personality disorder' (Kramer & Sachse, 2013; Snijders et al., 2015). The whole idea of there being identifiable 'mental disorders' has been challenged by many, including Sanders (2011) and Bohart (2017). Since the early 1990s, Margaret Warner has developed person-centred theory and practice for clients with what she terms 'difficult process'. She has described three types of processing – fragile, dissociated and psychotic – and suggests there may be more. Other, more diagnostic therapeutic approaches might refer to such clients as having borderline personality disorder, for example, or suffering dissociation, depersonalisation or psychosis. Warner (2016, 2017) has developed not only genuine new theory but also sensitive practice and a respectful vocabulary for describing clients' experiences. This positions her work in the person-centred tradition of critiquing the medical model of mental illness, eschewing symptom-led diagnostic categories, and letting understanding of distress be phenomenological, defined and led by client's lived experiences.

A research agenda

Earlier in this chapter we described how Carl Rogers was a pioneer in psychotherapy research. As previously mentioned, in 1956, he was awarded the first-ever Distinguished Scientific Contribution Award by the American Psychological Association. The citation read:

> For developing an original method to objectify the description and analysis of the psychotherapeutic process, for formulating a testable theory of psychotherapy and its effects on personality and behavior, and for extensive systematic research to exhibit the value of the method and explore and test the implications of the theory. His… flexible adaptation of scientific method in his attack on the formidable problems involved in the modification of the individual person have moved this area of psychological interest within the boundaries of scientific psychology. (Cited in Kirschenbaum & Henderson, 1990; p.201)

Rogers and his associates were the first to publish full transcripts of therapy sessions, using the then innovative technology of wax-disc recordings. They were the first to attempt to subject these and other data to scientific analysis (see Raskin, 2004). From the late 1940s to the mid-1950s, the University of Chicago Counseling Center was a world centre of excellence in Western psychotherapy research. Much more recently, Rogers' contribution was again acknowledged in the dedication of the interdivisional American Psychological Association publication *Psychotherapy Relationships That Work* (Norcross & Lambert, 2019). They wrote: 'Dedicated to Carl R. Rogers [and Edward S. Bordin]: pioneers in investigating and advancing the therapeutic relationship'.

However, if we look to the late 20th century, we find very little research into psychotherapy outcomes involving client-centered/person-centred therapy itself. Then, as the new millennium unfolded, a research agenda began to germinate and take root. Supported by WAPCEPC and the journal *Person-Centered & Experiential Psychotherapies*, awareness of and a new enthusiasm for research developed. This was best evidenced by the publication of an international collaboration, sponsored by WAPCEPC, with the confident title *Person-Centered and Experiential Therapies Work* (Cooper et al., 2010). Latterly, the meta-analyses of empathy (Elliott et al., 2019), positive regard and affirmation (Farber et al., 2019) and congruence (Kolden et al., 2019) have contributed to an interest and confidence in person-centred therapies. Throughout the pages of this book, you will find many references and details of research undertaken in the last 25 years.

Looking forward

Since the advent of WAPCEPC, the tribes have had an organisational meeting point where information exchange, challenging debate, support, project development and international representation can take place. WAPCEPC offers bursaries to new and established researchers, thereby supporting development and innovation.

The tribes of the person-centred nation continue to develop and diversify as the new millennium unfolds. There are now many variations of therapeutic approach that trace their origins back to the work of Carl Rogers, several of which feature in this book. 'Challenging debate' is still high on the agenda. Issues of definition still loom large as the tribes deliberate which criteria should determine whether a therapeutic approach falls within a broad definition of the term 'person-centred therapies' (or broader still, the 'person-centred approach'). The discussion continues to return to two core issues: directivity/non-directivity and the necessity and sufficiency of the therapeutic conditions. Historically, the parameters of this debate have been set by the position of the classical non-directive person-centred therapists, and arguably this continues to be the case. There is scant evidence that Rogers himself moved very far, if at all, from these basic principles during his life. However, one of the challenges of history is that it can look very different depending on where we are standing – on our experience, our cultures, our values and our beliefs. The publication of a third edition of this book adds to our history and to our debates. Although there is an argument that play therapy and pre-therapy have been a part of the person-centred nation from pretty much the 'beginning', the possible tribes included here have increased from five in the first edition to 11 in this third one. The next 20 years will be interesting times.

Recommended reading

Barrett-Lennard, G.T. (1998). *Carl Rogers' helping system: Journey and substance.* Sage.
A study of the history of the person-centred approach.

Kirschenbaum, H. (2007). *The life and work of Carl Rogers.* PCCS Books.
A comprehensive review of Carl Rogers and his development.

References

Baker, N. (2012). Experiential person-centred therapy. In P. Sanders (Ed.), *The tribes of the person-centred nation* (2nd ed.) (pp.71–101). PCCS Books.

Barrett-Lennard, G.T. (1998). *Carl Rogers' helping system: Journey and substance.* Sage.

Bohart, A.C. (2017). A client-centered perspective on 'psychopathology'. *Person-Centered & Experiential Psychotherapies, 16*(1), 14–26.

Burry, P. (2008). *Living with the Gloria films: A daughter's memory.* PCCS Books.

Cooper, M., Watson, J.C. & Hölldampf, D. (Eds.). (2010). *Person-centered and experiential therapies work.* PCCS Books.

Elliott, R., Bohart, A.C., & Watson, J.C. (2019). Empathy. In J.C. Norcross & M.J. Lambert (Eds.), *Psychotherapy relationships that work. Volume 1: Evidence-based therapist contributions* (3rd ed.) (pp.245–287). Oxford University Press.

Farber, B.A., Suzuki, J.Y. & Lynch, D.A. (2019). Positive regard and affirmation. In J.C. Norcross & M.J. Lambert (Eds.), *Psychotherapy relationships that work. Volume 1: Evidence-based therapist contributions* (3rd ed.) (pp.288–322). Oxford University Press.

Gendlin, E.T. (1962). *Experiencing and the creation of meaning* (2nd ed.). Free Press.

Gendlin, E.T. (1974). Client-centered and experiential psychotherapy. In D.A. Wexler & L.N. Rice (Eds.), *Innovations in client-centered therapy* (pp.211–26). John Wiley.

Gendlin, E.T. (1978). *Focusing.* Everest House.

Grant, B. (1990). Principled and instrumental non-directiveness in person-centered and client-centered psychotherapy. *Person-Centered Review, 5*(1), 77–88. Reprinted in D.J. Cain (Ed.). (2002), *Classics in the person-centered approach* (pp.371–377). PCCS Books.

Grant, B. (2003, July). *Client-centered therapy: Ethics, knowledge, and perfection.* PCE World Conference, Egmond-aan-Zee.

Hogan, R.A. (1952). A measure of client defensiveness. In W. Wolff & J.A. Precker (Eds.), *Personality monographs. Vol. 3: Success in psychotherapy* (pp.112–142). Grune & Stratton.

Horney, K. (1937). *The neurotic personality of our time.* W.W. Norton & Co.

Kirschenbaum, H. (1979). *On becoming Carl Rogers.* Dalacorte Press.

Kirschenbaum, H. (2007). *The life and work of Carl Rogers.* PCCS Books.

Kirschenbaum, H. & Henderson, V. L. (Eds.). (1990) *The Carl Rogers reader.* Constable.

Knox, R., Murphy, D., Wiggins, S. & Cooper, M. (Eds.). (2013). *Relational depth: New perspectives and developments.* Palgrave Macmillan.

Koch, S. (1959). *Psychology: A study of a science.* McGraw-Hill.

Kolden, G.G., Chia-Chiang, W., Austin, S.B., Chang, Y. & Klein, M.H. (2019). Congruence. In J.C. Norcross & M.J. Lambert (Eds.), *Psychotherapy relationships that work. Volume 1: Evidence-based therapist contributions* (3rd ed.) (pp. 323–350). Oxford University Press.

Kramer, U. & Sachse, R. (2013). Early clarification processes in clients presenting with borderline personality disorder: Relations with symptom level and change. *Person-Centered & Experiential Psychotherapies, 12*(2), 157–175.

Lietaer, G. (1990). The client-centred approach after the Wisconsin project: A personal view on its evolution. In G. Lietaer, J. Rombauts & R. Van Balen (Eds.), *Client-centered and experiential psychotherapy in the nineties* (pp.19–45). Leuven University Press.

Lietaer, G. (2002). The united colors of person-centered and experiential psychotherapies. *Person-Centered & Experiential Psychotherapies, 1*(1–2), 4–13.

Mearns, D. (1996). Working at relational depth with clients in person-centred therapy. *Counselling, 7*(4), 306–311.

Mearns, D. & Cooper, M. (2018). *Working at relational depth in counselling and psychotherapy* (2nd ed.). Sage.

Mearns, D. & Thorne, B. (2000). *Person-centred therapy today: New frontiers in theory and practice.* Sage.

Moon, K., Rice, B. & Schneider, C. (2001). Stanley W. Standal and the need for positive regard. In J.D. Bozarth & P. Wilkins (Eds.). *Rogers' therapeutic conditions. Volume 3: Unconditional positive regard* (pp.19–34). PCCS Books.

Norcross, J.C. & Lambert, M.J. (Eds.). (2019). What works in the psychotherapy relationship: Results, conclusions and practices. In *Psychotherapy relationships that work. Volume 1: Evidence-based therapist contributions* (3rd ed.) (pp.631–646). Oxford University Press.

Raskin, N.J. (1948). The development of nondirective therapy. *Journal of Consulting Psychology, 12*, 92–110.

Raskin, N.J. (1949). The development of the 'parallel studies' project. *Journal of Counseling Psychology, 13*, 206–219. Reprinted in N. Raskin (Ed.). (2004), *Contributions to client-centered therapy and the person-centered approach* (pp.33–53). PCCS Books.

Raskin, N.J. (Ed.). (2004). *Contributions to client-centered therapy and the person-centered approach.* PCCS Books.

Rice, L.N. & Greenberg, L.S. (1984). *Patterns of change: Intensive analysis of psychotherapy process.* Guilford Press.

Rogers, C.R. (1939). *The clinical treatment of the problem child.* Houghton Mifflin.

Rogers, C.R. (1942). *Counseling and psychotherapy: Newer concepts in practice.* Houghton Mifflin.

Rogers, C.R. (1951). *Client-centered therapy: Its current practice, implications and theory.* Houghton Mifflin.

Rogers, C.R. (1957). The necessary and sufficient conditions of therapeutic personality change. *Journal of Consulting Psychology, 21*, 95–103.

Rogers, C.R. (1959). A theory of therapy, personality, and interpersonal relationships as developed in the client-centred framework. In S. Koch, (Ed.), *Psychology: A study of a science. Vol. 3: Formulations of the person and the social context* (pp.184–256). McGraw-Hill.

Rogers, C.R. (1961). *On becoming a person: A therapist's view of psychotherapy.* Houghton Mifflin.

Rogers, C.R. (1969). *Freedom to learn: A view of what education might become.* Charles E. Merrill.

Rogers, C.R. (1970). *Carl Rogers on encounter groups.* Harper & Row.

Rogers, C.R. (1977). *Carl Rogers on personal power: Inner strength and its revolutionary impact.* Delacorte.

Rogers C.R. (1980). *A way of being.* Houghton Mifflin.

Rogers, C.R. (1986) A client-centered/person centered approach to therapy. In I.L. Kutash & A. Wolf (Eds.), *Psychotherapist's casebook* (pp.197–208). Jossey-Bass.

Rogers C.R. & Coulson, W.R. (Eds.). (1968). *Man and the science of man.* Charles E. Merrill.

Rogers, C.R. & Dymond, R.F. (1954). *Psychotherapy and personality change.* University of Chicago Press.

Rogers C.R. & Russell, D.E. (2002). *Carl Rogers, the quiet revolutionary: An oral history.* Penmarin Books.

Rogers C.R., Gendlin, E.T., Kiesler, D.J. & Truax, C.B. (1967). *The therapeutic relationship and its impact: A study of psychotherapy with schizophrenics.* University of Wisconsin Press.

Sanders, P. (2011). Schizophrenia is not an illness – A response to van Blaricom. *Person-Centered & Experiential Psychotherapies, 6*(2), 112–128.

Schmid, P.F. (2001a). Authenticity: The person as his or her own author. Dialogical and ethical perspectives on therapy as an encounter relationship. And beyond. In G. Wyatt (Ed.), *Rogers' therapeutic conditions. Volume 1: Congruence* (pp.213–228). PCCS Books.

Schmid, P.F. (2001b). Comprehension: The art of not-knowing. Dialogical and ethical perspectives on empathy as dialogue in personal and person-centred relationships. In S. Haugh & T. Merry (Eds.), *Rogers' therapeutic conditions. Volume 2: Empathy* (pp.53–71). PCCS Books.

Schmid, P.F. (2001c). Acknowledgement: The art of responding. Dialogical and ethical perspectives on the challenge of unconditional personal relationships in therapy and beyond. In J. Bozarth & P. Wilkins (Eds.), *Rogers' therapeutic conditions. Volume 3: Unconditional positive regard* (pp.49–64). PCCS Books.

Schmid, P.F. (2002). Presence: Im-media-te co-experiencing and co-responding. Phenomenological, dialogical and ethical perspectives on contact and perception in person-centred therapy and beyond. In G. Wyatt & P. Sanders (Eds.), *Rogers' therapeutic conditions. Volume 4: Contact and perception* (pp.182–203). PCCS Books.

Schmid, P.F. (2013). Dialogue as the foundation of person-centred therapy. In R. Knox, D. Murphy, S. Wiggins & M. Cooper (Eds.), *Relational depth: New perspectives and developments* (pp.155–174). Palgrave Macmillan.

Seeman, J. (1983). *Personality integration*. Human Sciences Press.

Seeman, J. & Raskin, N.J. (1953). Research perspectives in client-centered therapy. In H.O. Mowrer (Ed.), *Psychotherapy: Theory and research* (pp.205–234). Ronald Press.

Shlien, J.M. (2003). *To lead an honorable life: Invitations to think about client-centered therapy and the person-centered approach*. PCCS Books.

Shostrom, E.L. (1965). *Three approaches to psychotherapy I*. https://psychedfilms.com/films/three-approaches-to-psychotherapy-i/

Shostrom, E.L. (1977). *Three approaches to psychotherapy II*. https://psychedfilms.com/films/three-approaches-to-psychotherapy-ii/

Snijders, J.A. (Hans), Amons, P.J.T. & Dierick, P. (2015). Client-centered/experiential group psychotherapy with borderline clients: Specific processes and challenges. *Person-Centered & Experiential Psychotherapies, 14*(1), 18–31.

Standal, S.W. (1954). *The need for positive regard: A contribution to client-centered theory.* Unpublished doctoral dissertation. University of Chicago.

Thorne, B. (1991). *Person-centred counselling: Therapeutic and spiritual dimensions*. Whurr.

Thorne, B. (1998). *Person-centred counselling and Christian spirituality: The secular and the holy.* Whurr.

Thorne, B. (2002). *The mystical power of person-centred therapy: Hope beyond despair.* Whurr.

Thorne, B. (2012). *Carl Rogers*. (3rd ed.). Sage.

van Blaricom, J. (2006). A person-centered approach to schizophrenia. *Person-Centered & Experiential Psychotherapies, 5*(3), 155–173.

Warner, M. (2000). Person-centered psychotherapy: One nation, many tribes. *Person-Centered Journal 7*(1), 28–39.

Warner, M. (2016). Difficult process: Working with fragile and dissociated client experiences. In C. Lago & D. Charura (Eds.), *The person-centred counselling and psychotherapy handbook: Origins, developments and current applications* (pp.102–110). Open University Press/McGraw-Hill.

Warner, M. (2017). A person-centred view of human nature, wellness and psychopathology. In S. Joseph (Ed.), *The handbook of person-centred therapy and mental health* (pp.92–115). PCCS Books.

Zimring, F.M. (1974). Theory and practice of client-centered therapy: A cognitive view. In D.A. Wexler & L.N. Rice (Eds.), *Innovations in client-centered therapy* (pp.117–137). John Wiley.

2. Classical person-centred therapy

Tony Merry and Sheila Haugh

Introduction

Classical person-centred therapy developed from the work of Carl Rogers, the American psychotherapist, researcher and academic, and his colleagues, from about 1940 onwards (see Chapter 1, this volume). It offered a radical way of working with people that departed sharply from the Freudian and cognitive-behavioural approaches that were dominant in psychology at that time. With its emphasis on the qualities of the relationship between client and therapist, and its rejection of diagnostic assessment and labelling, it remains as radical today as it was in the 1940s. Currently, person-centred therapy (PCT) is one of the most widely used approaches to helping relationships in the UK and Europe, though not always the best understood.

Person-centred therapy has developed through a number of evolutionary phases and has been known by different terms at different times. These were, first, 'non-directive therapy', then 'client-centred therapy', and finally 'person-centred therapy' (see Chapter 1, this volume). The name changes are significant in that they illustrate some shifts of emphasis over the past 60 years or so.

According to Barrett-Lennard (1998), in his discussion of the history and international development of the person-centred approach, the 'non-directive phase', from about 1940 to 1950, emphasised the development of a non-judgemental atmosphere in the therapy relationship in which the accent was on the skills of the therapist to promote the therapy process. From the 1950s to the early 1960s (the 'client-centred phase'), the emphasis was on counsellor attitudes rather than skills, and on reflecting the client's feelings. The idea of the counsellor as a person involved subjectively in the therapy relationship began to take shape. From the 1960s to the present day (the 'person-centred phase'), the emphasis shifted again, this time towards therapist attitudes, values and relationship qualities.

Throughout this period, some basic philosophical and theoretical ideas have remained fairly constant, with new perspectives and understandings emerging over the years. The sections that follow explore these ideas and build up a comprehensive picture of the theory and practice of person-centred therapy in its classical form.

The person and 'human nature'

Rogers took an optimistic view of human nature. He described 'the person' as forward-moving, constructive, realistic and trustworthy, in contrast to those who favoured such terms as hostile, antisocial, destructive or evil. This positive, constructive view of the person is a recurring feature of Rogers' thinking. At the same time, he was not naïve about the existence of destructive, antisocial or other negative aspects of human behaviour. He did not, however, regard such negative aspects as inherent, or somehow a basic component of the human condition.

The term 'human nature', although an imprecise concept open to a variety of interpretations, is used in person-centred psychology to denote certain characteristics of persons that Rogers thought to be universal (see Merry, 2020; pp.19–24). He viewed individuals as constantly in the process of developing and, in Rogers' term, 'becoming'. Rogers regarded people as motivated by a tendency for growth and enhancement, and as constructive, trustworthy, responsive, creative and adaptive, or capable of becoming so.

Although Rogers is usually associated with one-to-one therapy, his concern was with the person in relation to others and to society at large, as well as with the individual's 'inner world'. His theory of personality (Rogers, 1959), for example, suggests how individuals build up pictures of themselves (their self-concepts) through early (and subsequent) relationships with others. In individual terms, what is 'real' to any person is what exists within their inner subjective world or internal frame of reference. This reality forms the basis for the way a person behaves in the world and responds to events and experiences. This phenomenological approach holds that the best way to understand a person's behaviour and feelings is to understand how that person experiences, perceives and interprets the surrounding world. For Rogers, then, the most important area of psychological study was the individual's subjective experience, because this experience informs and underpins all behaviour.

Rogers (1961) described his trust in human nature in the following terms:

> [T]he basic nature of the human being, *when functioning freely*, is constructive and trustworthy… When we are able to free the individual from defensiveness, so that he (sic) is open to the wide range of his own needs, as well as the wide range of environmental and social demands, his reactions may be trusted to be positive, forward moving, constructive… His total behavior… as he moves toward being open to all his experience, will be more balanced and realistic, behavior which is appropriate to the survival and enhancement of a highly social animal. (p.194, emphasis added)

The actualising tendency

The key to understanding Rogers' view of the person is his formulation of the theory of actualisation – one of the basic theoretical constructs in person-centred psychology. It is the tendency for an individual to fulfil their potential and is regarded as the sole motivation for human behaviour and development (Rogers, 1957, 1959).

This theory suggests that organisms, including humans of course, tend to develop positively and constructively in environments that support such development. Hostile or destructive environments, on the other hand, tend to inhibit development of constructive potential. The theory of actualisation is a biologically based theory that describes the interaction between an individual organism and its environment. It is not a 'moral theory' and does not ascribe values to particular kinds of behaviour or kinds of people.

To Rogers, the environment plays a central part in influencing how individuals develop, form self-concepts and acquire self-esteem. Actualisation occurs in physical, biological, social, cultural and psychological contexts, and this constitutes the environment in which the person lives. An interaction between genetic predisposition, the environment and individual experience shapes the specific ways in which actualisation is expressed. The process of actualisation is not regarded as a conscious 'activity' in which the individual makes choices between alternatives, but as a process in which the total organism is involved at both conscious and non-conscious levels. 'Consciousness' or 'self-awareness' enables a wide range of choices to be made, with the person's behaviour, values and attitudes open to change and reformulation in the light of learning and experience.

Behaviour is seen as 'goal directed' in that it represents attempts by the person to maintain and enhance themselves in response to whatever environmental conditions are being experienced. The theory of actualisation proposes that there is a 'growth tendency' that, in an ideal or perfect environment, would result in each individual fulfilling all their constructive, personal and pro-social potentials. Such an environment would, from the moment of a person's birth, be experienced as nurturing, safe and accepting of individual differences. In these circumstances, human capacities for constructive relationships, the understanding of others and creative action, for example, would be expressed. It is important to note that not all potentialities of individuals, such as the potential to commit violent acts towards others, are regarded as aspects of the directional nature of the actualising tendency. Humans have both constructive and destructive potentials. In an environment in which positive regard is lacking, the actualisation of destructive potential is more likely. Destructive potential includes destructive behaviours towards self or others. When such behaviour does occur, the concept of actualisation directs our attention for an explanation to the environmental conditions that have distorted or corrupted the pro-social direction of the actualising process.

However, for Rogers, the environment is never ideal or consistently constructive. There are always constraints to be confronted, many of which are likely to obstruct a person's capacity for growth towards the theoretical ideal of being fully functioning. These constraints might include poor physical conditions, and crucially they include unsatisfactory relationships with others, ranging from emotional neglect and the absence of love and nurturing to more severe degrees of abuse and deprivation. Nevertheless, each person interacts with their environment, including those aspects of the environment that tend to inhibit growth, in an effort to develop as fully as possible in whatever circumstances prevail. If, for example, the developing person experiences relationships with others that are only hostile or aggressive in some way, then the person's need for nurturing and emotional warmth will remain unmet. This is likely to have destructive or inhibiting effects on their emotional or psychological development, and these effects are likely to manifest themselves throughout the person's lifetime. Even so, the actualising tendency is still present, no matter how unsuitable the environment in which the individual finds themself. The only way to destroy the actualising tendency completely is to destroy the organism – the person.

Some aspects of behaviour that may be interpreted as 'negative' or 'self-destructive', when viewed phenomenologically (that is, from within the individual's own frame of reference), can be regarded as manifestations of the actualising tendency's capacity to defend the person against threat. For example, a person's apparent inability to form or sustain close, intimate relationships with others and to opt instead for a series of unfulfilling casual relationships seems to challenge the notion of actualisation always working towards the individual's enhancement. When viewed from within the person's inner subjective world, however, this behaviour is understandable if previous attempts at intimacy have resulted in significant emotional hurt. In this case, 'the tendency towards actualisation' is in the direction of self-defence because emotional and physical survival takes precedence over self-enhancement. This does not mean, however, that the self-destructive behaviour is not open to change, as we shall see later.

The actualising tendency is, then, viewed as a universal characteristic of living things, but its detailed expression in human beings is always unique to the individual. It is the motivation for all individual action, whether or not the circumstances at any one moment are favourable or unfavourable for growth and development. In unfavourable conditions the expression of the actualising tendency may become distorted, but even so the tendency remains as constructive as the environment allows. In Rogers' (1951) words, the human being 'has one basic tendency and striving – to actualize, maintain and enhance the experiencing organism' (p.487). The implications of this idea are profound: 'No aspect of the client is to be regarded conditionally, as [any] aspect is always an expression of the potential of the whole and trustworthy organism' (Levitt, 2008, p.229).

Self and the self-actualising tendency

The general tendency toward actualisation results in the differentiation of some experience into an 'I' or 'me' – in other words, a self or self-concept. Rogers (1961) viewed this self as fluid and changing, although at any one time it has certain consistent characteristics. Thus, the self is a particular part of the person's total experiencing (this total experiencing is sometimes referred to as 'organismic experiencing'). Self-actualisation is best thought of as a sub-system of the general actualising tendency. These two concepts are often confused. The function of self-actualisation is to maintain and enhance the self-structure; the actualising tendency refers to the organism as a whole.

The person as a whole, as an aspect of their growth, fulfils the potential to differentiate as a separate person with a specific identity. The process of self-actualisation appears after the development of a self-structure, and it is this process, self-actualisation, that maintains and develops the self-structure. The constructs of self and self-actualisation are very significant in Rogers' (1959) theory of the development of the person and how the person may become disturbed. In favourable conditions, the formation of a self-concept and the actualising of the self result in the person being open to experience with a self-concept that is in harmony with their organismic experiencing. On the other hand, unfavourable conditions may result in the actualising of a self that is in conflict with organismic experiencing. It is this conflict that results in psychological disturbance. For example, a child may have the experience that a particular situation is frightening, and they may react accordingly by showing fear and crying. In other words, the child's organismic experience is one of being afraid. In favourable circumstances, the child's fear would be responded to by an adult with understanding and reassurance. The child would continue to be held in positive regard and the fear accepted, both by the child and the adult, as a natural and spontaneous response to a perceived threat. The child's developing sense of themself and actual experience would be in harmony and no conflict would result. On the other hand, if the child's fear were responded to without understanding and in a way that tended to negate the experience of fear, the experience would be overridden and denied or distorted by the child's emerging self. The organismic experience ('I am afraid') would be denied by the self ('I am not afraid', or 'Fear is not an acceptable part of me').

In this way, the process of self-actualising will continue to express a self that contains conflicts between self-experience and organismic experiencing. Some experiencing will be accepted into awareness because it is consistent with the self-concept; other experiencing may be denied to awareness or distorted in some way because it conflicts with the self-concept. The extent to which such conflicts accumulate through experiences similar to the example given above determines, for Rogers, the extent to which the person is psychologically troubled.

Self theory

The concept of self is central in PCT. We can think of 'the self' as a consistent set of experiences and perceptions that we gradually differentiate into an 'I' or 'me', 'together with the values attached to those concepts' (Rogers, 1951, p.498). As the self develops, we begin to attach certain values to our experience and build up a picture of our selves through our interactions with our environment, and especially with others who have significance for us, such as early caregivers. The self becomes the inner, experiencing person, able to reflect consciously on experience and act in the world in ways that are consistent with our experience of it.

Rogers' (1951) personality theory is organised into a set of 19 statements (he called them 'propositions') that explain how an individual develops a sense of self and suggest the ways in which the person becomes either fully functioning or not. Rogers regarded each person as inhabiting a 'world' of which they are the centre. The individual is in a constant process of experiencing and perceiving the world and defining what is for them 'reality'. The actualising tendency provides the motivation for everything the person does, and every act reflects the tendency of the person to maintain and develop themselves in some way physically and psychologically. It follows from this that behaviour is the goal-directed attempts by the person to satisfy needs as they are experienced.

Feeling and emotion accompany and influence this goal-directed behaviour, and the intensity of the emotion being experienced is related to the significance of the behaviour. For example, an emotion will be very strongly experienced if a powerful need is being frustrated or satisfied, and less strongly experienced if the need is not so great.

Rogers' (1951) 19 propositions also describe how the person positively values the experiences that tend to maintain and enhance the person and negatively values those that do not. In other words, the self-structure consists both of experiences and the values attached to them. Some of the time, those values are experienced directly, but at other times experiences may become valued either positively or negatively because those values have been absorbed from others as if they had been experienced directly, often in a distorted fashion. This 'absorption' is described as introjection: the internalisation of material that is simultaneously ignored and acted upon. Introjection is the process whereby a person incorporates an external value into their psychological structure without modification and then believes, to some degree, that it originates from inside them.

This is key to understanding Rogers' (1951, 1959) theory of how people become emotionally disturbed. As experiences occur, the person may accurately perceive them and organise them into the self-structure, or the person may ignore them completely because they cannot perceive any relationship between the experience and the self-structure as it currently exists. Crucially, the person may distort or deny the experience because it is inconsistent with the existing self-structure and may threaten to undermine that structure if the experience is incorporated accurately. The example we gave above, where a child does not allow themself to experience fear because to do so would be inconsistent with a self-structure that is unable to admit fear into awareness, is an example of this kind of denial. Alternatively, the child may distort the experience of fear into a feeling of guilt, for example, if guilt were an acceptable component of the self-structure at that time. Another way of putting it is to think of a sequence:

1. At the beginning of life, the individual is fully congruent – able to admit all experience into awareness without distortion.
2. Later, the person meets disapproval, rejection or other threat, and experiences anxiety.
3. The formation of the self-concept becomes conditioned by these negative experiences, and the person internalises negative judgements about themself.
4. This conditioned self-concept becomes reinforced by further experiences, and the person becomes alienated from their 'true self'.
5. The person is now incongruent. They are no longer able to admit all experiences into awareness without distortion.

Psychological 'maladjustment', for Rogers (1951, 1959), results when a person denies or distorts experience and does not absorb it accurately into the self-structure. This is described as incongruence. On the other hand, adjustment (congruence) exists when the self is able to allow all experience into awareness without any distortion. Any experience that is inconsistent with the current self-structure may be perceived as a threat, and the more threat is perceived, the more rigid the self-structure becomes, in order to defend itself against the experience. If the individual finds themself in a relationship where there is little or no threat of negative judgement, the person is in a better position to allow hitherto denied or distorted experience more fully and accurately into awareness. When this happens, the person begins to reorganise their self-concept so that the introjected and distorted values that have been attached to experience become replaced by the person's own values. The person becomes more trusting of their own experience and less vulnerable to the values and judgements of others. Ultimately, they cease to behave in the world in ways they have learned are acceptable to others, and to deny and devalue their experience, and begin to behave more authentically, with greater confidence and trust in their own, internal valuing process.

The locus of evaluation

Rogers (1951, 1959) thought that when someone as making judgements about issues and people, they were guided either by the values they had previously introjected from others, or by their own valuing process. Where people relied too heavily on the values of others, Rogers described them as experiencing an *external locus of evaluation*, and when they were able to be more trusting and reliant on their own *organismic valuing process*, he described them as having an *internal locus of evaluation*. This is important because Rogers believed a characteristic of the healthy or fully functioning person is to have trust in the validity of their own values and judgements.

Conditions of worth and the self-concept

The term Rogers chose for introjected values was *conditions of worth* (1959). He argued that we are brought into the world with two related needs. The first need is to experience unconditional positive regard from those around us on whom we depend for survival. The second is to develop positive self-regard through the formation of a constructive self-concept. It is through experience and feedback from our environment that we develop a self-concept, and when this feedback is positive and constructive, it feeds our self-concept, which in turn enables us to value our self. In other words, if our experience, feelings and behaviour are accepted, understood and valued by those around us and on whom we depend, our needs for positive self-regard and for positive regard from others are met.

However, because the need to experience positive regard from others is so great (in an individual's perception, it is a survival need), we will sometimes accept the values and judgements of others, even when they contradict our own experience. In the child's perception of the world, thinking, feeling and behaving in ways that continue to attract positive regard then become more important than accepting and valuing our own experience. We will introject the judgements and evaluations of others into our self-concept as if they were our own.

As we gradually build up and refine our self-concept, we are unaware of which elements are the result of direct experience and which are introjected from others. The self becomes composed of a mixture of personal values and values derived from others. Whenever people of significance to us value some aspects of us as more deserving of positive regard than others, we begin to avoid or seek out certain self-experiences according to how worthy they are of our self-regard. This process of positively valuing only those experiences that contribute to positive self-regard and rejecting or avoiding those that do not are the result of us acquiring conditions of worth. If, throughout our life, we were only ever to experience unconditional positive regard from others, then no conditions of worth would develop. Self-regard would be unconditional, and the need for positive regard from others and positive self-regard would never conflict with our internal (i.e. 'organismic') valuing system.

However, it is unlikely that we would only ever experience unconditional positive regard, and it is therefore inevitable that we develop some conditions of worth. This makes us vulnerable to perceiving and making sense of our experiences somewhat selectively. We allow into our awareness those experiences that are consistent with our self-concept, and we deny or distort those that are inconsistent with it. This can become something of a circular process. We tend to regard experiences that are inconsistent or incongruent with our self-concept as threatening, and we tend to protect ourselves from such experiences by distorting or denying them. In this way, we reinforce the incongruence between experience and self, and we become even more defensive and less open to experience. More recently, the notion of 'significant others' has been widened to include the cultures we inhabit. While a culture might support the self-actualising tendency, at the same time 'environmental factors as oppressive forces can make it more challenging [for a person] to engage the full range of their innate self-actualizing force' (Swan & Ceballos, 2020, p.159).

Mearns (1999) and Mearns and Thorne (2000) advanced a modification of Rogers' theory of self that is still consistent with general person-centred theory. They suggest that the self can take on different configurations of the elements present within it, in response to the varying circumstances of a person's life. Feelings, thoughts and behaviour change as the person adapts and responds to the environment, but 'the self' remains consistent, no matter what circumstances are encountered. In this way, while a person may think, feel and behave in a particular way in one situation, their feelings, thoughts and actions may be very different in another. Certain configurations might exist as an adaptation to the introjection of particular conditions of worth. A person may, for example, regard themselves as 'bad' or 'worthless' when it comes to being a parent, but 'good' or 'of value' when it comes to being a teacher. Each configuration serves a purpose in maintaining the person's self-concept in different circumstances or in response to different experiences. Mearns and Thorne are careful to point out that this does not amount to a 'splitting' of the personality or any kind of 'dissociative state', because the person's fundamental values and level of self-esteem remain constant.

The fully functioning person

In person-centred theory the *fully functioning person* is synonymous with the fully congruent person. That is, a person's experiencing is available to their awareness without denial or distortion. As such, fully functioning is also the definition of optimal *congruence* – of optimal psychological health and optimal psychological 'maturity'. The fully functioning person is described as a hypothetical endpoint as, for Rogers (1959), the fully functioning person 'would be a person-in-process, a person continually changing' (p.235). He continues:

> Thus his (sic) specific behaviors cannot in any way be described in advance. The only statement which can be made is that the behaviors would be adequately adaptive to each new situation, and that the person would be continually in a process of further self-actualization. (p.235)

The notion of the fully functioning person brings into relief the process nature of person-centred theory more generally. Actualisation of the organism and actualisation of the self are understood as ongoing processes, hence the terms actualis*ing* tendency and self-actualis*ing* tendency. For Rogers (1961), the fully functioning person is a hypothetical endpoint, and it might be better to think of this person as always on the road to becoming rather than someone reaching a particular destination. As Rogers describes it (1959), this is an ever-developing 'process of functioning more fully' (p.191).

Counselling and psychotherapy

Rogers did not make a distinction between 'counselling' and 'psychotherapy', seeing them as essentially the same activity – an attitude that persists among many person-centred practitioners today. Whatever label is used, person-centred therapy is a form of therapy in which the relationship between client and therapist is the most significant factor in promoting change and development. While the therapeutic relationship is accepted as important in most forms of counselling and therapy, person-centred therapy is unique in viewing the relationship itself as therapeutic, aside from anything that may be said or done within it. The emphasis is almost exclusively placed on the qualities of the relationship between the client and the therapist. In other words, the formation and maintenance of a strong therapeutic relationship is not seen as a preparation for the implementation of any strategies or techniques. Rogers' (1942, 1951, 1957, 1959, 1961) view was that psychological or emotional healing was promoted within a relationship in which the client experienced being accepted, valued and understood. The motivation for healing is supplied by the person's tendency to actualise constructively in an environment that facilitates such development.

The six conditions

Rogers (Rogers & Dymond, 1954) was led to this view as a result of his clinical experience and his research into the factors that promote change within therapy and those that militate against it. In 1957, Rogers published his seminal scientific paper in which he outlined 'the necessary and sufficient conditions of therapeutic personality change'. He identified and described six of these necessary and sufficient conditions in the following way:

> 1. That two persons are in *contact*.
> 2. That the first person, whom we shall term the client, is in a state of *incongruence*, being *vulnerable* or *anxious*.
> 3. That the second person, whom we shall term the therapist, is *congruent* in the *relationship*.
> 4. That the therapist is *experiencing unconditional positive regard* toward the client.
> 5. That the therapist is *experiencing* an *empathic* understanding of the client's *internal frame of reference*.
> 6. That the client *perceives*, at least to a minimal degree, conditions 4 and 5, the *unconditional positive regard* of the therapist for him (sic), and the *empathic* understanding of the therapist. (pp.213–214; original emphases)

He further explained, in a chapter published in 1959:

> [I]t is hypothesized that [the process of therapy] never commences *without* these conditions being met… [and] the same conditions are regarded as sufficient for therapy, regardless of the particular characteristics of the client. (pp.214)

This theory of therapeutic relationships has become known as the 'conditions model'. However, three of the six conditions have generally received most attention, becoming known as 'the core conditions' – a phrase that is almost impossible to find in Rogers' own writings.

Condition 1: Two persons are in contact

The first condition seems so obviously a condition necessary for therapeutic change to take place that it is often missed as an area of exploration or consideration during training. Rogers regarded this first condition as so simple that it should, perhaps, be termed an assumption in, or precondition for, therapy (1959, p.222; see also 1957). He explicated this idea when he wrote in his later book that the two people (client and therapist) need to have the 'minimum essential of a relationship', and continued: '…which makes a perceived or subceived difference in the experiential field of the [each] other' (1959, p.207). *Subception* is the idea that we react to things outside of our awareness or non-consciously. In practice this means that, if a client and therapist are responding to each other in any way, there is contact, as each will be making a difference in the perceptual world of the other (see Wyatt & Sanders, 2002).

Garry Prouty's development of 'pre-therapy' (e.g. Prouty, 1994; Prouty et al., 2002; Sanders, 2007) evolved from his work with clients whose capacity for any form of contact seemed deeply impaired (see Chapter 11, this volume). Prouty explored ways in which contact can be made with those whose degree of psychological impairment seems to make it impossible. Such clients include those with some psychotic experiences, those in deep shock or in catatonic states, some people with learning disabilities, and those with autism (see Brooks & Paterson, 2011), dementia or brain injury. It was argued by Bozarth (1998) that 'pre-therapy' was not person-centred therapy, even if it was a major development of the principles of the PCA to therapy and their application to this group of clients. However, Prouty described pre-therapy as 'an integrated empathic attitude' (2001, p.157). It 'emphasizes empathic contact and a theory of psychological contact' (Prouty, 1999, p.28). The ideas developed in pre-therapy are extremely useful in developing a deeper understanding of this first condition.

Conditions 2, 3 and 4: The 'core' conditions

More familiar to trainees and practitioners of the person-centred approach are the conditions that have tended to be erroneously called the 'core' conditions. We can describe them as the attitudes or way of being of the therapist. They are, first, that the therapist is *congruent* in the relationship; second, that the therapist is experiencing *unconditional positive regard* toward the client, and third, that the therapist experiences *an empathic understanding* of the client's internal frame of reference. It needs to be remembered that these three conditions are only meaningful in the context of all the conditions taken together and that, in the absence of conditions 1 and 6, they do not constitute Rogers' theory of effective therapy.

Congruence/incongruence

The notion of congruence forms the second and third conditions of Rogers' theory of therapy. Congruence describes the state of being when a person is fully functioning, and is synonymous with optimal psychological health (Haugh, 2001). Feelings can be accessed at any moment and are 'not denied to awareness or distorted in awareness' (Haugh, 2000, p.62). A person is most likely to seek therapy if they are experiencing some sense of incongruence (condition 2). In other words, something doesn't feel quite right; they are unhappy or feeling depressed, for example. The underlying reasons, and even the feelings themselves, may be vague and unclear, but they sense something is wrong.

For the therapist (condition 3), congruence is described as the 'accurate matching of experience with awareness' (Rogers, 1961, p.282). Further, 'the therapist's *symbolization* of his (sic) own experience *in the relationship* must be accurate, if therapy is to be most effective' (Rogers, 1959; p.214; emphasis added). It is not necessary (or possible) that the therapist be fully functioning, only that they can be open to all feelings and experiencing in this particular relationship. Rogers' 'necessary and sufficient conditions' (as they are now commonly known) do not propose that congruence needs to be communicated to the client. Words like 'authenticity', 'realness' and 'genuineness' have been used to describe the therapist's capacity to enter into the therapy relationship as a self-aware person whose feelings are available to them. Rogers used these terms somewhat interchangeably in his own writings, and in the therapeutic context 'authenticity', 'realness' and 'genuineness' may be regarded not as definitions but as *outcomes* of congruence (Haugh, 2001). That is, the congruent (enough) therapist, is often experienced as authentic, real and genuine in their way of being.

Much debate has taken place over the years as to if, when and how to share 'congruence' with a client, even if it is not called for in the theory. In the first case, congruence describes a state in which feelings are not denied or distorted in awareness (they are accurately symbolised). In the second case, congruence refers to the therapist's behaviour being consistent with those feelings: for example, a congruent therapist who is afraid of, or intimidated by, a client would be able to admit those feelings to themselves and would acknowledge these feelings internally. The therapist may decide that directly communicating those feelings to the client would be the most honest and appropriate thing to do, especially if the feelings interfered or blocked the therapist's capacity to remain empathic. On the other hand, the therapist may decide to discuss and explore those feelings elsewhere (in supervision or their personal therapy, for example), before communicating them to the client. The therapist may also decide that it would not be appropriate to communicate them. The therapist would be fulfilling the condition of congruence in so far as the feelings were not being denied or distorted. If the therapist's behaviour were to become inauthentic, perhaps as a result of trying to cover up the feeling, then the therapist's behaviour would become incongruent.

It can be a matter of fine judgement in deciding whether or not to disclose a feeling or a thought to a client, not least in making the distinction between 'self-disclosure' and a congruent response (see Tudor & Worrall, 1994). It may depend on a number of factors, including the client's present state of vulnerability or anxiety, the current strength of the therapy relationship and the therapist's experience. Total congruence in both its 'internal' meaning and its 'communication' meaning is undoubtedly only a theoretical ideal linked to the ideal of the hypothetical fully functioning person. Rogers (1961, p.282) believed that the extent to which a therapist was able to experience congruence determined, in some measure, the extent to which the client experienced the relationship as therapeutic.

It is important to emphasise that congruence is not a skill or technique; rather, it is a fundamental value or attitude that contributes to a therapist's total 'way of being' in the world and with clients in therapy. Congruence requires a commitment to the development of authenticity and self-awareness, with those qualities being integrated expressions of the therapist's values and attitudes in relation to clients.

Unconditional positive regard

Unconditional positive regard (UPR) refers to the consistent acceptance, by the therapist, of a client's experience: their feelings, thoughts and the meanings they make of them (Rogers, 1961, p.282). Tudor and Worrall (2006) describe UPR succinctly thus: 'The message to the client is not that whatever he thinks or feels is OK, but that no one thing he thinks or feels is more or less valuable or acceptable than any other' (p.202).

It is neither necessary nor desirable for the therapist to be engaged in making moralistic evaluations of the client – positive or negative.

It is useful to remember the 'beginnings' of the notion of UPR. Rogers (1959) wrote of 'prizing' (p.208), and more recently Haugh (2014) has highlighted kindness as an important aspect of UPR. Tudor and Worrall (2006) strongly assert that UPR 'demands, legitimises and makes room for a kind of loving within the process of therapeutic relationships' (p.204). The commonplace (in counselling circles at least) use of the phrase 'unconditional positive regard' can lead us to forget the warmth and the compassion intended by the idea, and even more so when the acronym UPR is adopted. Rogers (1957) also thought that the term itself might be a little unfortunate as it had an absolute, 'all-or-nothing' ring to it, and remarked that:

> It is probably evident… that completely unconditional positive regard would never exist except in theory… I believe the most accurate statement is that the effective therapist experiences unconditional positive regard for the client during many moments of his (sic) contact with him, yet from time to time he experiences only a conditional positive regard – and perhaps at times a negative regard, though this is not likely in effective therapy. It is in this sense that unconditional positive regard exists as a matter of degree in any relationship. (Kirschenbaum & Henderson, 1990, p.225)

As with congruence, UPR cannot be considered a skill or one of a therapist's repertoire of techniques. It is part of a person's system of values and is an integrated aspect of that person, not something that can be adopted temporarily and, perhaps, inauthentically in order to fulfil the attitudinal conditions. It is also unlikely that UPR is often directly expressed by the therapist, and it does not usually take the form of 'supportive', 'encouraging' or 'approving' statements made by the therapist to the client (although such statements may, from time to time, be made). UPR is more likely to be conveyed through the therapist's close, empathic and non-judgemental following of the client's experiencing as they express it.

Bozarth (2001) views UPR, 'as the curative factor for the pathological development of personality', and asserts that:

> This has to be true, given Rogers' conceptualisation of personal dysfunctions being predicated upon the introjection of conditional positive regard by significant others and by society. Conditional regard is countered by the unconditional positive regard of the therapist. (p.16)

This position is echoed by Wilkins (2000), who states that, 'if any condition is more important than another, it is the communication of unconditional positive regard' (p.46). Merry (2020) has similarly highlighted the particular prominence person-centred therapy theory gives to the communication of UPR through close empathic attending to the client as a person.

Condition 5: Empathic understanding

The fifth condition is the notion of empathy. For Rogers, empathy, or empathic understanding, is primarily an attitude or, in Rogers' terms (1975), 'a way of being' (p.2). It is not a skill that can be modelled and taught in a structured or methodical way as a particular kind of communication process.

Central to this condition is the philosophy of phenomenology. Contemporary phenomenology is an approach in which understanding of the world is rooted in the immediate experience of the individual. Each individual perceives events and gives them meaning and, in order to understand the behaviour of another, we need to understand the meanings they give to events. Hence Rogers proposed empathy as a core factor in effective therapy. This contrasted, for example, with the behaviourists' search for meaning in external, objective categories of events and the psychoanalysts' search for meaning in Freud's categories of symbols in order to allow expert analysis by the therapist.

Empathic understanding involves an active process of reaching out to another person. It means trying to capture something of the feeling and meaning of a person's experience. It is not 'just listening'. Empathy involves a process of 'being with' another person – that is, attempting to 'step into the other person's shoes' and 'see the world through the other person's eyes', laying aside one's own perceptions, values, meanings and perspectives as far as possible (Merry, 2020, p.153).

The term 'internal frame of reference' is useful here (Rogers, 1959, p.210). It refers to the need for the therapist to understand the experiences of the client from the client's point of view, rather than by comparing a client's experiences with their own and assuming some degree of shared meaning. It is useful to distinguish empathy from sympathy. A sympathetic response to another person's distress – welcome and human though that often is – is not necessarily accompanied by any significant degree of understanding. It tends towards a cognitive appreciation of how a situation might be for someone. It is this component, understanding, that begins to differentiate an empathic response from a sympathetic one. A helpful way to conceptualise empathic understanding is to think of it as an internal experience of the therapist, followed by the sensitive and skilful communication of that experience to the client. We can then regard empathy as a process in which the client's feelings, thoughts and other experiences are received by the therapist, who then checks or tests their understanding in an intentional and purposeful way. This enables the client to experience being heard and, to some degree, understood, and to correct any misunderstanding or incomplete understanding, allowing the process to continue. It is useful to remember that empathy is not only about a person's feelings; it encompasses all parts of their way of being, all the ways they are experiencing the world in any given moment – cognitively, emotionally and experientially.

A further aspect of empathy should be emphasised here – the 'as if' quality of empathic understanding. This refers to the idea that one can enter the frame of reference of another person to the extent that events, feelings, and thoughts can be experienced, to some extent, as if they were one's own – but without losing the 'as if' quality. The empathic therapist maintains their separate identity, 'resonates' with the client's experience and engages with the client as a person but does not become overwhelmed by any strong feelings that may be expressed.

The following is an example of the unfolding process of empathic understanding. The full transcript of this session between the therapist (Carl Rogers) and the client (Ms G) can be found in Merry (1995/2006):

Ms G: I … er … For a long time I've felt like there, there is this thing in me and I don't know what it is… and… sometimes when I hear other people talking I… and it's not so much the words that they're using but the feelings that I can sense in them… of … um … I feel heavy and I know that their feelings are touching the same kind of feelings in me.

Carl: They're touching that secret part of you that you don't quite know what it is.

Ms G: Mm a lot of the time that is hurt or pain and sometimes it's anger as well.

Carl: But you feel that whatever this is that is sort of frightening within, is of negative feelings of pain and hurt and possibly anger.

Ms G: [*Nods*] And if I get in touch with them that they will overwhelm me and there's a fear of getting lost in them somehow and of not being able to find my way back to the joy that I can feel.

Carl: That if you ever let yourself really live in or feel those feelings, maybe you'd never find your way back to pleasantness and happiness and joy.

Ms G: 'Cos I feel like I can't let go of things like hurt and I can't let go of things like resentment… I want to, want to let go of those things, but I don't know how, how to do that, so I don't want to explore them, I feel that if I explore them, they will always be with me and I've kind of learnt to experience joy… but having said that to you I'm questioning whether that joy is real.

Carl: Makes you wonder whether maybe the joy would be more real if you were able to explore some of those frightening feelings. (pp.141–142)

This is empathic because Rogers is attending very closely to Ms G's internal world, with its mixture of thoughts and feelings that she cannot, as yet, express completely. Rogers does not attempt to guide or direct his client, or give advice, or make suggestions about what Ms G should do or what she should focus her attention on. Instead, Rogers concentrates on careful listening to what Ms G is trying to express and the way she expresses it, and he checks with her the extent of his understanding of her world as she is currently experiencing it.

Empathic responses of the kind illustrated above have often been misunderstood as a 'technique' or 'strategy'. Empathy is neither of these things. Nor is it simply a sophisticated form of 'active listening'. It is a genuine dedication on the part of the therapist to understanding the internal, subjective world of another person without the value judgements that normally accompany such an activity. Rogers objected to the term 'reflection of feelings', based on his dislike of empathy being misrepresented as the 'technique' of reflection. John Shlien (cited in Rogers, 1986) saw real advantages in the use of the term 'reflection of feeling', as it transformed a 'philosophy' of being empathic into constructive action. Unfortunately, this distinction is often lost and can lead to the caricature of a person-centred therapist as just a 'nodding head' or one who simply repeats what the client has just said.

For a 'classical' person-centred therapist, empathic understanding, also known as 'empathic understanding responses' (Brodley, 2011), is not used in order to achieve any particular effect or outcome. It is not about encouraging clients to focus on selected aspects of experience, or bringing issues or problems to the client's attention, or helping a client towards insight or 'personal growth'. Paradoxically, however, any of these (and others) may be outcomes of the client's experience of being understood with empathy and without judgement. This is a subtle and often overlooked point, which may become clearer on reading the brief discussion of 'the principled non-directive attitude' later in this chapter. The classical person-centred therapist is not trying to produce a particular effect, or achieve a set of specific therapeutic goals, other than the creation of a relationship in which the client's internal resources become released for the purposes of bringing about psychological change. This is not a haphazard process or one left to chance. The empathic (principled) non-directive attitude of the counsellor is viewed as contributing to the building of a relationship in which the actualising tendency of the client becomes available to reorganise the client's internal world to one that is less defended and more open to experience without the same defences that have hitherto prevailed. 'Skills' and 'techniques' in classical person-centred therapy are confined to the skilled ways in which counsellors communicate their non-judgemental empathic understanding (see condition 6).

It is important to recognise that Rogers did not say that a therapist had to fully experience empathic understanding, congruence and UPR in order for therapy to be effective. It is closer to the spirit of Rogers' words to suggest that it is the extent to which the therapist is able to experience these things that determines the extent to which the relationship is experienced as constructive by the client. In other words, therapy can proceed even if the therapist experiences these conditions only partially at times, and even not at all at others, provided the overall experience of the relationship by the client is one of significant empathy, authenticity and non-judgemental respect that is effectively communicated to the client.

Condition 6: Client perception

Rather like the first condition, for a long while there was little concentration on the sixth condition, the client's perception of the therapist's UPR and empathic understanding. This is largely, of course, about the therapist's ability to communicate those attitudes, and the lack of attention in the literature may have been due to a reluctance among person-centred theorists and practitioners to focus on skills in an approach that is predominantly attitudinal rather than based on expertise or cleverness. Nevertheless, if the empathic, congruent therapist who is full of unconditional positive regard is unable to communicate these attitudes effectively, it is unlikely that therapy will be particularly useful. This is crystalised in the work of pre-therapy (Chapter 11, this volume) with people who find it unusually difficult to engage with psychological contact.

In the late 1990s and early 2000s, the Institute for Person-Centred Learning ran a number of workshops titled 'Advanced Communication Skills'. These workshops took the position that, while person-centred therapy may be an attitudinal approach, there are certainly skills that can be learned by a therapist to enable them to 'communicate' the attitudes of empathy and UPR effectively and sensitively. Since that time, much has been written about the different ways in which therapists might approach this (for example, Mearns & Thorne, 2013; Merry, 2020; Tolan, 2017). Wyatt and Sanders (2002) have helpfully compiled a collection of papers on Rogers' therapeutic conditions that deal both with 'contact' and the way in which Rogers' therapeutic attitudes may be perceived and experienced by clients.

The six conditions work together

While it can be useful to separate the six conditions, particularly in order to understand their meaning, it is important to emphasise that together they form a coherent whole, or Gestalt, of interdependent elements. In terms of the therapist's observable behaviour, it is likely that the communication of empathic understanding will appear to be the therapist's main activity. However, it is probable that deep empathic understanding cannot be experienced by a therapist who is to some significant extent incongruent or lacking in positive regard. The 'conditions' constitute the therapist's total 'way of being' with the client and, from a classical standpoint, it is this way of being that establishes the psychological environment in which the client's actualising process will tend to be expressed in positive and constructive ways.

Unlike many other approaches to counselling and psychotherapy, including many of those within the person-centred family, classical person-centred therapy has not developed a set of associated techniques, strategies or methods, or a system of diagnostic classification of psychological problems. This is not an oversight, and there are a number of good theoretical reasons for it.

First, 'the necessary and sufficient conditions' theory is about the characteristics of all constructive human relationships and can be applied beyond the therapy relationship to other aspects of human experience. It is not a 'how to do it' method. The theory requires therapists to develop a particular set of values and attitudes towards others that are reflected consistently in their behaviour. For example, the person-centred therapist regards the change process as one involving the client's internal resources for growth and development and believes that these resources become increasingly available in a psychological environment that is free of threat and rich in positive regard and empathic understanding. It is not so much a question of what the therapist *does*, but how they *are* in relation to clients.

Detailed research has shown that Rogers characteristically made empathic following responses most of the time when in therapy with a client (e.g. Brodley & Brody, 1990; Merry, 1996; Moon et al., 2011). He can be seen as dedicating himself to gaining as deep an understanding of his clients as possible for him, and continually checking out or testing his understanding. The essentially non-judgemental and non-directive nature of his responses varied very little, if at all, from one client to another. There is no sense when reading Rogers' work, or that of other published person-centred practitioners, that they put into operation a set of predetermined skills, or that their underlying values varied with the kind of problem or issue the client was expressing.

Second, Rogers (1951) did not regard diagnostic categories as helpful. In fact, he thought they were more likely to be damaging, and certainly did not view them as useful in determining specific 'treatment plans'. For him, all manifestations of psychological disturbance are regarded as having a single 'cause' – corruption or damage to the actualising tendency created by destructive or 'negative' experiences, resulting in the introjection of self-destructive conditions of worth.

This can also be said of the process of 'assessment'. Most therapeutic approaches require the client's current state of emotional or psychological functioning to be assessed by the therapist prior to the initiation of therapy itself. This process, it is argued, will enable the therapist to plan, devise and apply the strategies and techniques most likely to 'fit' with the client's apparent 'treatment needs'. Assessment, in this scenario, becomes an aspect of diagnosis and, in the view of classical person-centred theory, thereby shifts attention away from the individual client to some theoretical label that has been assigned to them.

'Necessary and sufficient'

The theory that the six conditions are both necessary and sufficient is a topic of some disagreement among the person-centred tribes discussed in this book. The contentious area is the sufficiency of the six conditions – there is more general agreement about their necessity. In the classical position, the sufficiency of the six conditions is considered axiomatic. In this view, the therapist cannot both be attending empathically to the client's internal world and simultaneously engaged in making decisions about that experiencing or the manner of it with a view to intervening with any kind of technical instruction, suggestion, advice or other therapist-framed response. To put it most bluntly, any intervention that changes the client's experiencing away from its current process towards one considered by the therapist to be of more benefit is considered counter-therapeutic and a compromise of the essential non-directive nature of person-centred therapy.

The necessary and sufficient conditions also challenge the notion of the need to diagnose clients – something present-day healthcare systems see as an imperative: assess → diagnose → treat. Some person-centred therapists have found a way to reconcile person-centred practice with these demands. Paul Wilkins and Martin Gill (2003), for example, argue that the necessary and sufficient conditions and the seven stages of process (see Rogers, 1961, pp.125–159) introduce a form of assessment. They enable the person-centred therapist to decide the likelihood of establishing a successful therapeutic endeavour, monitor its progress and, to a lesser extent, determine what they, the therapist, does. They believe that this is both legitimate in terms of person-centred theory and essential to good practice. Person-centred experiential counselling for depression (PCE-CfD) (see Chapter 6, this volume) has similarly tailored a classical person-centred approach to meet the demands of a contemporary healthcare environment.

Non-directivity: A characteristic of classical person-centred therapy

From a classical standpoint, person-centred therapy is perhaps best regarded as comprising a coherent and consistent set of basic values and attitudes that a therapist brings to their relationships with others. Implied in the 'conditions theory' is a deep respect for a person's uniqueness and individuality, together with a trust in the person's capacity for ongoing change and personal development. It stands on the belief that people have the right to their own psychological self-determination. In other words, each person has the right to establish their own identity and to express their unique being in the world in ways that respect the right to self-determination of others.

More explicitly stated in classical person-centred theory are the values, attitudes and personal qualities of the therapist that need to exist in order for the relationship to initiate and maintain the client's change process. A further characteristic of the relationship that is implied by the conditions theory is that it is a non-directive one. This is such an important principle that it needs some further discussion.

Although Rogers did not use the term 'non-directive' in his theory statement of 1957 and 1959, he did use it elsewhere, and person-centred therapy was for a time known as 'non-directive therapy' (see Chapter 1, this volume). 'Non-directivity' refers to the general attitude that change is a naturally occurring process driven by the actualising tendency and its content is uniquely determined by the needs of each individual (Tudor & Worrall, 2006). Rogers (1961) noted that the change process displays its own direction in that it tends to be away from reliance on the evaluations and judgements of others and towards increasing reliance on the individual's own valuing system (i.e. from an external towards an internal locus of evaluation). Rogers also noted that, among other things, change involved a dissolving of conditions of worth so that the person becomes less inhibited by introjected values and attitudes and increasingly free to respond to experience in novel and creative ways, with less internal conflict. Person-centred theory views these general developments as being outcomes of changes in the client's psychological environment provided by the person-centred therapy relationship. In other words, the environmental factors (relationships with others, cultural and social environments) that lead to the internalisation of conditions of worth and the development of an external locus of evaluation can be corrected for by the client's immersion in a more constructive environment. The absence of threat in this environment, together with the experiences of being understood empathically by a congruent therapist who holds an attitude of UPR, enables a client to allow more experience into awareness without the associated distortion and denial of internalised conditions of worth.

Person-centred theory regards this process as being unpredictable in its specifics and likely to be idiosyncratic for each client. The principle of non-directivity is important because it enables each client's change process to unfold as more denied or distorted experience becomes accurately available to awareness. Since the content of this experience cannot be predicted, the therapist cannot assume to know what direction the therapy should take or what 'issues' may or may not prove to have significance for the client (see Keys, 2003).

In 2002, Merry and Brodley wrote:

> The process of change in client-centered therapy is predictable only in very general terms. It is idiosyncratic and, in detail, unpredictable for each individual. It is this

> unpredictability, and the person-specific unique processes that it represents, that makes therapist attempts to direct the process both unnecessary and countertherapeutic. Directivity implies foreknowledge both of the destination and of the most efficient way of arriving there. Because each client's 'journey' is personal and idiosyncratic, direction needs to emerge from within the client, supported by the understanding relationship, rather than imposed by the therapist. (p. 72)

Susan Stephen (in press) states simply and clearly that non-directivity:

> is fundamental to person-centred practice: an attitude held by the therapist from which they trust and relate to their client as a person with agency, autonomy, and the capacity to grow in response to their own unique experience in the world.

From a classical standpoint, this non-directive attitude minimises the possibility that the therapist behaves, either knowingly or not, in ways that assume power over the client or expertise on the client's behalf. Barry Grant, in his seminal 1990 paper, made the useful distinction between *instrumental* and *principled* non-directiveness. Instrumental non-directiveness he regards as a kind of technique: a decision actively made by the therapist to be non-directive on the basis it will be helpful to the client. Principled non-directiveness, in Grant's view, is a moral choice: i.e. a choice to respect clients as autonomous individuals. Principled non-directiveness is thus an expression both of respect for the client's own self-resources and of the determination on the therapist's part not to control the course of the therapy and to follow the client's individual process as it emerges. Simply, it 'implies being responsive to the client's direction' (Levitt, 2008, p.*i*).

From this position, it can be understood that the principle of non-directivity does not mean repeating what the client has just said, and nor does it mean sitting in a tormenting silence waiting for the client to say something, out of fear of being directive. And if the therapist's approach is tormenting for the client, then it is probably not very empathic (see Stephen (in press) for a discussion of non-directivity in practice). Principled non-directivity does not mean the adoption of a laissez-faire attitude of non-involvement, or one of leaving the therapeutic process to the vagaries of chance. Rather, it is an ethical stance taken towards the complex processes involved in human psychological growth and development, most of which are poorly or incompletely understood. Empathic following of an individual's idiosyncratic and unpredictable journey into the roots of their sense of 'self' requires an active, involved and non-judgemental concentration. The source of change is assumed as residing within the individual, and the imposition of externally located technical expertise is regarded as counter-productive in locating and activating the individual's self-healing resources. In this writer's experience (SH), an increasing number of person-centred practitioners are choosing to use 'principled non-directivity' to describe how they work. They see it as a better description of their ethical intent to trust the client's inner resources and direction than 'being non-directive because that's how a person-centred therapist works'.

For Grant (1990, p.77), 'Instrumental non-directiveness is expressed by empathic responses and by encouraging clients to find solutions within themselves.' It is 'essentially a means of facilitating growth' that is 'often helpful and sometimes unhelpful'. Principled non-directiveness on the other hand:

> is an ideally unwavering expression of respect that is manifested in many and unpredictable ways, but usually in the form of empathic responses. Many of the same behaviors are consistent with both versions of nondirectiveness, but they are done for different reasons, in different spirits (p.86)

As Grant acknowledges, of course, there are times in any therapeutic relationship where the client's resources seem unavailable or the process becomes stuck and little observable change takes place. The temptation in such circumstances is for the therapist to provide the direction, or to assume responsibility, for the client's process rather than for the therapist's own empathic resources and ability to remain immersed in the client's inner world. Such experiences of 'stuckness' are not confined to classical person-centred therapy but are common in all therapeutic traditions. In the 'classical' position, these experiences are regarded as acceptable (if somewhat frustrating) realities of the process of personal development that may often be essential components of it. The change process is commonly not a straight-line progression, but more usually one of moments of therapeutic movement and periods of retreat, consolidation and stasis. Classical person-centred therapists regard these static moments as important parts of an ongoing process and respect them as manifestations of a client's current limited capacity to confront personal issues. In such circumstances, the therapist is more likely to evaluate their own ability to remain empathically attuned to the client and their own (the therapist's) experiencing, than to consider ways of directly intervening into the client's process.

Principled non-directivity is a subject that throws into relief the differences between classical person-centred therapy and most (if not all) other approaches to therapy, including some of those discussed in this book. It is an issue that finds description in Margaret Warner's (2000) five 'levels of interventiveness'. Level 2 is where the therapist is simply trying to communicate their understanding of the client's frame of reference; level 3 is where the therapist 'brings material into the therapeutic relationship, doing so in ways that foster the client's choice as to whether and how to use such material' (p.32). Classically orientated person-centred therapists will, most often, be working non-directively, at level 2.

Research

In Chapter 1 (this volume), Pete Sanders and Sheila Haugh note that Rogers and his colleagues at Ohio State and Chicago were the first to research psychotherapy sessions using emerging audio-recording technology. From the early 1950s to the 1970s, they developed methodologies and measuring instruments to conduct small- and large-scale studies. Classical person-centred therapists were also at the front of developments in qualitative as well as quantitative research. That first flush of involvement has since subsided, and the classical position has been largely absent from quantitative research in recent years.

The late 1900s and the early 2000s saw a surge in research in person-centred therapies, mainly in Canada and Northern Europe. A number of extensive 'meta-analyses' of various types of person-centred therapies were conducted, including client-centered/non-directive therapy. These meta-analyses included outcome studies, studies comparing person-centred therapies with other approaches (notably cognitive behaviour therapy) and studies of the effectiveness of person-centred therapies with people experiencing different psychological problems, such as depression (Cuijpers et al., 2012), 'borderline personality disorder' (Kramer & Sachse, 2013; Snijdere et al., 2015) and social anxiety (MacLeod & Elliott, 2014).

Three meta-analyses are of particular interest to person-centred therapists. Elliott and colleagues (2019) found 'empathy to be a medium-sized predictor of outcome in psychotherapy, with the best outcome being associated with clients' reports of therapist empathy' (p.276). Looking at congruence and genuineness, Kolden and colleagues (2019) concluded that congruence/genuineness is 'consistently associated with and predictive of client change' (p.246). Finally, Farber and colleagues (2019), while noting the 'difficulties in the agreement of the phrase "positive regard and affirmation"' (p. 290), report that the 'provision of positive regard or affirmation significantly predicts and is related to therapeutic success' (p.314). Issues of diversity are woefully absent in the data available to the researchers in these meta-analyses.

More recently, there has been an increasing number of small, qualitative research projects emerging from master's programmes in person-centred psychotherapy (for example, Blowers & Haugh, 2021; Peacock, 2023). Wendy Traynor's doctoral thesis (2019) looked at person-centred therapy and pre-therapy for people who hear voices or have unusual experiences or psychotic processes, and explored practitioner and client perceptions of helpful and unhelpful practice and client changes. Her findings support the value of non-directive person-centred therapy with this particular group of people. It is to be hoped that more of these studies find their way into publication.

Recent large-scale randomised control trials (RCTs) (Nye et al., 2019; Cooper et al., 2021) have researched person-centred experiential therapy (PCET) in comparison with cognitive behavioural therapy (CBT) in counselling for depression (CfD) (see Chapter 5, this volume) and humanistic counselling in schools, respectively. Robert Elliott's (2016) summary of the research over the past 60 years is generally favourable toward person-centred experiential psychotherapies.

However, in truth, there are few studies in recent years that have been dedicated to classical person-centred therapy. It may be that some classical person-centred therapists have an aversion to the measurements and assessments required by RCTs and the depersonalisation they involve. That said, the financial support and infrastructures needed for RCTs are usually only available within the university sector and, in the UK at least, there are not many classical person-centred therapists to be found in these arenas. It is clear that there remains an urgent need both to demonstrate the effectiveness of classical person-centred therapy with specific psychological problems and explore its comparative effectiveness with other person-centred therapies and other modalities.

Resources

Further reading

For complete beginners or as a refresher:

- Sanders, P. (2006). *The person-centred counselling primer*. PCCS Books.
- Tudor, K. & Merry, T. (2006). *Dictionary of person-centred psychology.* PCCS Books.

For an accessible introduction including some recent developments:

- Merry, T., with Haugh S. (2020). *Learning and being in person-centred counselling* (3rd ed.). PCCS Books.

For a collection of the works of Carl Rogers:

- Kirschenbaum, H. & Henderson, V.L. (Eds.). (1996). *The Carl Rogers reader.* Houghton Mifflin.

For a biography of Carl Rogers:

- Kirschenbaum, H. (2007). *The life and work of Carl Rogers.* PCCS Books.

For a list of all Carl Rogers' articles:

- https://scholar.google.co.uk/citations?user=d4rhVqEAAAAJ&hl=en&oi=sra

Organisations

There are no organisations dedicated exclusively to a classical approach to PCT. **The Person-Centred Association (tPCA)** welcomes everyone with an interest in the PCA, whether their interest is in therapy or the wider applications of the approach:
https://www.the-pca.org.uk/

tPCA also includes a number of special interest groups: www.the-pca.org.uk/community/communities-of-practice-and-special-interest-groups.html

tPCA also offers various types of membership including free membership to students during their pre-qualifying training.

The **World Association for Person-Centered and Experiential Psychotherapies (WAPCEP)** offers a reduced student rate. It supports the biennial PCE World Conferences and publishes the quarterly journal *Person-Centered & Experiential Psychotherapies.*
www.pce-world.org

References

Barrett-Lennard, G.T. (1998). *Carl Rogers' helping system: Journey and substance.* Sage.

Blowers, D. & Haugh, S. (2021). Health anxiety and the self-concept: A person-centered/experiential study. *Person-Centered & Experiential Psychotherapies, 20*(3), 266–281.

Bozarth, J.D. (1998). Remembering Eleanor: A different way of contact. *The Person-Centered Journal, 5*, 36–38.

Bozarth, J.D. (2001). Client-centred unconditional positive regard: A historical perspective. In J.D. Bozarth & P. Wilkins (Eds.), *Rogers' therapeutic conditions: Evolution, theory and practice. Volume 3: Unconditional positive regard* (pp.5–18). PCCS Books.

Brodley, B.T. (2011). The empathic understanding response process. In K.A. Moon, M. Witty, B. Grant & B. Rice (Eds.), *Practicing client-centered therapy: Selected writings of Barbara Temaner Brodley* (pp.173–179). PCCS Books.

Brodley, B.T., & Brody, A.F. (1990). *Understanding client-centered therapy through interviews conducted by Carl Rogers.* Paper presented to the panel: 'Fifty Years of Client-Centered Psychotherapy: Recent research'. American Psychological Association Annual Conference, Boston MA.

Brooks, S. & Paterson, G. (2011). Using contact work in interactions with adults with learning disabilities and autistic spectrum disorders. *British Journal of Learning Disorders, 39*, 161–166

Cooper, M., Stafford, M.R., Saxon, D., Beecham, J., Bonin, E.-M., Barkham, M., Bower, P., Cromarty, K., Duncan, C., Pearce, P., Rameswari, T., & Ryan, G. (2021). Humanistic counselling plus pastoral care as usual versus pastoral care as usual for the treatment of psychological distress in adolescents in UK state schools (ETHOS): A randomised controlled trial. *The Lancet Child & Adolescent Health, 5*(3), 178–189.

Cuijpers, P., Driessen, E., Hollon, S. D., Van Oppen, P., Barth, J. & Andersson, G. (2012). The efficacy of non-directive supportive therapy for adult depression: A meta-analysis. *Clinical Psychology Review, 32*(4), 280–291.

Elliott, R. (2016). Research on person-centred/experiential psychotherapy and counselling: Summary of the main findings. In C. Lago & D. Charura (Eds.), *The person-centred counselling and psychotherapy handbook: Origins, developments and current applications* (pp.223–232). Open University Press.

Elliott, R., Bohart, A.C., Watson, J.C. & Murphy, D. (2019). Empathy. In J.C. Norcross & M.J. Lambert (Eds.), *Psychotherapy relationships that work. Volume 1: Evidence-based therapist contributions* (3rd ed.) (pp.245–287). Oxford University Press.

Farber, B.A., Suzuki, J.Y. & Lynch, D.A. (2019). Positive regard and affirmation. In J.C. Norcross & M.J. Lambert (Eds.), *Psychotherapy relationships that work. Volume 1: Evidence-based therapist contributions* (3rd ed.) (pp.288–322). Oxford University Press.

Grant, B. (1990). Principled and instrumental non-directiveness in person-centered and client-centered psychotherapy. *Person-Centered Review, 5*(1), 77–88.

Haugh, S. (2000). Congruence: A confusion of language. In T. Merry (Ed.), *The BAPCA reader* (pp.62–67). PCCS Books.

Haugh, S. (2001). A historical review of the development of the concept of congruence. In G. Wyatt (Ed.), *Rogers' therapeutic conditions: evolution, theory and practice. Volume 2: Empathy* (pp.1–17). PCCS Books.

Haugh, S. (2014, April). *Kindness, concern and love.* [Presentation]. Czechia/Slovak PCA Symposium, Praha, Czechia.

Keys, S. (Ed.). (2003). *Idiosyncratic person-centered therapy: From the personal to the universal.* PCCS Books.

Kirshenbaum, H. & Henderson, V.L. (Eds.) (1990). *The Carl Rogers reader.* Constable.

Kolden, G.G., Wang, C.-C., Austin, S. B., Chang, Y. & Klein, M.H. (2019). Congruence/genuineness. In J.C. Norcross & M.J. Lambert (Eds.), *Psychotherapy relationships that work: Volume 1: Evidence-based therapist contributions* (3rd ed.) (pp.323–350). Oxford University Press.

Kramer, U. & Sachse, R. (2013). Early clarification processes in clients presenting with borderline personality disorder: Relations with symptom level and change. *Person-Centered & Experiential Psychotherapies, 12*(2), 157–175.

Levitt, B.E. (2008). Beyond fiefdoms. In B.E. Levitt (Ed.), *Reflections on human potential: Bridging the person-centered approach and positive psychology* (pp.227–235). PCCS Books.

MacLeod, R. & Elliott, R. (2014). Nondirective person-centered therapy for social anxiety: A hermeneutic single-case efficacy design study of a good outcome case. *Person-Centered & Experiential Psychotherapies, 13*(4), 294–311.

Mearns, D. (1999). Person-centred therapy with configurations of the self. *Counselling, 10*(2), 125–130.

Mearns, D. & Thorne, B. (2000). *Person-centred therapy today: New frontiers in theory and practice.* Sage.

Mearns, D. & Thorne, B. (2013). *Person-centred counselling in action* (4th ed.). Sage.

Merry, T. (1995/2006). *Invitation to person-centred psychology* (2nd ed.). PCCS Books.

Merry, T. (1996). An analysis of ten demonstration interviews by Carl Rogers: Implications for the training of client-centred counsellors. In R. Hutterer, G. Pawlowsky, P. Schmid & R. Stipsits (Eds.), *Client-centered and experiential psychotherapy: A paradigm in motion* (pp.273–283). Peter Lang.

Merry, T. & Brodley, B.T. (2002). The nondirective attitude in client-centered therapy: A response to Kahn. *Journal of Humanistic Psychology, 42*(2), 66–77.

Merry, T. with Haugh, S. (2020*). Learning and being in person-centred counselling* (3rd ed.). PCCS Books.

Moon, K.A., Witty, M., Grant, B. & Rice, B. (Eds.). (2011). *Practicing client-centered therapy: Selected writings of Barbara Temaner Brodley.* PCCS Books.

Nye, A., Connell, J., Haake, R. & Barkham, M. (2019). Person-centred experiential therapy (PCET) training within a UK NHS IAPT service: Experiences of selected counsellors in the PRaCTICED trial. *British Journal of Guidance & Counselling, 47*(5), 619–634.

Peacock, R. (2023). Encountering sexuality difference: The experiences of person-centered counselors and psychotherapists who self-describe as heterosexual and have worked with lesbian, gay, bisexual and queer clients. *Person-Centered & Experiential Psychotherapies,* 1–19. DOI:10.1080/14779757.2022.2161005

Prouty, G. (1994). *Theoretical evolutions in person-centered/experiential therapy: Applications to schizophrenic and retarded psychoses.* Praeger.

Prouty, G. (1999). Pre-therapy: Is it person-centered? A reply to Jerold Bozarth. *The Person-Centred Journal, 6(1)*, 28–31.

Prouty, G. (2001). A new mode of empathy: Empathic contact. In S. Haugh & T. Merry (Eds.), *Rogers' therapeutic conditions: Evolution, theory and practice. Volume 2: Empathy* (pp.155–162). PCCS Books.

Prouty, G., Van Werde, D. & Pörtner, M. (2002). *Pre-therapy: Reaching contact-impaired clients.* PCCS Books.

Rogers, C.R. (1942). *Counseling and psychotherapy: Newer concepts in practice.* Houghton Mifflin.

Rogers, C.R. (1951). *Client-centered therapy.* Houghton Mifflin.

Rogers, C.R. (1957). The necessary and sufficient conditions of therapeutic personality change. *Journal of Consulting Psychology, 21*, 95–103. Reprinted in H. Kirschenbaum & V.L. Henderson (Eds.). (1990). *The Carl Rogers Reader* (pp.219–235). Constable.

Rogers, C.R. (1959). A theory of therapy, personality, and interpersonal relationships as developed in the client-centered framework. In S. Koch, (Ed.). *Psychology: A study of a science, volume 3.* McGraw-Hill.

Rogers, C.R. (1961). *On becoming a person: A therapist's view of psychotherapy.* Constable.

Rogers, C.R. (1975). Empathic: An unappreciated way of being. *The Counseling Psychologist, 5*(2), 2–10.

Rogers, C.R. (1986). Reflection of feelings. *Person-Centered Review, 1*(4), 375–377. Reprinted in H. Kirschenbaum & V.L. Henderson (Eds.). (1990), *The Carl Rogers reader* (pp.127–129). Constable.

Rogers, C.R. & Dymond, R.F. (1954). *Psychotherapy and personality change: Co-ordinated research studies in the client-centered approach.* University of Chicago Press.

Sanders, P. (ed.) (2007). *The contact work primer: A concise, accessible and comprehensive introduction to pre-therapy and the work of Garry Prouty.* PCCS Books.

Snijdere, J.A.H., Amons, P.J.T. & Dierick, P. (2015). Client-centered/experiential group psychotherapy with borderline clients: Specific processes and challenges. *Person-Centered & Experiential Psychotherapies, 14*(1), 18–31.

Stephen, S. (In press). The non-directive attitude. In G. Di Malta, M. Cooper, M. O'Hara, Y. Gololob & S. Stephen (Eds.), *The handbook of person-centred psychotherapy and counselling* (3rd ed.) (In press). Bloomsbury.

Swan, A.M. & Ceballos, P. (2020). Person-centered conceptualization of multiculturalism and social justice in counseling. *Person-Centered & Experiential Psychotherapies, 19*(2), 154–167.

Tolan, J., with Cameron, R. (2017). *Skills in person-centred counselling and psychotherapy* (3rd ed.). Sage.

Traynor, W. (2019). *Person-centred therapy and pre-therapy for people who hear voices, have unusual experiences or psychotic processes: Practitioner and client perceptions of helpful and unhelpful practice and perceived client changes.* PhD thesis. University of Strathclyde]. https://stax.strath.ac.uk/concern/theses/pg15bd892

Tudor, K. & Worrall, M. (1994). Congruence reconsidered. *British Journal of Guidance & Counselling, 22*(2), 197–206.

Tudor, K. & Worrall, M. (2006). *Person-centred therapy: A clinical philosophy.* Routledge.

Warner, M.S. (2000). Person-centered psychotherapy: One nation many tribes. *The Person-Centred Journal, 7*(1), 28–39.

Wilkins, P. (2000). Unconditional regard reconsidered. *British Journal of Guidance and Counselling, 28*(1), 23–36. Reprinted in J. Bozarth & P. Wilkins (Eds.) (2001), *Rogers' therapeutic conditions: Evolution, theory and practice. Volume 3: Unconditional positive regard* (pp.35–48). PCCS Books.

Wilkins, P. & Gill, M. (2003). Assessment in person-centered therapy. *Person-Centered & Experiential Psychotherapies, 2*(3), 172–187.

Wyatt, G. & Sanders, P. (2002). *Rogers' therapeutic conditions: Evolution, theory and practice. Volume 4: Contact and perception*. PCCS Books.

3. The relational approach to person-centred therapy

Gina Di Malta, Mick Cooper, Rosanne Knox and Steve Cox

Relational refers to the relationship between things or beings. 'Relational' can be considered as an umbrella term that describes a breadth of ways of being together. This includes being 'dialogical', and the relational approach to person-centred therapy is sometimes referred to as the 'relational/dialogical', or just 'dialogical', tribe. *Dialogue* refers to an exchange of words between people that can help to develop new meaning. Dialogical describes, therefore, a particular aspect of relating (Cox, 2016). A relational approach would see therapy as bi-directional or multi-directional, co-created through the dialogue of therapeutic interconnection (see Cox 2016; Murphy, 2013).

The classical person-centred approach is based on the view of humans as individual, autonomous beings who, through their interactions with others, may be changed but still retain their separateness (Chapter 2, this volume). Rogers developed his theories within a wider individualistic socio-historical context. The concept of the *actualising tendency,* for example, is an essentially individualistic construct (e.g., Holdstock, 1993). While Rogers' classical model contained all the bases for a relational model to emerge, his original writing was less focused on the first and sixth conditions – the two conditions that speak the most to the relational and dialogical (Gaylin, 2002). The first condition, *psychological contact*, describes the relational basis of the encounter, and the sixth condition, *client perception*, deepens meaning that is made through dialogue (Cox, 2016). With the exception, perhaps, of Wyatt and Sanders (2001), these two conditions have received comparatively little consideration in person-centred literature.

Following Rogers' publication of *On Becoming a Person* in 1961 (Rogers, 1961a), Ellingham (2011, p.153) described a 'development shift in the formulation of therapy' where

Rogers made the relational nature of his approach more prominent. By the time *A Way of Being* was published in 1980 (Rogers, 1980), Rogers had further revised his original thinking concerning the actualising tendency to include a more expansive 'formative tendency'. Therapy was not, then, simply a relational activity between client and therapist; it was also a relationship that routinely explored the dynamics of other relationships. As Rogers (1980) wrote: 'relationship transcends itself and becomes a part of something larger' (p.129).

Despite this progression, there was little adjustment made to person-centred theory that accommodated this relational shift. As a result, wider relational thinking fits less well within classical theoretical constructs. Yet over time, increasing numbers of person-centred thinkers have paid attention to this issue. Holdstock (1990, 1993, 1996), for example, has argued that the organism is formed by its social context and should not be separated from it. Barrett-Lennard (2005) writes:

> Our inner and outer relational experiences are so closely interwoven in the total tapestry of life's process that the warp and weft almost disappear. (p.15)

In this chapter, we focus on the evolution of a relational approach to person-centred therapy. This focuses on what it means to be human through a relational lens, and through this lens revisits Rogers' psychological foundations for person-centred therapy. This focus on the relational encourages a therapeutic practice of mutuality, reciprocity and intimacy. Mearns and Cooper's (2005/2018) work on *relational depth* exemplifies these aspects, as does Schmid's (2002) concept of *encounter* – being with and being counter to the other. A relational paradigm focuses not only on depth but also on breadth of relating and the various relational dynamics (e.g. O'Hara, 1995; Natiello, 2001; Proctor, 2006). These influences have led to the relational paradigm being envisaged as an inter-relational dynamic encompassing not only our relationship with the other but also the co-created relationship between people, our relationship with our world and social context, and the relationship with self.

The relational approach to person-centred therapy is not a radical departure from the classical person-centred approach (Chapter 2, this volume), and, unlike emotion-focused therapy (Chapter 5, this volume) or pre-therapy (Chapter 11, this volume), is not a stand-alone community of person-centred practitioners. Some of the authors of this chapter identify the relational approach as a particular tribe of person-centred therapy, and others view the relational shift as a natural evolution that affects all the tribes. Nevertheless, we all agree that it is a distinctive understanding of what it means to be person-centred, and one that is influential in the UK and internationally.

From individualism to intersubjectivity: Theoretical foundations

Ontology is the study of what it means to *be:* the nature of being and existence (including human existence). Classical person-centred therapy is founded on the assumption that each human being comes into the world – and exists – as an individual, separate organism (see Chapter 2, this volume). From this classical perspective, individual human growth is derailed by the conditional positive regard of significant others (Rogers, 1951, 1959). Yet, in Rogers' classical model of human personality and development, the organism retains its essential discreteness (Cooper, in press). Indeed, a return to its own, individual beliefs, judgements and experiences – an 'internal locus of evaluation' – is considered the *sine qua non* of healthy, full functioning.

This assumption, however, that human beings are like 'self-encapsulated "shells" or monads' (Bohart, 2003, p.112) has been robustly criticised over the past century – from both within and outside of the person-centred field. This is for a number of reasons.

First, there is the ethics of such an individualised model of the person. If we start with the assumption that human beings are separate, independent and discrete, then what of human caring, giving and compassion? No doubt, Rogers' classical theories and practices are highly relational, with empathy and acceptance of others at their core (Rogers, 1957). But if the natural state of human beings is to be separate and apart, then this can lend itself to a worldview in which *self*-achievement and *self*-gain become prioritised, rather than collaboration, relationality and being-ness with others.

This is, perhaps, the underlying concern of many cross-cultural and feminist theorists, who have challenged the assumption that individuality is the natural state of human being. From these standpoints, individualised ontologies are not simply 'value-free' truths but ideological assumptions that legitimise a very specific set of social relations: Western, patriarchal and capitalist (Mearns & Cooper, 2005/2018). From these critical standpoints, if everyone is seen, first and foremost, as an individual – and if our individuality is considered the most essential thing about us – then human striving and competing for individual gain can be legitimised as the 'normal' state of affairs. Market capitalism is the norm because, if we do not make profit, another individual will; gun ownership is the norm in some countries such as the US because we each have to protect ourselves from predatory others. And, it can be argued, the assumption of individuality is so engrained here that we do not even recognise it as an assumption: it is just 'how things are'. So critics of this individualistic perspective have tried to show that such a way of seeing the world is not the only one possible. Feminist critics, for instance, have argued that women tend to see the world in more relational and interdependent ways than men (e.g., Gilligan, 1993; Jordan et al., 1991). And cross-cultural theorists have shown that many non-Western cultures have a more 'interdependent' view of the self (see, for instance, Ratts & Pedersen, 2014).

Such critiques open up alternative ways of understanding the essence of human being: ways that may lend themselves towards more relational and prosocial practices. Closely related to this ethical critique, across the 20th century, individualistic assumptions have been challenged from a philosophical standpoint. Key here is the 'existential' philosopher Martin Heidegger (1926/1962) who, drawing on phenomenology (the study of human experiencing), set out to understand the nature of the ever-changing flux of human existence. For Heidegger, others are integral to our existences because, at the level of lived-being, we are constantly doing things with others, or using tools that have emerged from an interpersonal matrix. For example, let us take your being right now, which we might describe phenomenologically as a 'you-reading-this-book' – an integrated, holistic experiencing. Here, what we can note is that the 'book' part of this experiencing is something that others have been fundamentally involved in: authors, publishers, editors, printers. So a whole community of people is there in your experiencing. And, perhaps most fundamentally, the language that you are using to make sense of these words – which transmit ideas from our brains to yours – are not your own personal creation, but a system of communication that has evolved across millennia of human being. So, in this sense, the very essence of your being is infused with the beingness of others, and this is not something we can stand 'outside' of and view 'objectively'. As Derrida (1974) writes: 'all that desire had wished to wrest from the play of language finds itself recaptured by that play' (p.337).

From a developmental perspective, a range of psychologists and psychoanalysts have also argued that human infants do not begin life as separate, isolated individuals, but as part of a fundamentally relational matrix (Mearns & Cooper, 2005/2018). Best known here, perhaps, is the thinking of psychoanalyst D.W. Winnicott, who stated that 'there is no such thing as a baby, only a nursing couple' (quoted in Curtis & Hirsch, 2003, p.73). What he meant by this is that the infant is inextricably and inevitably bound up in relationships to others from the very start of its existence. Closely related, research in the field of social neuroscience shows that, when people interact, they are continually impacting on each other's internal biological states, 'influencing the long-term construction of each other's brains' (Cozolino, 2014, p.xv). This influence is particularly significant during infancy, where the 'external foetus' (Gerhardt, 2014) – thrust into the world at a still early stage – needs to complete its growth.

This understanding of human being as inextricably tied in with the being of others is termed an *intersubjective* perspective (see, for instance, Crossley, 1996). Figure 3.1 is an attempt to illustrate how this perspective differs from an individualistic standpoint. In Figure 3.1, each human entity – the shaded circles – is separate and discrete from other human entities, like balls on a snooker table. By contrast, from an intersubjective standpoint, human being, the dashed semi-circles, exists as an 'opennesses' to other human being. Here, rather than fixed and definite boundaries, there is a fluidity and flow from person to persons. Human existence is in the space 'in between', a 'dialogical existence', as conceptualised by the existential philosopher Martin Buber (1947). As Peter Schmid emphasises throughout his work, however, these individualistic and intersubjective positions should not be understood in opposition, as 'either/or'. Rather, for Schmid, the essence of the person-centred approach is that it embraces *both* of these positions: that is, it understands people as *both* separate *and* in relation to others. He writes: 'Only in the dialectic of both interpretations, not in an either-or but in a both-and, does the mystery of the person become accessible' (Schmid, 2002).

So what relevance does this 'intersubjective turn' have for the practice of person-centred therapy? The answers here are subtle but perhaps profound. First, if human beings are not understood as discrete, separate organisms, then the notion of being 'non-directive' and 'non-invasive', as emphasised by a classical person-centred perspective (see Chapter 2, this volume), becomes more problematic. How is it possible to be *non*-directive when we are always, inevitably, in relation with the other? Say, for instance, a client is asking for advice. From a relational standpoint, it would indeed be influencing the client to give advice, but, from this relational standpoint, to *not* give advice would also be influencing (for instance, the client might feel hurt or annoyed that we were not responsive to them).

Figure 3.1: Individualistic and intersubjective models of the person

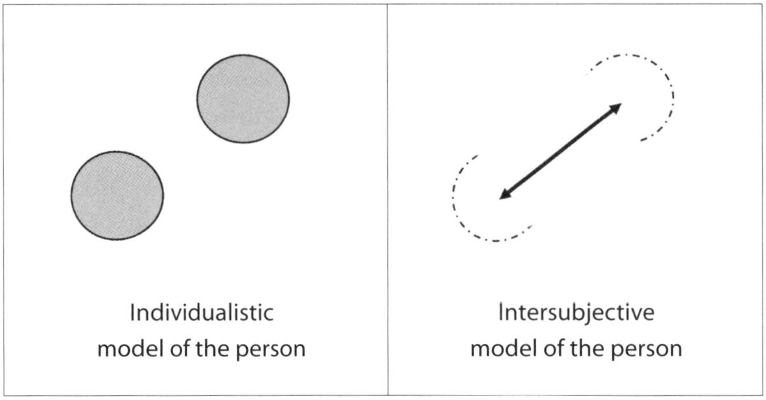

From this intersubjective position, then, there is no possibility of acting in a 'neutral', non-influencing way, and that means non-directivity has a less dominant place in a relational, dialogical person-centred approach (as with, for instance, emotion-focused therapy or motivational interviewing; see respectively, Chapters 5 and 7, this volume). Rather, the emphasis is more on how we can establish a positive, relational encounter with the client: one that can influence them in helpful ways. This, then, opens up an emphasis on relational depth, as well as a wider range of potential therapist activities, above and beyond the classical 'empathic unfolding response' process (Freire, 2013). Second, and closely related, from a relational standpoint (in contrast to a classical one), wellbeing is less about having an autonomous, self-determined way of being and more about the capacity to engage in healing and rewarding relationships. That is, an in-depth relationship is not simply something that *adds* to clients' lives, a 'bonus' to their natural state of individual wellbeing (Mearns & Cooper, 2005/2018). Rather, it is a means of returning clients to their natural state of connectedness with others: 'Like a fish out of water, the client who is isolated from others cannot breathe, cannot take in the nutrients they need to sustain life' (Mearns & Cooper, 2005/2018, p.5).

Key practices

As with a classical model, the relational approach sees Rogers' (1957) six conditions as necessary for therapeutic change to occur. However, in a relational practice, there is a greater emphasis on the importance of 'making contact' and 'being received' by the client. A relational practice, therefore, can be seen as the therapist making more of an active endeavour to achieve a genuine and mutual encounter with the client in therapy.

Here we view and present aspects of such practice through four inter-linked relational lenses:

- The relationship with another – in practice the therapist is active in communicating their congruence and positive regard to the client, and free to offer a broader range of responses to meet their client.

- The co-created relationship – the therapist relates with an openness to being impacted and changed as a result of what is co-created in the relationship.
- The self-relationship – the therapist is able to come forward to this encounter with the client because of their commitment to developing their own self-awareness and self-acceptance.
- The world and universal relationship – the therapist's encounter is rooted in an openness to difference that also necessitates some awareness and a curiosity about the world and other cultures.

Although we present these facets of practice separately, it is important to recognise that the relationship with another, the co-created relationship, self-relationship, and world and universal relationship simultaneously co-exist as aspects of one dynamic whole. They demonstrate the breadth of our relating and the importance of being open to the multi-directional tapestry of our relationships. O'Hara (1995) states that, whenever she expressed herself authentically, 'I also expressed my gender, class, ideology, and cosmology' (p.133).

Relationship with another

Within a relational practice, establishing and maintaining a relationship with the client is seen as the therapist's responsibility. This is achieved through the therapist taking an active stance and endeavour towards achieving contact and being received by the client. This endeavour is reflected in Schmid's writing (1994; 1998a, 1998b, 1998c, 2002). Schmid proposed a basis for the ethical foundation of a relational practice and introduced the philosophy of Levinas' reversing of Buber's 'I-Thou' to 'Thou-I'. In other words, instead of the other gaining meaning through the acknowledgment of me or I, the dynamic is turned around: the client calls the therapist into service. Therapy responds to the suffering of the other and their cry for help and is seen as 'a responsibility rooted in fundamental ethics' (Schmid, 2002, p.84). Seeing the person-centred encounter as an ethical act has profound implications for the practice of person-centred therapy because responding to another's need establishes a moral necessity that is both personal and political. For example, a client's distress is valued in terms of authenticity and relationship rather than a medicalised disease. This means acknowledging the authority and value of a person over any institution (e.g. Sanders, 2005).

Key practices to actively encounter the client include active congruence and active positive regard, leading to a co-created relationship.

Active congruence

Active congruence departs from a classical definition of congruence in that the therapist more freely and proactively lets themselves respond and be seen by the client. With active congruence, the therapist trusts, more fully, that their transparency about who they are – and open display of their own self-acceptance and self-trust – would be healing for the client. With this openness, the therapist not only demonstrates that they trust themselves but also that they have trust in the client. In addition, the therapist trusts that a full range of responses available to them has the potential to be helpful to the client.

In their book, *Working at Relational Depth in Psychotherapy*, Mearns and Cooper (2005/2018) view realness as central to experiencing moments of profound encounter: 'There's something about being absolutely there just as a person' (Cooper, 2005, p.91). Such realness or active congruence is the opposite of being artificial or contrived, or play-acting the role of 'psychotherapist' in the relationship. Mearns and Cooper describe that quality of realness as letting the other person know what is genuinely going on inside oneself. This aspect of realness can also be termed *self-disclosure* or *transparency*.

In the following case example (adapted from Mearns & Cooper, 2018), Fatima, the therapist, demonstrates a form of active congruence by being aware of her own experiencing and being transparent about it, and so encountering the client at a deeper level.

> Fatima is finding it hard to follow what Jane, her client, is saying in the therapy. Fatima 'sits' briefly on this awareness because she is aware that Jane could feel as if she is not explaining her story properly. However Fatima trusts her intention of wanting to really understand Jane, and from this grounded place she is able to communicate this intention to Jane, as well as her felt sense of what might be happening for Jane in that moment: 'Please can you slow down a bit, Jane. I really want to understand what you're wanting to say to me, but I find that I am getting lost. It feels a bit like… like a jigsaw puzzle but that there are missing pieces.' Jane is able to receive Fatima's transparent communication grounded in her genuine care and intention to help her. She replies: 'Yes, exactly. I feel like I'm grasping at pieces and don't even have the box cover to know what it looks like.' After this, the dialogue moves from a surface-level narrative and Fatima and Jane begin to explore how Jane really feels. By sharing her own, deeper experiences and responses, Fatima has helped Jane to access hers.

In this scenario, we can see that Fatima could have felt too anxious to tell Jane that she was not following her story. She could have thought that she was not a good enough therapist because she couldn't follow Jane's story; she might not have wanted to risk hurting Jane's feelings by implying Jane could not explain herself properly; she may have been worried that Jane would get angry, thinking that her therapist was incompetent and not listening to her properly. However, Fatima chose to be transparent in the relationship, which opened the possibility of a genuine and deepened encounter.

Mearns and Cooper (2018) argue that, from a relational person-centred standpoint, an encounter between therapist and client must happen between two human beings who hold on to their uniqueness and individuality. Such an encounter requires difference (Schmid, 2002). Thus, therapists are in no way required to shed their personality or merge with their client. Instead, they come as themselves, with their 'personal signature' (Stern, 2004). They come as people who behave naturally and respond spontaneously to their clients – as 'the unique, genuine human being that they are: a solid and grounded "otherness" with which the client can interact' (Mearns & Cooper, 2018, p.48).

Active congruence also involves offering a fuller range of possible responses in the service of the client. For instance, it is likely that, as part of seeking to encounter the other, a therapist providing the core condition of empathy is necessary, but it may not necessarily be sufficient when seeking to consistently meet the client and their needs (see, for example, Cooper et al., 2023). Sometimes the client may need advice, psychoeducation, the phone number of a physiotherapist, or even for the therapist to share just a little bit about their holiday (if, for instance, the client asks at the beginning of a session). Of course, the latter may not be about meeting a fundamental need, but it is about meeting the client where they are and acknowledging their need to relate socially or satisfy a little curiosity, or their desire to know their therapist, and these are all equally valid parts of being human. By contrast, withholding a benign piece of information could leave an unnecessary relational void and create a moment of disconnection between the client and therapist.

A therapist's active congruence may lead to responses that are unique and personal to each client at each moment. Mearns and Cooper (2005/2018) view responsiveness as the therapist having no pre-decided or formulaic strategy. Such responsiveness is found to be important in the development of closeness and intimacy (Laurenceau et al., 2004). With this, the client comes to appreciate their own uniqueness through a relationship with the therapist that feels unique.

Active congruence does not mean that the therapist should disclose whatever they think or feel whenever they think or feel it. Research indicates that therapist self-disclosures should be judicially used, and not overly personal (Hill et al., 2019). The therapeutic space is for the client, and it is essential that the therapist does not hijack this for their own, personal agenda. Sometimes, too, therapists' 'intuitive' responses or reactions will be more about them than their clients (as the psychodynamic theory of countertransference teaches us), so it is important that therapist disclosures – or desires to disclose – are critically reflected on – for instance, in supervision. But active congruence is about having that potential to be open and real and disclosing, and to meet the client – at all times – as just one genuine human being with another. Relationally, we and our clients are all in one complex inter-personal nexus. Our focus, as therapists, is on the client's experiencing and being within that realm, but by being fully real in that encounter – rather than striving to 'extract' ourselves – we can help to elucidate that process.

Active positive regard

Within a relational practice, active congruence is inseparable from active positive regard: a deep valuing, prizing and appreciation of the client that is both felt and openly communicated. Within a relational and dialogical perspective, Mearns and Cooper (2005/2018) have called this 'affirming the other' or the 'therapist's genuine care' (Knox, 2013; Knox & Cooper, 2011; Knox et al., 2013; McMillan & McLeod, 2006). This is something 'over and above' the therapist's non-judgemental acceptance. Rather, it is a sense that the therapist is genuinely interested and concerned with the client's wellbeing: that the client matters to the therapist and impacts on them. Buber (1958) termed this *confirmation*: 'an act of love through which one acknowledges the other as one who exists in his [sic] own peculiar form and has the right to do so' (Friedman, 1985, p.134).

It is this care that provides the safe grounding from which the therapist is able to be freer and real in the relationship. In such relating, there is no space for judgement or criticism; instead, every challenge or perspective comes from a place of acceptance (Knox, 2013, p.25).

Active positive regard departs, to some extent, from classical unconditional positive regard. Rogers (1957) emphasised the importance of attitudes that positively value the other; that confirm, respect and trust the totality of the client's experience. However, a relational practice requires more deliberate and outwardly communicated positive affirmation of the client, their strengths, their achievements and their uniqueness (e.g. Mearns & Cooper, 2005/2018). Active positive regard goes beyond just refraining from judgement, or holding an attitude that 'However you are is alright by me'. It is a positive prizing of the client. In this context, the term 'acceptance' might also be considered insufficient to describe the therapist's attitude to their client. Rather, the term 'honouring' might be a more adequate reflection (Tangen & Cashwell, 2016).

In classical person-centred theory, the need for positive regard is not seen as an inherent expression of the organism but as a 'secondary' need (Rogers, 1959; Standal, 1954). But from a relational standpoint, the need for positive regard is considered integral to the organism: a part of their innate desire for relatedness and connection (Mearns & Cooper, 2005/2018). Buber (1988) writes:

> The human person needs confirmation because man as man needs it… Sent forth from the natural domain of species into the hazard of the solitary category, surrounded by the air of chaos which came into being with him, secretly and bashfully he watches for a Yes which allows him to be and which can come to him only from one human person to another. It is from one man to another that the heavenly bread of self-being is passed. (p.61)

From this standpoint, then, actively prizing and positively regarding a client is not a means of derailing their 'inner' growth process, but the offering of an essential nutrient to their growth. It is the 'yes' that allows them to be – the 'bread' through which clients can return to their true, relational home.

In the following example (adapted from Mearns & Cooper, 2005/2018), in the context of trauma-informed practices, the therapist Malika is deeply touched by her client Jen as Jen shares her pain of being abused by a family friend in childhood. In this moment, as she witnesses Jen's pain and deep vulnerability, Malika is both sitting with Jen's pain and also affirming her strength and being.

> As Malika hears Jen's story, she experiences a wave of emotion coming over her body. She senses and recognises a mixture of anger, rage and helplessness in her. Then tears start falling down her cheeks. Malika and Jen weep together silently for a few moments as they experience this deep pain. Then Malika shares with Jen about the wave of anger, rage and helplessness that just came over her and the sadness that came afterwards for them both, and recognises that Jen has had to live with these feelings and this pain since she experienced the abuse. Malika says from a place of awe and care how much she is amazed and inspired by Jen's courage to be able to be with and share these feelings, and

> for the life that Jen has been able to live, her successful career, and the raising of her two children, despite having lived through a horrifying trauma. Malika's heartfelt warmth is deeply felt and communicated through the emotions that transpire in her words and her eye contact and posture.

Here Malika's emotional response is used in service of the client. Not only is she actively congruent and transparent with her emotions, but she is also connected with the part of herself that actively values Jen and sees her strengths, her resources and her potential as she shares her vulnerability. Sometimes, and only if it is coming from a genuine place, it can be helpful for a client to hear that it is not frightening for the therapist to witness their vulnerability or that what the therapist sees from their perspective is deeply valued.

Co-created relationship

Relational practice is 'deeply rooted in the empathic co-experiencing with the client and the relationship' (Schmid, 2013, p.170). In this section, emphasis is placed on what is co-created and co-experienced between the therapist and client in the therapeutic process of a relational practice. From a co-creative process involving both client and therapist, it is possible that personal resonance emerges from client and therapist, and, importantly, from between the two (Schmid & Mearns, 2006; Mearns & Cooper, 2005, 2018). This process is poetically articulated by Buber (1958) when he says:

> The human being that emerges from the act of pure relation that so involves his being has now in his being something more than has grown in him, of which he did not know before and whose origin he is not rightly able to indicate. (p.40)

The potential for mutual connection and exchange requires an ability and willingness to engage in relationship by both the therapist and client. This ability and willingness can unfold naturally for the therapist as a result of the active congruence and positive regard described in the section above. In addition, the therapist can 'invite' or facilitate the client to relate more deeply (Mearns & Cooper, 2005/2018).

A key aspect of the co-created relationship is relational depth (Mearns & Cooper, 2018), and this is now seen as central to relational practice (Di Malta et al., 2023; Kim et al., 2020). In the following example (a summary of data from several cases, adapted from Knox, 2011), we see how a moment of relational depth unfolds for a client:

> Initially clients are aware of a sense of slowing down, or as some describe it, as if they are entering a space of timelessness. As they slow down, they also feel themselves delving deeper, being aware of an acute sense of vulnerability, and they find that they feel comfortable in bringing that vulnerability. If they continue to feel safe in relation to the therapist, they begin to open up both towards their therapist, and to previously hidden parts of themselves, giving them a feeling of self-connection and wholeness. They then seem to experience a feeling of aliveness, energy and excitement. This

> experience appears to be central to the event, leading to feelings of self-acceptance and self-worth, and ultimately a sense of relief, calm, and peace. At this point clients feel most connected, and remember this most vividly. (p.286)

For such moments to occur, the therapist (and client) must be able to be vulnerable and open to what unfolds in the relationship. For instance, the therapist needs to let go of any aims and desires to *do* something for the client (McMillan & McLeod, 2006). In addition, Schmid and Mearns (2006) have stressed that the therapist (as well as the client) needs to be open to the risk of being hurt, touched, loved or rejected by another. The therapist and client must also, at some level, make a conscious decision to engage at depth. Clients have reported that, immediately before they had such an experience, they had reached a state of readiness, and felt that they themselves made a decision to bring their vulnerability to the fore in the therapeutic relationship and engage more deeply with their therapist (Knox & Cooper, 2010).

Therapist factors that were perceived by clients as inviting a willingness to relate at relational depth pertain to active congruence and active positive regard. These were the clients' perceptions of their therapist's trustworthiness and realness, emotional warmth and earnest desire to understand (Knox & Cooper, 2010). Clients also described a personal, human approach on the therapist's part, and a willingness to be open and transparent. They also reported that they felt better able to connect when they sensed that their therapist truly cared about them and was providing something 'over and above' their professional role (Knox & Cooper, 2010). In contrast, factors that clients highlighted as inhibitive of relational depth included a cold, formal attitude and their experience of their therapist as distant, powerful, interpreting, misunderstanding or seeming to be saying the right words without really meaning them (Knox & Cooper, 2010; McMillan & McLeod, 2006).

It is possible that, as part of a relational approach to person-centred therapy, the co-created relationship is where most of the healing occurs. As discussed, such a co-created relationship is viewed as unfolding from the relationship with the other, with the therapist actively seeking to encounter the client. We will now turn to discussing how the self-relationship may also be seen as a precursor to being able to encounter the other.

Self-relationship

The therapist's relationship to themself is an essential part of relational practice. It is built similarly on *active positive self-regard* and an openness to and curiosity about all parts of the self. The development of self-awareness and the practice of self-inquiry have been fundamental requirements of person-centred therapy practice. Rogers articulated the significance of self-relationship throughout his writing, and even indicated that his degree of success in creating a therapeutic relationship was 'measure of the growth I have achieved myself' (Rogers, 1961b, p.56). Rogers also illustrated the need for the ongoing personal development of the therapist, commenting: 'If I am interested in creating helping relationships I have a fascinating lifetime job ahead of me, stretching and developing my potentialities in the direction of growth' (1961b, p.56).

In addition, the idea of the personhood of the therapist being a major contributor to the process of change is also articulated in Rogers' (1957, 1959) third condition for therapeutic change:

> The third condition is that the therapist should be, within the confines of this relationship, a congruent, genuine, integrated person. It means that within the relationship he is freely and deeply himself, with his actual experience accurately represented by his awareness of himself. It is the opposite of presenting a facade, either knowingly or unknowingly. (Rogers, 1957, p.97)

A relational practice puts particular emphasis on an active practice of self-relationship. Although Rogers made it clear that, for the therapist, a developing self-relationship is important, he said little about how this was to be achieved. Over time, many relational person-centred therapists have contributed to an ongoing exploration of this necessity. In a comprehensive examination of person-centred training, Mearns (1997) described personal development as 'the "Self" of the counsellor that is the central ingredient in the endeavour' (p.xi). He also identified numerous ways in which the therapist can pursue self-exploration, as part of their personal development, through 'awareness, understanding and experimentation with Self' (Mearns, 1997, pp.97–108).

In an interview with Stillwell (1998), Villas-Boas Bowen talks about cultivating her inner self and spirit: 'When your own internal frame of reference is in place you experience self-comfort, self-trust, and a realistic self-acceptance' (p.32). To get in touch with your inner self, Villas-Boas Bowen explains:

> A person can do it for herself. She directs inward Carl's three conditions. She practices empathy to quiet her conscious thought, order her emotions, cultivate a relationship with her indwelling spirit; she practices unconditional positive regard towards her own dark side and her contradictory nature; she practices congruence in facing as-it-is-ness. (p.32)

Similarly, Mearns and Cooper (2005/2018) suggest that an awareness of one's own self-experiences and a willingness to access one's personal 'existential touchstones' may support a personal freedom that makes deep relating possible (Tangen & Cashwell, 2016). This refers to an awareness of the elements within a person from which they draw strength and find their own depths. This awareness is accompanied by self-acceptance, which is the precursor to accepting the other. If the therapist is not comfortable with all parts of their own self, even the 'not so nice' parts, then there is less likelihood that they will be able to relate to the parts of the client that the client might not like.

The list of possible developmental activities is vast. It includes offering the core conditions to oneself, meditating, practising mindfulness, participation in encounter or other group work, and personal therapy or supervision. Honing our relationship with our own self may be considered mandatory for an ethical therapist, but how this is achieved is a matter of personal choice. It might include, for example, self-witnessing, self-dialogue, self-understanding, self-acceptance, and being in tune with our felt sense (Chapter 4, this volume). Mearns and Cooper (2005/2018) suggest creating contexts where the therapist genuinely meets their self and experiences themselves meeting others in a direct and immediate fashion.

In the following case example, Gina, the first author of this chapter, shares her own process of developing a self-relationship.

> Aside from exploring my thoughts and feelings in my own personal therapy and discussing my clinical practice in supervision, I develop my self-relationship by sometimes going on solo trips to new places. When I do this, I am committed to caring for myself in the same way that I would a child. I have an internal dialogue: I listen to my body, my feelings, and my thoughts. I give myself some loving reassurance in moments of anxiety by thinking to myself, 'It's okay, it's normal to feel anxious in this completely new place. Perhaps I am a little tired. Would I like to rest?' Part of the growth for me comes from being confronted by the world, with its beautiful and scary parts, my own internal highs and lows in response to this, and being the only friend I can rely on as I go through it. In these circumstances, where there is no distraction, having active positive self-regard and being responsive to one's own needs can more easily come into focus, and the value of these interventions in the service of the self becomes very clear.

In this example, the self-dialogue is what Cooper (2003a) called an *I-I mode* of relating. This is a transposition of Buber's (1958) I-Thou to the intrapersonal level, where a person communicates with themself in an empathic, affirming and compassionate way. Cooper (2003b) suggests that, in this mode of self-relating, the person recognises different feelings, thoughts and behaviours as valid and legitimate and is open to their own 'otherness' – that is, they are in touch with the unknown in them (Rogers, 1986/1990). This contrasts with an *I–Me* self-relational stance – equivalent to Buber's I–It attitude – where the person makes little attempt to try to understand and empathise with themselves or how they came to act in a particular way (Cooper, 2003a). Instead, aspects of themselves are treated as objects – 'things' to be dealt with and, often, eradicated.

Mearns and Cooper (2005/2018) offer a description of what true self-acceptance might look like. They view it as the degree to which a person sees themself as a 'reasonable' human being, capable of a range of actions but fundamentally reliable to themself and others. They add that this should not be confused with self-aggrandisement over others, as it does not rely on comparison; rather, it is about sustaining one's own positive self-view. Such a self-view is not threatened by relationships and the person can entertain the other person's difference and even criticism without needing to protect themselves against the impact that it might have on a fragile self.

World and universal relationship

A dimension no less central to a relational practice is a focus on the wider environment – a mode of relating that is of particular importance at this time of impending climate catastrophe. Scholars from across the person-centred community recognise that all organisms, human or otherwise, can be truly understood only within the context of their environments (Barrett-Lennard, 2005; Mearns & Cooper, 2005/2018; Schmid, 2013; Tudor & Worrall, 2006). Cox (2016) reminds us that: 'If therapists are to truly meet their clients, then there is an imperative to meet the world of the client and not just the client's feelings and thoughts' (p.36).

In addition, therapists must explore their own worlds: their cultural and political landscapes, their prejudices, hurts, ignorance, fears, privileges and drives, all within social contexts.

Ignoring social context limits therapy. For example, Chantler (2004) demonstrates that, when Rogers counsels a client who is Black (Whiteley, 1977; Moodley et al., 2004), his empathy and connection are significantly impaired because he does not reference his client's race, even though his client repeatedly speaks of it as being of major personal importance. Although we bring our worlds into the therapeutic space, the decision to illuminate them, or not, is another matter.

The following case study by the fourth author of this chapter, Steve Cox, of an encounter with a client, 'Rob', demonstrates the benefit of seeking social context – context that was hitherto absent from the dialogue.

> Rob's wife had died. When he talked about her, it was clear that she had been the centre of his world. Rob felt lost without her. Not only was his heart well and truly broken but he also felt ill-equipped and unable to function in life without his wife's instruction. With each session, Rob appeared to be more and more depressed. Steve was used to the intensity of grief getting stronger in the initial months of bereavement, but this was different. Rob was shutting down. Although Steve had done his best to connect with Rob and to communicate his understanding and valuing of him, he also started to sense an unknown – something missing, not being said. After a while, the volume of the unsaid became such that Steve felt he had to say something:
>
> Steve: Rob we have talked about your love for Liz, your feelings of heartbreak and about the hopelessness in your life since her death. But it occurs to me that I don't know much about you and the things in your life that perhaps didn't involve Liz.
>
> As Steve said these words, he was acutely aware of Rob's deep felt sense of grief and his fragility. He could sense these things within his own body and that the expression of his words voiced something of Rob's pain. When Rob replied, Steve could sense that he was starting to respond in a different way, from a different aspect of himself.
>
> Steve: What are your passions, Rob?
>
> Although Rob wasn't saying anything at this point, Steve could see that something within him was stirring. Rob seemed to be somehow interested. His affect was less flat and something was awakening.
>
> Rob: I don't really have any, anymore.

There was something in Rob's response that seemed incomplete. Something inside of Steve didn't fully believe that Rob didn't still have passions, even if they were submerged. Steve persisted.

Steve: Apart from Liz, what was it that lit your fire?

Rob: I used to be an internationally acclaimed landscape gardener.

Steve: Wow.

Steve's interest was palpable. In the moments that followed this revelation, Rob's demeanour changed and he became animated. He went on to describe his life working on large landscape projects, travelling the world, going from one exotic location to the next. From a narrow, inward, locked-in survival mindset, Rob started to make tentative outward explorations.

Rob: I've just had a thought: I might ring up my stepson, John, to see if he wants a hand with his garden.

Two sessions later, Rob had turned his life around. Of course, he was still grieving, but he was also regularly meeting up with his stepson (Liz's son). From isolation, he was interacting and was regaining a sense of purpose. Listening to what was not said, particularly concerning the social context of Rob's life, gave necessary breadth to Rob's living.

Research evidence

The relationship with another

The evidence base for the relational approach to person-centred therapy consists primarily of evidence in support of relational factors (see Norcross & Lambert, 2019). There are no trials of effectiveness that directly compare a relational person-centred approach with another form of therapy – person-centred or otherwise. Research, however, indicates that a range of relational factors are associated with positive therapy outcomes (Norcross & Lambert, 2019), including all three of the 'core conditions' (Elliott et al., 2018; Farber et al., 2018; Kolden et al., 2019). Furthermore, a recent meta-analysis has highlighted that both therapists' and clients' expressions of authentic emotions in psychotherapy contribute to good outcomes (Peluso & Freund, 2018). This finding offers evidence for the benefits of active congruence, in particular realness and transparency, as a contributor of outcomes.

The co-created relationship

More recently, research looking at relational factors as experienced within the therapy dyad or as a shared experience points to direct evidence in favour of the co-created relationship. Research on mutuality and relational depth are key developments of research in this area.

Mutuality

Research on the reciprocity or *mutuality* of relational factors is a new area of psychotherapy research (e.g. Cornelius-White et al., 2018; Murphy & Cramer, 2014). This shifts the focus from a unilateral perception of the therapeutic relationship to a perception of the therapeutic relationship within the therapist/client dyad.

Murphy and colleagues (2012) were the first to define mutuality as the co-experiencing of the core conditions and suggest that this might be an under-researched area. Murphy and Cramer (2014) explored associations of treatment progress at the third session of therapy with both clients' and therapists' ratings of the core conditions using the Barrett-Lennard (2015) Relationship Inventory (a measure of the core conditions). They found that the association between positive client ratings of therapist-provided conditions and treatment progress was stronger when both client and therapist rated each other as providing high levels of the therapeutic conditions. These findings suggested that the mutual experiencing of Rogers' therapeutic conditions may have led to improved progress in therapy.

Flückiger and colleagues (2020) similarly explored the reciprocity of the therapeutic bond of the working alliance within therapeutic dyads. They found that, when clients and therapists gave similar scores on the bond scale, higher bond ratings predicted lower levels of symptoms in the next session.

A meta-analysis of quantitative and qualitative studies has corroborated these findings, indicating the positive association between mutuality and therapeutic progress (Cornelius-White et al., 2018). In this study, the authors used a broader definition of mutuality: therapist and client co-experiencing relational qualities including, but not restricted to, mutual empathy, mutual positive regard and a perception of congruence in the other.

Relational depth and outcomes

Relational depth experiences, as described in qualitative research, appear intertwined with psychological growth (e.g. Mearns & Cooper, 2005/2018; Knox & Cooper, 2011; McMillan & McLeod, 2006). Clients, for instance, described that 'their eyes had been opened' or that something 'had shifted' (Knox & Cooper, 2011, p.143). Other impacts included greater self-understanding; more clarity of thought; improved relationships with family and friends, and feeling more alive, happy or at ease (Knox & Cooper, 2011). Many clients saw the experience as a catalyst for change and reported an enduring increased connection to self, others and the world. One client in Knox's (Knox & Cooper, 2011) study, for instance, said:

> I've come away today… able to stand in the garden again and be in the world, and know that I'm not alone and I don't know what makes me know I'm not alone… but that empathy that I felt, and that connection that I felt, it gives me nourishment. (p. 238)

An additional benefit described by clients was the greater level of authenticity experienced within the continuing therapeutic relationship. Descriptions also consistently included a wide range of self-experiences and emotions, such as feeling 'relief', 'whole', 'validated' and 'energised'. It was often referred to as an empowering experience.

A small body of quantitative research also points to associations of greater relational depth with improved therapeutic outcomes, including reduced psychological distress (Leung, 2008; Wiggins et al., 2012). A recent study by Kim and colleagues (2020) of 55 psychotherapy clients in a clinical setting suggests associations between relational depth – as measured with the Relational Depth Inventory (Wiggins, 2011) – and increased unconditional self-regard and authenticity. In another recent study (Di Malta et al., 2023), the frequency of relational depth moments in psychotherapy clients – as measured by the Relational Depth Frequency Scale (Di Malta et al., 2020) – was also associated with increased satisfaction with psychotherapy and the psychotherapist.

Self-relationship

Recent evidence has turned to evaluating and developing counsellor training to support relational depth experiences within a relational approach. A study by Tangen and Cashwell (2016) first pointed to the role that training can have in supporting the development of counsellors to engage at relational depth. They highlighted the importance of personal counselling for student counsellors, and of educators developing strong supervisory and mentoring relationships with their students. Their findings also suggested that students could be taught how to structure sessions and use counselling skills with the aim of inviting depth.

Ray and colleagues (2021) explored responses from 10 doctoral students before and after a semester involving relational depth training. The training consisted of reading teaching material, clinical experiential activities and a cohort process group. Trainees deepened their reflections around relational depth and appeared to give a more personal response in terms of the mutuality of experiences. They also talked about the impact on them personally and professionally. Trainees also seemed to put more emphasis on the importance of counsellor authenticity in therapy.

A recent meta-synthesis that explored factors that facilitate relational depth suggests that potential areas of self-development for counsellors could be the following:

- establishing dialogue with one's inner world
- working with attachment
- responding sensitively to beliefs and values
- deepening each other's understanding
- addressing ruptures
- understanding the client's role in meeting at relational depth (Wilcox & Almasifard, 2023).

The world and universal relationships

This is perhaps the most under-researched area in respect of the relational approach and one that needs further development. Lago and Christodulidi (2013) have pointed to potential barriers to engaging at relational depth with people from culturally diverse backgrounds, highlighting obstacles such as the therapist's lack of knowledge, communication difficulties, and power imbalances. Further research on relational factors and co-created experiences with specific culturally diverse groups is vitally needed to inform culturally sensitive ways of engaging with them. In addition, research is also needed on how bringing culture and issues of power into the therapy room impacts on the co-created relationship.

To date, however, there is evidence that relational depth can be experienced in a range of therapeutic contexts and with a few different client groups where it could have nuanced therapeutic benefits. In the context of sex addiction treatment, relational depth supports a more holistic conceptualisation of treatment and facilitates addressing issues of shame and attachment insecurities (Woehler et al., 2018). With patients receiving treatment for cancer, experiences of relational depth were associated with normalising patients' heightened vulnerability and emotionality (Anderson, 2021). With young people, significant relational events in therapy were similar to adults' descriptions of relational depth events (Gurvitz, 2017; Knox, 2008). Most clients also report experiencing relational depth during online therapy, offering similar descriptions to those described in face-to-face therapy, such as 'beyond words', 'unforgettable', and 'life-changing' (Treanor, 2017).

Summary

This chapter details the theoretical and clinical foundations for a relational approach to person-centred therapy. It covers its evolution, philosophical and psychological roots and practice. This approach has evolved from classical person-centred therapy by giving a new emphasis to the first and sixth conditions: contact and client perceptions of connectivity with the therapist. The relational approach has four interlinked dimensions from which to derive relational practice: the relationship to another, where the therapist has an ethical responsibility to encounter the client; the co-created relationship, where healing occurs through moments of relational depth; the self-relationship, as an ongoing commitment to developing self-acceptance, and the relationship to the social world and contexts.

Evidence for the benefits of the relational approach is growing. It comes from research into factors that touch on relationship with the other, and more recently from evidence for the links between relational depth and mutuality, which reflect the co-created relationship. There is also some evidence on the importance of the self-relationship and relationship with the world. Further research is needed in each of these areas, and most importantly on integrating cultural sensitivity into relational person-centred practices.

Resources

Key books

- Mearns, D. & Cooper, M. (2018). *Working at relational depth in counselling and psychotherapy.* (2nd ed.). Sage. A key resource on all elements of relational depth

- Schmid, P.F. (2006). The challenge of the other: Towards dialogical person-centered psychotherapy and counseling. *Person-Centered & Experiential Psychotherapies, 5*(4), 240–254. This is one of Schmid's many papers that detail his philosophical relational perspective. See more at http://pfs-online.at

Training resources

- For a series of self-development exercises and reflections to support a therapist's ability to relate at depth, see Cooper, M. (2013). Experiencing relational depth: self-development exercises and reflections. In R. Knox, D. Murphy, S. Wiggins & M. Cooper M. (Eds), *Relational depth: New perspectives and developments* (pp.137–152). Palgrave Macmillan.
- Another set of trainee activities for relational depth can be found in: Ray, D.C., Lankford, C.T., McCullough, R. & Woehler, E. (2019). Meeting at relational depth: The transformative responsibility of counselor education. *Journal of Professional Counseling: Practice, Theory & Research*, *46*(1-2), 77–90.

Websites

- Resources for working at relational depth can be found on Mick Cooper's website at: www.mick-cooper.squarespace.com/relational-depth
- A video of a session between Mick Cooper and 'Julie' demonstrating humanistic/person-centred skills in listening, empathising, and helping clients to deepen their emotional processing and awareness can be seen at: www.youtube.com/watch?v=Md3rdQssxxE

References

Anderson, R. (2021). *A qualitative exploration of cancer patients' experiences of moments of relational depth with their therapist during psychological therapy*. Unpublished doctoral dissertation. University of Roehampton, London.

Barrett-Lennard, G.T. (2005). *Relationship at the centre: Healing in a troubled world*. Whurr Publications

Barrett-Lennard, G.T. (2015). *The Relationship Inventory: A complete resource and guide*. John Wiley.

Bohart, A.C. (2003). Person-centered psychotherapy and related experiential approaches. In A.S. Gurman & S.B. Messer (Eds.), *Essential psychotherapies: Theory and practice* (2nd ed.) (pp.107–148). Guilford Press.

Buber, M. (1947). Dialogue (R.G. Smith, Trans.). In M. Buber, *Between man and man* (pp.17–59). Fontana.

Buber, M. (1958). *I and thou* (R.G. Smith, Trans.; 2nd ed.). T&T Clark Ltd.

Buber, M. (1988). The knowledge of man: Selected essays (M. Friedman & R.G. Smith, Trans.). Humanities Press International Inc.

Chantler, K. (2004). Double-edged sword: Power and person-centred counselling. In R. Moodley, C. Lago, & A. Talahite (Eds.), *Carl Rogers counsels a black client: Race and culture in person-centred counselling* (pp.116–129). PCCS Books.

Cooper, M. (2003a). 'I-I' And 'I-Me': Transposing Buber's interpersonal attitudes to the intrapersonal plane. *Journal of Constructivist Psychology, 16*(2), 131–153.

Cooper, M. (2003b). Between freedom and despair: Existential challenges and contributions to person-centered and experiential therapy. *Person-Centered & Experiential Psychotherapies, 2*(1), 43–56.

Cooper, M. (2005). Therapists' experiences of relational depth: A qualitative interview study. *Counselling and Psychotherapy Research, 5*(2), 87–95.

Cooper, M. (In press). Developmental and personality theory. In G. Di Malta, M. Cooper, Y. Gololob, M. O'Hara & S. Stephen (Eds.), *The handbook of person-centred psychotherapy and counselling* (3rd ed.) (In press). Bloomsbury.

Cooper, M., Di Malta, G., Knox, S., Oddli, H.W. & Swift, J.K. (2023). Patient perspectives on working with preferences in psychotherapy: A consensual qualitative research study. *Psychotherapy Research*, 1–15.

Cornelius-White, J.H., Kanamori, Y., Murphy, D., & Tickle, E. (2018). Mutuality in psychotherapy: A meta-analysis and meta-synthesis. *Journal of Psychotherapy Integration, 28*(4), 489.

Cox, S. (2016). Relational and dialogical aspects of person-centred therapeutic practice. In P. Wilkins (Ed.), *Person-centred and experiential therapies: Contemporary approaches and issues in practice* (pp.32–46). Sage.

Cozolino, L. (2014). *The neuroscience of human relationships* (2nd ed.). W.W. Norton.

Crossley, N. (1996). *Intersubjectivity: The fabric of social becoming*. Sage.

Curtis, R.C. & Hirsch, I. (2003). Relational approaches to psychoanalytic psychotherapy. In A.S. Gurman & S.B. Messer (Eds.), *Essential psychotherapies: Theory and practice* (2nd ed.) (pp.69–106). Guilford Press.

Derrida, J. (1974). *Of grammatology* (G.C. Spivak, Trans.). John Hopkins University Press.

Di Malta, G., Evans, C. & Cooper, M. (2020). Development and validation of the Relational Depth Frequency Scale. *Psychotherapy Research, 30*(2), 213–227.

Di Malta, G., She, Z., Raymond-Barker, B. & Cooper, M. (2023). Extended validation of the Relational Depth Frequency Scale: Retest reliability, divergent and criterion validity, and measurement invariance in UK-and US-stratified samples. *Journal of Clinical Psychology, 79*(9), 2040–2052.

Ellingham, I. (2011). Carl Rogers' fateful wrong move in the development of Rogerian relational therapy: Retitling 'relationship therapy' 'non-directive therapy'. *Person-Centered & Experiential Psychotherapies, 10*, 181–197.

Elliott, R., Bohart, A.C., Watson, J.C. & Murphy, D. (2018). Therapist empathy and client outcome: An updated meta-analysis. *Psychotherapy, 55*(4), 399–410.

Farber, B.A., Suzuki, J.Y. & Lynch, D.A. (2018). Positive regard and psychotherapy outcome: A meta-analytic review. *Psychotherapy, 55*(4), 411–423.

Flückiger, C., Rubel, J., Del Re, A.C., Horvath, A.O., Wampold, B.E., Crits-Christoph, P., ... & Barber, J.P. (2020). The reciprocal relationship between alliance and early treatment symptoms: A two-stage individual participant data meta-analysis. *Journal of Consulting and Clinical Psychology, 88*(9), 829.

Freire, E. (2013). Empathy. In M. Cooper, P.F. Schmid, M. O'Hara & A.C. Bohart (Eds.), *The handbook of person-centred psychotherapy and counselling* (pp.165–179) (2nd ed.). Palgrave.

Friedman, M. (1985). *The healing dialogue in psychotherapy*. Jason Aronson, Inc.

Gaylin, N.L. (2002). The relationship: The heart of the matter. In J.C. Watson, R.N. Goldman & S. Warner (Eds.), *Client-centred and experiential psychotherapy in the 21st Century: Advances in theory, research and practice* (pp.339–347). PCCS Books.

Gerhardt, S. (2014). *Why love matters: How affection shapes a baby's brain* (2nd ed.). Routledge.

Gilligan, C. (1993). *In a different voice: Psychological theory and women's development*. Harvard University Press.

Gurvitz, S. (2017). *Young people's experience of important moments of change in the therapeutic relationship*. Unpublished PsychD dissertation. University of Roehampton, London.

Heidegger, M. (1926/1962). *Being and time*. (J. Macquarrie & E. Robinson, Trans.). Blackwell Publishing.

Hill, C.E., Knox, S. & Pinto-Coelho, K.G. (2019). Self-disclosure and immediacy. In J.C. Norcross & M.J. Lambert (Eds.), *Psychotherapy relationships that work. Volume 1: Evidence-based therapist contributions* (3rd ed.) (pp.379–420). Oxford University.

Holdstock, L. (1990). Can client-centred therapy transcend its mono cultural roots? In G. Lietaer, J. Rombauts & R. Van Baten (Eds.), *Client-centered and experiential therapies in the nineties* (pp.109–121). Leuven University Press. Holdstock, L. (1993). Can we afford not to revision the person-centred concept of Self? In D. Brazier (Ed.), *Beyond Carl Rogers* (pp.229–252). Constable.

Holdstock, L. (1996). Discrepancy between the person-centred theories of self and of therapy. In R. Hutterer, G. Pawlowsky, P.F. Schmid & R. Stripots (Eds.), *Client-centered and experiential psychotherapy: A paradigm in motion* (pp.47–52). Peter Lang.

Jordan, J.V., Kaplan, A.G., Miller, J.B., Stiver, I.P. & Surrey, J.L. (Eds.). (1991). *Women's growth in connection: Writings from the Stone Centre*. Guilford Press.

Kim, J., Joseph, S. & Price, S. (2020). The positive psychology of relational depth and its association with unconditional positive self-regard and authenticity. *Person-Centered & Experiential Psychotherapies, 19*(1), 12–21.

Knox, R. (2008). Clients' experiences of relational depth in person-centred counselling. *Counselling and Psychotherapy Research, 8*(3), 182–188.

Knox, R. (2011). *Clients' experiences of relational depth*. PhD dissertation. University of Strathclyde. https://www.researchgate.net/profile/Rosanne-Knox/publication/233445567_Clients'_experiences_of_relational_depth_in_person-centred_counselling/links/56192d1308ae044edbaf8a66

Knox, R. (2013). Relational depth from the client's perspective. In R. Knox, D. Murphy, S. Wiggins & M. Cooper (Eds.), *Relational depth: New perspectives and developments* (pp.21–35). Palgrave.

Knox, R. & Cooper, M. (2010). Relational qualities associates with moments of relational depth: The client's perspective. *Person-Centered & Experiential Psychotherapies, 9*(3), 236–256.

Knox, R. & Cooper, M. (2011). A state of readiness: An exploration of the client's role in meeting at relational depth. *Journal of Humanistic Psychology, 51*(1), 61–81.

Knox, R., Murphy, D., Wiggins, S. & Cooper, M. (Eds.). (2013). *Relational depth: New perspectives and developments.* Palgrave Macmillan.

Kolden, G.G., Wang, C.-C., Austin, S.B., Change, Y. & Klein, M.H. (2019). Congruence/genuineness. In J.C. Norcross & M.J. Lambert (Eds.), *Psychotherapy relationships that work. Volume 1: Evidence-based therapist contributions* (3rd ed.) (pp.323–350). Oxford University.

Lago, C. & Christodulidi, F. (2013). Client-therapist diversity: Aspiring towards relational depth. In R. Knox, D. Murphy, S. Wiggins, & M. Cooper M. (Eds.), *Relational depth: New perspectives and developments* (pp.137–152). Palgrave Macmillan.

Laurenceau, J.-P., Rivera, L.M., Schaffer, A.R. & Pietromonaco, P.R. (2004). Intimacy as interpersonal process: Current status and future directions. In D.J. Mashek & A.P. Aron (Eds.), *Handbook of closeness and intimacy* (pp.61–78). Lawrence Erlbaum.

Leung, J. (2008). *A quantitative online study exploring the factors associated with the experience and perceived importance of relational depth.* Unpublished DPsych dissertation. University of Strathclyde, Glasgow.

McMillan, M. & McLeod, J. (2006). Letting go: The client's experiences of relational depth. *Person-Centered & Experiential Psychotherapies, 5*(4), 277–292.

Mearns D. (1997). *Person-centred training.* Sage.

Mearns, D. & Cooper, M. (2005/2018). *Working at relational depth in counselling and psychotherapy* (2nd ed.). Sage.

Moodley, R., Lago, C. & Talahite, A. (Eds.). (2004). *Carl Rogers counsels a black client.* PCCS Books.

Murphy D. (2013). Mutuality and relational depth in counselling and psychotherapy. In R. Knox, D. Murphy, S. Wiggins & M. Cooper (Eds.), *Relational depth: New perspectives and developments* (pp.185–195). Palgrave Macmillan.

Murphy, D. & Cramer, D. (2014). Mutuality of Rogers' therapeutic conditions and treatment progress in the first three psychotherapy sessions. *Psychotherapy Research, 24*(6), 651–661.

Murphy, D., Cramer, D. & Joseph, S. (2012). Mutuality in person-centered therapy: A new agenda for research and practice. *Person-Centered & Experiential Psychotherapies, 11*, 109–123.

Natiello P. (2001). *The person-centred approach: A passionate presence.* PCCS Books.

Norcross, J.C. & Lambert, M.J. (Eds.) (2019). *Psychotherapy relationships that work. Volume 1: Evidence-based therapist contributions* (3rd ed.). Oxford University.

O'Hara, M. (1995). Streams: On becoming a postmodern person. In M.M. Suhd (Ed.), *Positive regard: Carl Rogers and other notables he influenced* (pp.105–155). Science and Behavior Books.

Peluso, P.R. & Freund, R.R. (2018). Therapist and client emotional expression and psychotherapy outcomes: A meta-analysis. *Psychotherapy, 55*(4), 461.

Proctor, G. (2006). Therapy: Opium for the masses or helps those who least need it? In G. Proctor, M. Cooper, P. Sanders & B. Malcolm (Eds.), *Politicising the person-centred approach: An agenda for social change* (pp.66–79). PCCS Books.

Ratts, M.J. & Pedersen, P.B. (2014). *Counseling for multiculturalism and social justice: Integration, theory, and application* (4th ed.). American Counseling Association.

Ray, D.C., Lankford, C.T., Malacara, A.B., Woehler, E. & McCullough, R. (2021). Exploring counselor experiences of training in relational depth: An interpretative phenomenological inquiry. *Journal of Counseling & Development, 99*(1), 84–95.

Rogers, C.R. (1951). *Client-centered therapy*. Houghton and Mifflin.

Rogers, C.R. (1957). The necessary and sufficient conditions of therapeutic personality change. *Journal of Consulting Psychology, 21*(2), 95–103.

Rogers, C.R. (1959). A theory of therapy, personality and interpersonal relationships as developed in the client-centered framework. In S. Koch (Ed.), *Psychology: A study of science, vol. 3.* (pp.184–256). McGraw-Hill.

Rogers, C.R. (1961a). *On becoming a person: A therapist's view of psychotherapy.* Houghton Mifflin.

Rogers, C.R. (1961b). Ellen West and loneliness. *Review of Existential Psychology and Psychiatry, 1*(2), 94–101.

Rogers, C.R. (1980). *A way of being*. Houghton Mifflin.

Rogers, C.R. (1986/1990). A client-centered/person-centered approach to therapy. In H. Kirschenbaum & V. Henderson (Eds.), *The Carl Rogers reader* (pp.135–152). Constable.

Sanders, P. (2005). Principled and strategic opposition to the medicalisation of distress and all of its apparatus. In S. Joseph & R. Worsley (Eds.), *Person-centred psychopathology: A positive psychology of mental health* (pp.21–42). PCCS Books

Schmid, P.F. (1994). *Personzentrierte Gruppenpsycherapic. Ein Handbuch, Vol I: Solidarität und Autonomie.* Edition Humanistische Psychologie.

Schmid, P.F. (1998a). *Im Anfang ist Gemeinschaft, Peronzentrierte Gruppenarbeit in Seelsorge und Praktischer Theologie. Vol III: Beitrag Zu einer Theologie der Gruppe.* Kehlhammer.

Schmid, P.F. (1998b). Face to face the art of encounter. In B. Thorne & E. Lambers (Eds.), *Person-centred therapy: A European perspective* (pp.74–90). Sage.

Schmid, P.F. (1998c). On becoming a person-centred approach: A person-centred understanding of the person. In B. Thorne & E. Lambers (Eds)., *Person-centred therapy: A European perspective* (pp.38–52). Sage.

Schmid, P.F. (2002). Knowledge of acknowledgement? Psychotherapy as 'the art of not-knowing' – prospects on further developments of a radical paradigm. *Person-Centered & Experiential Psychotherapies, 1*(1&2), 56–70.

Schmid, P.F. (2006). The challenge of the Other: Towards a dialogical person-centered psychotherapy and counselling. *Person-Centered & Experiential Psychotherapies, 5*(4), 240–254.

Schmid, P.F. (2013). The anthropological, relational, and ethical foundations of person-centred therapy. In M. Cooper, P.F. Schmid, M. O'Hara & G. Wyatt (Eds.), *The handbook of person-centred psychotherapy and counselling* (2nd ed.) (pp.66–83). Palgrave.

Schmid, P.F. & Mearns, D. (2006). Being-with and being-counter: Person-centered psychotherapy as an in-depth co-creative process of personalization. *Person-Centered & Experiential Psychotherapies, 5*(3), 174–190.

Standal, S.W. (1954). *The need for positive regard: A contribution to client-centered theory.* University of Chicago.

Stern, D.N. (2004). *The present moment in psychotherapy and everyday life.* W.W. Norton.

Stillwell, W. (1998). *Questing voices.* Center for Studies of the Person.

Tangen, J.L., & Cashwell, C.S. (2016). Touchstones of connection: A concept mapping study of counselor factors that contribute to relational depth. *The Journal of Humanistic Counseling, 55*(1), 20–36.

Treanor, A. (2017). *The extent to which relational depth can be reached in online therapy and the factors that facilitate and inhibit that experience: A mixed methods study.* Doctoral dissertation. University of Roehampton.

Tudor, K. & Worrall, M. (2006). *Person-centred therapy: A clinical philosophy.* Routledge.

Whiteley, J.M. (Dir.). (1977). *Carl Rogers counsels an individual: 'The right to be desperate' and 'On anger and hurt'.* American Personnel and Guidance Association.

Wiggins, S. (2011). *Relational depth and therapeutic outcome.* Paper presented at the 17th Annual BACP Research Conference, Edinburgh.

Wiggins, S., Elliott, R. & Cooper, M. (2012). The prevalence and characteristics of relational depth events in psychotherapy. *Psychotherapy Research, 22*(2), 139–158.

Wilcox, H. & Almasifard, S. (2023). Facilitating the client's experience of relational depth in counselling and psychotherapy: A thematic review. *Counselling and Psychotherapy Research, 23*(3), 603–616.

Woehler, E.S., Giordano, A.L. & Hagedorn, W.B. (2018). Moments of relational depth in sex addiction treatment. *Sexual Addiction & Compulsivity, 25*(2–3), 153–169.

Wyatt, G. & Sanders, P. (Eds.). (2001). *Rogers' therapeutic conditions: Evolution, theory and practice. Volume 4: Contact and perception.* PCCS Books.

4. Focusing-oriented therapy

Campbell Purton

Focusing-oriented therapy developed from the work of the Austrian-American philosopher and psychotherapist Eugene Gendlin. Gendlin was a close colleague of Carl Rogers at the University of Chicago Counseling Center in the 1950s, and Rogers acknowledged the importance of Gendlin's influence in developing his ideas during that period (Rogers 1958/1961).

Gendlin came to the United States from Austria at the age of 12. His family was one of the last Jewish families to escape from the Nazis in Vienna in 1938, and one particular experience during this terrifying episode is relevant to his discovery of focusing. The family had crossed Nazi Germany as far as Cologne and had been given an address where they could ask for help in continuing their journey. In a letter to Lore Korbei (Korbei, 1994), Gendlin gave this account:

> We found the right house and an apartment on the upper floor. There, my father went into a room with a man, and I waited maybe for a quarter of an hour. When my father came out, he was pale and said: 'Let's go.' Outside he explained that he could not trust this man. My father said that his feeling had said 'no' to him. My father had already said this many times: 'I follow my feeling.' But at this time I did not understand what he meant when he said he trusted his feelings. We were in a strange city and without any way out. We had put all our hopes on 'the address', and now this hope was destroyed, only because of what he had 'felt'.
>
> I was surprised then and also often asked myself later what kind of feeling it must be that tells you something. Sometimes I tried to find such a feeling within myself, but I could not. But that I started to look for it had its effect in the end. Forty years later, when I was asked how I could explain focusing, I remembered these circumstances. (p.179)

Focusing is concerned with the overall 'feel' of a situation, or of a problem, and with how a person expresses this feeling. 'Therapeutic focusing', as Gendlin called it, is best understood, I think, as a version of person-centred therapy that, along with Rogers' 'therapist conditions' of empathy, acceptance and congruence, emphasises the importance of what the *client* does in effective therapy. For Gendlin, this 'client aspect' of therapy involved something that he sometimes called 'resonating', meaning that, regardless of what the therapist says or does, the client needs to 'check' that it 'resonates' with what *they* actually feel or think. A very simple example would be where a therapist says, 'You feel ashamed' and the client pauses for a moment, and then says, 'Well, not exactly ashamed... more like embarrassed... but there's also something else that I can't quite get hold of yet.' It is this 'resonating' that lies at the heart of focusing. We can do such 'resonating' on our own if we want to be clearer about what we really feel about a situation, so that, as well as being an aspect of person-centred therapy, focusing can also be a kind of self-therapy. In fact, Gendlin's best-known book, *Focusing* (1978/2003), is a self-help book, rather than a book for counsellors.

It is worth making this point at the beginning because when counsellors first hear of 'focusing' and then look at Gendlin's book, it can seem that he is recommending that therapists should use their time with clients to teach them how to focus. This can be especially troubling for trainees in person-centred therapy, who rightly believe that explicit teaching is not what is involved in the approach. A much better introduction to focusing-oriented *therapy* can be found in Gendlin's chapter 'The small steps of the therapy process: how they come and how to help them come', in Lietaer and colleagues' (1990) book *Client-centered and Experiential Psychotherapy in the Nineties.*

Gendlin's first book on focusing-oriented therapy (Gendlin, 1996) appeared 18 years after his self-help book, but although Gendlin had written much on therapy in the intervening years, the image many therapists have of the approach derives from a book that is *not* itself about therapy. Lack of clarity about this distinction has caused much misunderstanding among the 'tribes of the person-centred nation'.

Historical background

This chapter is about focusing-oriented *therapy* (FOT), although I will need to refer later to what Gendlin says about self-help. First, I will outline how FOT developed out of Rogers' early work. More details of the historical background can be found in Chapter 1 (this volume), and in Judy Moore's (2021a, 2021b) more detailed account in Kypriotakis and Moore's two-volume compendium *Senses of Focusing* (2021). Here I will concentrate on Gendlin's place in the story.

Gendlin's background was in philosophy, and about half of his publications are in that field, but the philosophical theme that mainly concerned him relates very closely to what is involved in psychotherapy. It is the theme of how our lived *experiences* are related to the way we *talk* about them. In other words, much of what goes on in therapy – especially person-centred therapy and psychodynamic therapy – has to do with helping clients to find authentic ways of expressing themselves. In Rogers' terminology, the therapist is helping the client to be more 'congruent'; in Freud's terminology the therapist's aim is to 'help make the unconscious conscious'. However we put it, it does seem that a major aim of therapy is to help clients to become 'more themselves' – more authentic; to help them to express themselves more adequately, and hence to live more fully.

Gendlin – at that time a philosophy PhD student at the University of Chicago – wanted to join Rogers' group at the University Counseling Center in 1953 (see Chapter 1, this volume) because he saw that what Rogers and his colleagues were working with was exactly the theme that most interested him: the relationship between what we experience and how we express it. He says in an interview (Gendlin & Lietaer, 1983):

> [I]ndeed they were doing this; they were letting a person have directly this experience and slowly to work at how to express that, how to symbolise that, how to say that. (p.78)

He was interviewed by Rogers for a place on Rogers' counselling training course, and relates how, knowing that Gendlin was a philosopher (Gendlin, 2002):

> [Rogers] looked at me intently, and asked 'But are you obtuse about people?' (This seemed to be his observation of philosophers). I said no, I didn't think so; people talked to me about their problems, sometimes all night. I just didn't know how to help them. He accepted me for the year-long practicum. (p.4)

On completion of the practicum, Gendlin began to work with Rogers and his colleagues at the Chicago Counseling Center. With Fred Zimring (Gendlin & Zimring, 1955/1994), he developed a 'process scale' designed to measure the extent to which clients were trying to express what they were experiencing. This scale was subsequently developed into the Experiencing Scale that was used in the later Wisconsin study of schizophrenia (see Chapter 1, this volume). At the same time, Rogers (1958/1961) was working on a very similar 'process conception' of psychotherapy, involving a process scale with seven stages. In the first stage, clients mainly report on external events, but say little about themselves. In the subsequent stages, there is increasing expression of feeling, which is associated with therapeutic change.

Rogers gives many examples of the ways in which clients talk when they are making progress in therapy. Here are three, taken from a discussion of Rogers' 'fifth stage' in his process scale (1958/1961):

> Example: 'That kinda came out and I just don't understand it. (*Long pause*). I'm trying to get hold of what that terror is.'
>
> Example: 'Client is talking about an external event. Suddenly she gives a pained, stricken look. Therapist: 'What – what's hitting you now?' Client: 'I don't know. (*She cries*). I must have been getting a little too close to something I didn't want to talk about, or something.'

> Example: 'I feel stopped right now. Why is my mind blank right now? I feel as if I am hanging on to something, and I've been letting go of other things; and something in me is saying, "What more do I have to give up?"' (1958/1961, p.140)

The language here is more expressive than descriptive: something 'comes out', or the client expresses something that has 'hit them', or they express their 'stoppedness', or how they are 'hanging on to something'. The way I would put this is that in such examples the client is articulating their responses rather than describing their 'inner sensations'. I will come back later to the significance of this distinction.

During the period when Rogers and Gendlin were working on a process conception of therapy, Rogers was also stressing the importance of what later came to be called the 'core conditions' of effective therapy: empathy, acceptance and congruence (Rogers, 1957) (see Chapter 2, this volume). However, Rogers tended to see these conditions as combining into a single condition. In an address to the American Academy of Psychotherapists, he said: 'I believe I can state this condition in one word… that the client experiences himself as being fully received' (Rogers, 1956).

By the late 1950s, the theory emerging from Rogers' group was that, when clients are 'fully received' by the therapist, they gradually become able to give more spontaneous expression to what they experience. What they say now 'comes directly from their feelings' rather than from 'what most people would say here', or 'what is reasonable' or 'what must be so'. The crucial difference, I think, is that in the first kind of case the client is *expressing* their feelings, while in the second they are doing something else, such as reporting, deducing, concluding or speculating. The receptive attitude of the therapist encourages such client expression.

There were, however, some empirical results that were puzzling if the crucial element in therapy is simply the receptive attitude of the therapist. Two members of Rogers' group, William Kirtner and Desmond Cartwright, had obtained results that suggested it was often possible to predict from the first few sessions whether a client was likely to benefit from therapy. It seemed that, although the core conditions were important, much also depended on the personality of the client (Kirtner & Cartwright, 1958a), and on how the client related to what they were experiencing (Kirtner & Cartwright, 1958b).

Gendlin worked with clients in the way that he had been taught by Rogers. That is, he did his best to 'receive' clients and, like Rogers, he was actively engaged with them through careful empathic reflection. 'Reflection' has always been important in the tradition of therapy that runs from Rogers' early 'client-centered therapy' through to the later developments in person-centred therapy. In fact, around 90% of Rogers' interventions in therapy were reflections, or what Tony Merry (2000) calls 'verbal empathic following responses' (see Chapter 2, this volume). However, there was a difference in emphasis between Rogers and Gendlin about what the purpose of reflecting is.

Rogers originally saw it as a way of making sure that he had understood what the client had said. When Rogers reflected a client's words, the client would frequently say, 'That's not quite it – it's more like this.' Then Rogers would reflect this new way of putting it, and the client might 'correct' him by saying, 'Yes… it is that, but not *just* that… also *this...'* In that way, Rogers was able to reach an understanding of what exactly the client meant, and so was able to empathise more fully with them. Therapist empathy has been shown by much recent research to be one of the strongest correlates of therapeutic effectiveness (Wampold & Imel, 2015; Cooper 2008), but Rogers later came to accept that there is also the *client's* side to what is going on when the therapist reflects what the client has said.

There was an interesting discussion of this issue in the very first volume of the *Person-Centered Review,* published shortly before Rogers' death in 1987. 'Reflection' had come to be criticised by some therapists as a mockery of person-centred responding, but Rogers' friend and former colleague John Shlien wrote to him (Rogers, 1986/1990):

> 'Reflection' is unfairly damned. It was rightly criticised when you described the wooden mockery it could become in the hands of insensitive people, and you wrote beautifully on that point. But you neglected the other side. It is an instrument of artistic virtuosity in the hands of a sincere, intelligent, empathic listener. It made possible the development of client-centered therapy, when the philosophy alone could not have. (pp.127–129)

Around the same time, one of Rogers' clients had written (Slack, 1985):

> It was like Dr Rogers was a magic mirror. The process involved my sending rays towards that mirror. I looked into the mirror to get a glimpse of the reality that I am [...] This experience allowed me an opportunity to get a view of myself that was untainted by the perception of outside viewers.

In replying to these two points, Rogers (1986/1990) wrote:

> I have come to a double insight. From my point of view as therapist, I am not trying to 'reflect feelings'. I am trying to determine whether my understanding of the client's inner world is correct [...] On the other hand, I know that from a client's point of view we are holding up a mirror of his or her current experiencing. (pp.127–129)

The important point here is that Rogers' activity of reflecting enabled or encouraged clients to become more fully aware of what they were really feeling, or how exactly they were responding, and from each moment of fuller awareness further responses would come. Rogers (1961) called these 'moments of movement' (p.130); Gendlin (1996) called them 'change steps' or 'felt shifts' (p.20). Rogers (1954) held that an effective therapy session consisted of a sequence of such 'moments of movement', in the course of which the client comes to have a different perspective on their trouble. Rogers was not *guiding* his clients. Rather, within an atmosphere of genuine acceptance and empathy, he was helping clients attend to their situation and to their responses to it in a way that led to steps of change.

From Gendlin's perspective, what clients are doing in effective therapy is learning to attend to how they are responding and opening themselves to alternative ways of formulating those responses in the light of their situation as a whole. In Gendlin's (1984) way of putting it, the therapist facilitates this process by encouraging the client to attend to the 'edges' of what they are experiencing – those spots at which the client senses something that they can't yet articulate. Through attending to these faint 'whispers' or intimations, the client gradually comes to appreciate aspects of their situation that they hadn't previously appreciated. Then their situation feels different, and if it feels different, it *is* different.

Gendlin concluded from the study of thousands of recorded sessions that the more successful clients tend to talk in a different way from the less successful ones. Rather than report on external events or analyse their problems in an intellectual fashion, they often pause in a characteristic way and search for words that will express their responses. It is this kind of difference that Gendlin and his colleagues noticed in recordings of sessions and in the transcripts. If recordings are accurately transcribed, including the spaces where the client pauses [...], then it often can be seen at a glance whether the client is talking in the way that we are interested in. For example (Gendlin 1984):

> Client: (*Silence*)... (*Breath*)... Feels sort of heavy... like it *wants* to stay angry...
>
> Therapist: Something there *wants* to stay angry.
>
> Client: Mhm... (*Silence*)... Oh... (*Breath*)... yah... if I stop being angry I won't do anything about it... Yes... I'd love just to say it's OK and not have to cope with the situation. I've done that so often. (p.77)

It is this pausing, this attending to the 'edge' of our experiencing, and letting further feelings (or thoughts, bodily sensations, images or memories) come, that Gendlin calls 'focusing'. It involves attending to one's problem as a whole, letting old, familiar thoughts and feelings go by and waiting for something new, something fresh, to emerge. Then we check: 'This new thing that has come... Does that feel right...? Is it relevant...?' We are not to think about the answers to these questions, but to notice what spontaneously comes in response to them. We are opening ourselves to the wider reaches of our problem, to aspects or facets of the problem that we have not previously noticed or considered. Psychodynamic therapists might see this procedure as 'helping to make the unconscious conscious,' but Gendlin sees it rather differently. It is not necessarily that the 'new things' are 'just there, waiting to come out'. It may rather be that a new possibility dawns on us, something that would not have come to us if we had not been open to the problem as a wider whole.

Some clients do something like focusing spontaneously. It was largely through observing such clients that Gendlin 'discovered' focusing. Others are inclined to spend much of the session reporting events or feelings, and here the focusing-oriented therapist will from time to time encourage them to pause and give some attention to the whole difficulty that they have been talking about. The therapist may do this especially where clients have themselves expressed some kind of response to their difficulty, rather than simply describing what happened. For example, a client talks about their week, but at one point remarks, rather hesitantly, that they were a bit ashamed of something they said to a friend. They are then about to go on with their story, but the therapist says something like,

'You just said you felt ashamed… Is that the right word…?' thereby encouraging the client to articulate their response more fully.

Other clients spend a lot of time caught up in their emotions. They repeat again and again how depressed or angry or helpless they are. They are, we might say, 'acting out' their emotions – living them in the session. If this is the first time a client has really lived an emotion, the experience will probably be valuable for them, but some clients become stuck in their emotions or, as Freud (1936) put it, they suffer from 'repetition compulsion' (p.105). This is different from expressing one's feelings. In expressing one's feelings one is, in the moment, finding words that articulate the feeling, finding words that freshly 'come from' the feeling. In 'acting out', the words are just part of a repetitive response: that the client is saying these things is all of a piece with their habitual inarticulate response. Where a client is 'caught in' their feelings in this way, the focusing-oriented therapist may try to help them 'create a distance' from the feelings. Instead of simply being angry, for example, the client will be encouraged to give attention to their anger. The therapist may model this by saying such things as, 'You are really angry' or 'There is a lot of anger there.' The point of this is to help the client express or articulate their anger – to move from responding in a non-linguistic, inarticulate way (just being angry) to an articulate, linguistic way ('I really am angry'). Once the response becomes articulate, there is the possibility of modifying or refining the articulation, so that the client may now say, 'I feel angry… but it's a peculiar sort of anger… more like outrage… There is sort of self-righteous feel… and also… there's something of *hurt* in all this.' This, of course, is a focusing process, but it cannot begin until the client has begun to articulate their response rather than merely live it.

Focusing, we might say, is the client's side of effective person-centred therapy. It is what the client needs to do if they are to benefit fully from the therapist's 'receiving' of them. It is something that may happen quite spontaneously in the course of the therapeutic engagement, and if it does, the role of the therapist is to support it, or at least not interfere with it. All that may be required is the therapist's attentive presence. Where nothing of a focusing nature naturally occurs, there is the possibility of therapeutic moves that may encourage the client to focus a little, but such moves need to be tentative. Focusing will only be effective in an atmosphere in which the client feels free to follow their own path. It would be contradictory to suppose that a client could be *made* to focus; the possibility for encouraging focusing arises from the fact that it is a completely natural human activity – everyone at times pauses, and wonders, 'What's wrong?, 'Is that what I really want?', 'Do I really feel that?' or 'Is that quite what I meant to say?' The possibility for such reflective activity is always there, so the skill of the therapist lies largely in finding ways of stimulating it, encouraging it and facilitating it.

Gendlin always emphasised that focusing constitutes only one element in the therapeutic process, and that it is not the most important element. The most important element, he held, is simply to be with the client in the kind of way Rogers referred to when he wrote of 'receiving' the client. Gendlin (1990, pp.205–206) gives a vivid account of what he meant by this. The second most important thing then is to listen and reflect, as Rogers did. The encouragement of focusing comes third.

A focusing example

The following example (Gendlin, 1996) may help to indicate the kind of client–therapist interaction that is central to FOP:

> C: I'm mad at Tom [her new husband] for doing that. I want to push him away.
>
> T: What does that pushing away feel like?
>
> C: Hmmm... Like I want to shove him into that big black case my cello is in. *I think I must* want to shape and cut him to some mould of mine. I do that to people.
>
> T: Well, sense it a little longer.
>
> C: Hmm... Oh! (*Surprise*) It's like putting him away just now, but knowing that I will want him back later – keeping him in a safe place like a precious object. (p.40; emphasis in original)

The client begins by noticing that she wants to push her husband away. The therapist responds in a way that encourages her to give more attention to her response. Then comes the first pause as she attends: 'Hmmm…' Following the pause, her response becomes more articulated, more specific. She uses the metaphor of wanting to shove her husband into her cello case – *that* sort of pushing away. Then she does something different – she begins to analyse or speculate about what is going on: '*I think I must* want to shape him and cut him to some sort of mould. I do that to people.' The therapist realises that this is likely to be unhelpful, so rather than engaging with her analysis, he again encourages her to attend to her response. Then comes the second pause, followed by a further change in the way she is responding to her husband – a change that surprises her. She isn't trying to cut him to some sort of mould; she is putting him away safely for a while.

What is happening here is not an intellectual analysis of her situation, and the result is not primarily an 'insight'. What has happened is an actual change in her responding – a change in how she is in relation to her husband. It is the sort of change that Rogers (1961, p.130) called a 'moment of movement'. She is a little different now from the way she was before this moment.

In the focusing process, what the client says comes spontaneously, in the way that tears or laughter may come. It is a new expression of how things now are for them. The client's words are not of the nature of a report or conclusion. Rather, the client is responding in a new way, and the new words articulate that response. The therapeutic change is happening *there*, in the session; it is not a matter of the client having discovered an interesting new fact that is helpful for them to know in approaching their difficulty.

The notion of a 'felt sense'

Gendlin's (1993) way of putting it is that in the pauses (…) the client gives attention to their 'felt sense' of their difficulty. He invented the phrase 'felt sense' because he considered that there is no word in the English language that captures what he is concerned with. However, in some places he does suggest words that are used in very similar ways, such as 'having an inkling of something' or 'pondering over something'. For example, we might say that someone has 'just an inkling' of what to do, but can't yet say more. So they ponder over what they are feeling, asking themselves questions such as, 'What's this really all about?' Having a hunch, or an intuition, about something is very similar (Gendlin, 1993, 2000). In such cases, we attend to a situation that is troubling, puzzling or unclear, and then cast around for ways to articulate what we are feeling.

Gendlin always emphasised the importance of attending to the problem *as a whole*. In his first paper on focusing (1969), he wrote:

> People rarely let the crux of the problem come freshly to them from their feel of the problem as a whole. They already know what the crux is, or they decide what it is. (p.5)

He continued:

> [D]on't decide what is so important about it. Feel it all and don't decide anything. Wait and let the main crux come to you freshly. (p.5)

However, talking of 'the feel of the problem' can sometimes cause confusion. We may be inclined to think of this 'feeling' as some kind of bodily sensation, and Gendlin himself often puts the matter in that way. But at other times he expresses himself differently. In explaining what he means by a 'felt sense' Gendlin (e.g. 1993, p.28) often used the example of a poet who is trying to complete a poem. As they search for the line that will round it off, the poet's hand rotates in the air. This gesture tells us that they haven't yet got the final line, but that they soon will. It is different from simply not knowing how on earth to finish the poem.

I think we might say that to have a felt sense is to sense that something is 'on its way', or that one is 'on the edge' of something. Gendlin (1996, p.18) himself says something to this effect. He discusses an example where a person is talking about their fear of approaching an attractive person at a party: They say, 'I think I know what goes into that fear; it's that I've always been scared just to make a decision on my own. I'm scared it will be wrong. But… uhm…' This person, Gendlin writes, 'has a sense of the edge. "Uhm" is the felt sense.'

When Gendlin says '"Uhm" is the felt sense', we know what he means, but clearly he is not saying that the felt sense is the utterance of a word. In the same way, the felt sense is not the rotation of the poet's hand in the air. I would say – and Gendlin sometimes says – that nor is it the churning sensations the poet might have in their stomach. If the felt sense is a sensation, it is a very special kind of sensation (Gendlin, 1996, p.18): something distinct from ordinary body sensations, so that, while it is easy to say what a felt sense is *not*, it is – as Gendlin recognises – hard to say what it *is*.

My view of the difficulty here is that we are thinking of a 'felt sense' as a curious kind of *inner thing* – something we can locate if we look carefully enough. But that is not how the phrase is actually used. To have a felt sense is to be in a particular kind of situation – namely, one in which we are aware of a difficulty that we have but can't yet put it into words. I will say a bit more about this later.

Focusing and self-therapy

Gendlin wondered whether clients could be encouraged to do more of what the successful clients naturally do, and further work suggested that this was indeed possible. It was at this point in the development of FOT that misunderstandings began to arise. In his 1969 focusing paper, Gendlin raised the question of whether counselling clients might usefully be taught how to focus, and he suggested ways in which therapists might approach such teaching. As part of his research on focusing, he set out steps that could be followed in teaching it, but he didn't normally use the steps with clients. In this same early paper he wrote:

> Experiential interaction comes spontaneously from both persons. As therapist I often don't teach or help with focusing. Focusing, as deliberate silent instructed effort, must occur in the wider context of a therapeutic relationship. In presenting focusing I would not like to give rise to its being practised exclusively, but only in the context of one's preferred broader frame of therapy.

If there was to be teaching in connection with therapy, it would take place outside the therapy hour, since otherwise it would interfere with the flow of therapy. On the other hand, Gendlin saw that there could be value in teaching focusing as a self-help procedure. This was in the early 1970s, during the later stages of the Vietnam war, and with his wife Mary Hendricks, Gendlin wanted to make some contribution to alleviating people's suffering beyond the boundaries of psychotherapy. Together they produced the *Focusing* book, published in 1978 – the book for which Gendlin is best known. It has sold more than half a million copies and was undoubtedly of great help to many people. Mary (Hendricks, 2002) wrote that they received many notes of thanks from grateful readers, sometimes scribbled in pencil on scraps of paper.

The other side of the success of the book was that it resulted in focusing coming to be seen primarily as a taught procedure, and inevitably many person-centred therapists were wary of it. The resulting separation of FOT from classical person-centred therapy has to some extent continued until the present. I remember Gendlin saying once – not entirely seriously, I think – 'I wish I had never written that book!'

The 'six steps' and 'the bodily felt sense'

Gendlin's 1978 book sets out focusing instructions in a way that can be used by anyone, together with many suggestions on how to deal with difficulties that can arise in working with oneself in this way. As Gendlin describes it in this book, the focusing procedure involves six steps. The following is an abbreviated summary of Gendlin's words in which I have bracketed his references to 'the body', which I will discuss shortly.

1. Clear a space: How are you? What's between you and feeling fine? Don't answer; let what comes [in your body] do the answering. Greet each concern that comes.

2. Felt sense: Pick one problem to focus on. What do you sense [in your body] when you recall the whole of that problem? Sense all of that, the sense of the whole thing, the murky discomfort or the unclear [body-]sense of it.
3. Get a handle: What word, phrase or image comes out of the felt sense?
4. Resonate: Go back and forth between word (or image) and the felt sense. Is that right? When you get a perfect match, the words or images being just right for this feeling, let yourself feel that for a minute.
5. Ask: 'What is it about the whole problem, that makes me so ----?'
6. Receive: Welcome what came. Protect it from critical voices that interrupt. (pp.173–174)

The present chapter is not concerned with self-therapy, but if we are to understand why classical person-centred therapists have often been wary of focusing, we need to be clear about two things in connection with Gendlin's 1978 book. The first is that it does not describe a technique that therapists can use to work with clients. Rather, it is an instruction manual for working with oneself. Of course, the book *can* be used, and often is used by focusing teachers, to teach focusing outside any therapy context, and the person who is taught may well benefit therapeutically from the teaching. Gendlin does sometimes discuss this possibility (e.g. Gendlin 1969), but he emphasises that there is much more to therapy than focusing – especially the relationship between client and therapist. He makes clear his view that teaching focusing in therapy sessions would inevitably upset the dynamics of person-centred therapy.

The other thing that can cause confusion when reading Gendlin's 1978 book is connected with the issue I discussed earlier about how exactly we are to understand the phrase 'felt sense'. The book quite strongly emphasises the idea that a felt sense is a special kind of bodily sensation, usually to be found in the central part of the body. Gendlin notes that people vary a great deal in how aware they are of their bodily sensations, and suggests, in the context of self-help, that people who have little body awareness should practise noticing what sensations they have in particular parts of the body. This has been taken up by some focusing teachers as a standard preliminary when teaching focusing. It is similar to the 'body scan' that is taught in mindfulness training. You first give attention to your feet, noticing any sensations you feel there and moving them if necessary to bring attention to them. Then you bring your attention to the legs, arms, back, shoulders and so on, finally coming to rest in the central part of the body 'where we feel our emotions'. You can then begin focusing by saying to yourself something like, 'How am I feeling – in there – today? Am I okay? What stops me from being completely fine?'

This can work for some people, but it can also lead to problems. I have found that, when focusing is taught in this way, students often become very aware of their bodily sensations, but at the same time they may lose touch with the difficulties in their *lives*. In any case, this kind of practice doesn't fit well into the person-centred approach to *therapy.*

Over the years, a number of other focusing practitioners have expressed some unease with Gendlin's emphasis on the bodily nature of a felt sense. For example, the well-known focusing teacher Ann Weiser Cornell observed that many students find it hard to be sure whether what they feel is a felt sense or not. She wrote (Cornell, 1996): 'The biggest barrier to successfully finding a felt sense is wondering if you are doing it right – if you "really" have one' (p.29). And I remember, when I was first learning focusing, Ann's colleague Barbara McGavin saying that students often spent so much time locating felt senses in their body that there was no time for any focusing! And again, as we saw in the extract at the start of this chapter, Gendlin himself initially 'tried to find such a feeling within myself, but I could not'.

I have found when reading Gendlin that what he says nearly always still makes sense when we leave out the references to 'the body'. In the case of the 'six steps' above, for example, leaving out the words that I put in brackets doesn't ruin the meaning of what he is saying. It's the same in the following passage (Gendlin 1978/2003):

> Suppose you have been listening to a discussion and are about to say something relevant and important… Now suppose that, as you wait for your chance to speak, your attention is distracted for a moment and you lose hold of what you were about to say. The others are now giving you your turn, waiting for you to say what you wanted to say, but you cannot… What do you do to regain the sense of what you were going to say? [Where do you look for it? You look within the body… you grope within yourself. There you do have a felt sense… you have that feeling of what you forgot.] You might try simply becoming quiet, receptive, hoping that 'it' will open and what it was will come flooding back by itself. Or you can ask yourself questions: 'Was it something about…?' Or you can try to trace logical connections: 'They were talking about such-and-such, so it must have had to do with…' Or you can try to create the lost meaning by surrounding it with events like a lost piece of jigsaw puzzle: 'It came to me right after Carol said… and then, before I opened my mouth, Lou said…' Any of these processes might help lead you to 'it' but 'it' must respond. When it does, when it opens and what you wanted to say comes back…at that moment, when you again 'know' what you wanted to put across to these people, you still don't have it in words. (p.86)

I find that, if I read this through, omitting the section in brackets, it seems a perfectly adequate account of what many people would do. The section in brackets *assumes* that people also 'grope within themselves', and while some people might want to say this, others would not. As I'll suggest shortly, people vary a great deal here.

Rob van Woerden (1990) relates that, in a question to Gendlin at the Leuven person-centred conference in 1988, he said:

> You emphasised the 'body-sense'. However, I experience many times with myself and my clients that there is no body-sense at all, even when I or they have this 'it' and can point to it. If this is the case, I think emphasising the bodily aspect might be more confusing than helpful. (p.223)

To which Gendlin responded:

> I do not want to close down any other channels… I am sure that there is an entrance through the literal body… There might be other entrances.

Indeed, it is not hard to see what these 'other entrances' might be. When a person is giving attention to their difficulty as a whole, they may well become aware of bodily sensations such as a tightness in the chest, a sinking feeling in the stomach and so on. They then gently ask themselves something like, 'What's *this* about?' and often a new facet of their difficulty will emerge. Then they go back to the sensations in their body and check, 'Is that it…?' And so the focusing process continues. For such a person, focusing is very much a matter of working with bodily sensations, or 'working with the body'. But for other people, what usually comes to them when they focus are images. The image of a fallen tree comes to them, and they ask, 'What's *that* about?' and this brings to mind a possible aspect of their difficulty that they had not previously been aware of. And they also check what has come to mind – is that really it? – and further imagery comes. For them, focusing is largely about imagery, or 'working with the imagination'. For yet others, it is mainly emotions that come, or words and phrases. For musical people, it might be snatches of tunes. The important thing is not the 'mode' in which people focus but the *resonating,* as Gendlin calls it, between 'all that' and the particular sensations, images, words and so forth that come. And as Gendlin emphasises, it is important not simply to stay with the sensations, images and so forth, as if watching a movie. There needs to be a zigzag back and forth between them and how the situation feels now that they have come.

Unlike Gendlin, I would like to add that 'how the situation feels now' is not to have another (special sort of) sensation. Rather, it is to say that the situation now strikes me rather differently; that now I want to say, 'Oh, it's more like *this*!' Some of the issues involved here derive, I believe, from different background assumptions about how language works. This is not the place to go into them, but if we think of language as separate from the world, then we will be inclined to say that the meaning of a word is the corresponding thing in the world. 'Cat' means *those* things – cats; 'felt sense' means *those* things – felt senses. But if we think of language as part of the world, as much a part of our *behaviour* as running and jumping, then we will think of the meaning of a word as how we use it in certain contexts. We use 'cat' to pick out and distinguish certain kinds of animal. And we use 'felt sense' like 'hunch' or 'intimation', to express the fact that we can't yet find the words to say what we feel or why we feel it. These issues reflect ongoing debates in philosophy, especially between what are called 'ordinary language philosophy' and 'phenomenology'. A little more discussion of these issues can be found in Purton (2014a, 2014b, 2021), Luczaj (2021) and Puc (2022).

Difficulties in focusing

A common problem is that the client can be distracted from focusing on one problem by the pressure of other problems. For example, the client may have not just this particular anxiety in their life, but many anxieties. Here the therapist might suggest that the client gives a little attention to each problem – enough to register that it is there – and then invites the client to consider which problem they would like to work with in the present session. Gendlin refers to this procedure as 'making an inventory'. Just as, when we feel overwhelmed by the number of things we have to do, it can help to make a list, so it can help just to list our problems. We can't possibly work with them all at once.

Another difficulty is that, as soon as some new way of responding begins to emerge, a client's 'inner critic' may intervene and disparage the new way. For example, a client might have just begun to feel that they have some right to object to how they are being treated. They are for the first time inclined to respond in a new way, and they articulate their response as, 'I'm not having this!' But immediately a 'critical voice' says, 'You can't say that to him! You *can't!*' and the new response is smothered. Here, the focusing-oriented therapist might draw the client's attention to their inclination to smother the new response. Perhaps that inclination can also be given more articulation. What is that 'part' of the client so afraid of?

Gendlin (1996, Ch.9) and other focusing-oriented writers (e.g. Purton, 2004), have written about a number of such difficulties and possible ways of dealing with them. The focusing-oriented therapist, partly through their own experience of focusing, gradually becomes familiar with such difficulties and becomes more experienced in how to work with them. Of course, no two clients are alike, so that what works with one may not work with another, but that is always so in therapy.

Focusing and person-centred therapy

In what follows I will be understanding 'client-centred therapy' to mean roughly the kind of therapy referred to as 'classical person-centred therapy' in Chapter 2 of this volume. Rather more specifically, I will use the phrase to indicate the way of working that Barrett-Lennard (1998) called 'non-directive reflective therapy', which was characteristic of Rogers' method of therapy in the 1950s, when he and Gendlin were working closely together. What is now called 'person-centred therapy' developed rather later, together with still later developments such as emotion-focused therapy and the wider network of other 'tribes' that form the other chapters of this book.

In trying to understand the place of FOT within the 'person-centred nation', it is important to see that it is rooted more in Rogers' early (though continuing) work than in these subsequent 'person-centred' developments. As mentioned earlier, FOT retains Rogers' emphasis on the importance of 'receiving' the client, and also his emphasis on 'reflection'. These are not things that Rogers abandoned; he continued with them until the end of his life, and they have remained crucial elements in person-centred training ever since.

In person-centred therapy, and in focusing, the person is trying to find better ways of articulating what exactly their difficulty involves. Although focusing can be used in contexts other than therapy, it was discovered in the context of person-centred therapy and is not something distinct from person-centred therapy. Focusing is that element of effective person-centred therapy where, within the safe environment created by the core conditions, the client struggles to find a way of articulating their responses.

FOT and the procedures of the other schools

Gendlin (1996, Ch.11) suggests that it may be helpful to distinguish between the different *schools* of therapy and the different *procedures* that are used by therapists. Among the procedures are, for example:

- listening to the client
- reflecting what the client says
- empathising with the client
- therapist self-disclosure
- encouraging the client to free-associate
- interpreting what the client says in terms of past experiences
- reflecting on dreams
- intensifying what the client says
- reframing what the client says
- encouraging the client to role-play their situation
- encouraging the client to collect evidence for their beliefs
- encouraging the client to 'stay with' the way they respond to a situation.

Some of these practices are associated more with one school of therapy than with the others, but there is also considerable overlap. Listening is, of course, fairly universal; reflection is employed not only in person-centred therapy but also in some forms of psychodynamic therapy (such as Kohut and Winnicott). Therapist self-disclosure is found in several strands of person-centred therapy that emphasise the importance of 'congruence'. Reflection on dreams is used in both Jungian and Freudian therapy, but also in the person-centred tradition. Role-play is used in both Gestalt therapy and in emotion-focused therapy (see Chapter 5, this volume). Modern CBT strongly emphasises the importance of empathy (see, for example, Watson et al., 2014).

Sometimes the procedures are not exactly the same but have some similarity. Tentative interpretation is not quite the same as 'empathising in depth', but it is not utterly different either. A Gestalt therapist encouraging a client to role-play a 'part' of themself is not doing quite what a person-centred therapist does when encouraging a client to 'stay with how they are responding to this', but there is surely *some* likeness. When the CBT therapist suggests reframing a situation ('You could think of it not as rudeness but as honesty'), that is a more cognitive and 'directive' approach than when the psychodynamic or focusing-oriented therapist encourages a client to allow new spontaneous feelings to arise ('What else do you feel as you stay with her "rudeness"?'). But the distinction between thoughts and feelings is often not as sharp as it looks ('I don't think much of what he did' means much the same as 'I don't feel very good about what he did'), and whether a therapist's remark counts as 'directive' depends a lot on whether the client is directed by the remark (Mearns & Thorne, 2000). In short, the differences are often not as significant as they initially seem.

Gendlin (1996) suggests that the different schools of therapy form institutional unities, each with their own preferred philosophies, psychological theories, primary texts, training courses, certification procedures and so on, but that the broad procedural categories, which he terms 'avenues of therapy', cut across the institutional boundaries.

Each of the procedures that form part of an avenue of therapy can be incorporated into the focusing-oriented approach. There is no objection in principle to a therapist using any procedure so long as it is presented and employed in a way that is sensitive to the client's response. For example, if a client is caught between two opposing impulses and feels 'stuck', an FOT therapist might suggest the use of a two-chair procedure in order to help the client experience more fully the opposed tendencies. If the client is a drama student, this approach might strongly appeal to them and they might find it very effective. However, another client might find the suggestion alarming or irrelevant. Further, if this approach were used, it would not be in the spirit of 'a helpful technique that will sort out the client's difficulty'. It would be used more as a stimulus to help the client find a fresh way to respond to their situation. The hope would be that it could allow the client to express things that they have not so far been able to express. After employing any sort of procedure, the FOT therapist will want to check with the client how the client now feels and if their responses to their situation are different in any way. Has what was done helped them to move on a little, to become a little more 'themself'? At this point, there may be a return to something like focusing: how exactly are things different now? What has shifted? Is something more still needed? The therapist will not want to move quickly on to the use of another procedure, but is more likely now to listen, reflect and check that the use of the procedure has not disrupted their relationship with the client.

After a while, but perhaps not in the same session, the client may again reach a point where they feel stuck. Perhaps the client now feels that they have gone as far as they can in articulating their responses, and that they now need to go out into the world and try out a new way of responding to people. The therapist will support them in that, and then, when the client has tried out their new move in the outside world, the therapist will check with them whether there has been a change in how they are dealing with things. What sort of difference has this made? What do you sense to be at the root of this change? Where does this leave you now? Does it feel that there could be a next step? What might that be? Whatever procedures are used, focusing-oriented therapy remains person-centred, returning again and again to how the client is responding, while allowing the therapist to offer procedures that may be stimulating or supportive for the client.

FOT is then, in a sense, an 'integrative' therapy (see Chapter 9, this volume), but it does not attempt the impossible task of integrating the different schools of therapy, with their diverse philosophies and theories. It is open to bringing in procedures from any school, but the therapist brings them in in a way that respects the individuality of the client and repeatedly checks how the client is responding to the intervention in question. In this way it echoes what Rogers said many years ago: 'If a therapist has the attitudes we have come to regard as essential, probably he or she can use a variety of techniques' (Warner 2000, p.28). Or as Gendlin (1990) put it: 'The client-centred reflecting method is the central thing *with which* to use everything else' (p.207; emphasis in original).

Research

There is not a great deal of research devoted to FOT as such. This is largely because the number of therapists who identify as 'focusing-oriented' is very small compared with the numbers of person-centred, cognitive-behavioural and psychodynamic therapists. The principles of FOT tend be taught mainly as modules within person-centred training courses, and trainees completing such courses seldom set up explicitly as FOT therapists.

Elliott and colleagues' (2021) review of research on humanistic-experiential psychotherapies in the seventh edition of *Garfield & Bergin's Handbook of Psychotherapy & Behavior Change* includes focusing-oriented therapy in the list of humanistic-experiential therapies, but does not actually discuss any work on FOT. Their list of references includes just one study on FOT dreamwork (Ellis, 2016).

Hendricks (2002), in the first edition of the *Humanistic Psychotherapies* handbook, discussed a number of studies involving the Experiencing Scale (EXP) developed by Rogers and Gendlin, and Krycka and Ikemi (2016) in the second edition discuss more recent studies of this kind, together with studies involving more recent scales developed by FOT practitioners in Japan. However, Watson and Bedard (2006) and Parker (2014) raise doubts about whether the Experiencing Scale is as relevant to the study of FOT as it has usually been taken to be. Their point is that it is only at higher experiencing levels that anything like focusing can be said to be occurring, yet many of the studies are concerned with lower levels. Krycka & Ikemi (2016) also draw attention to studies that investigate some of the 'microprocesses' in FOT, such as 'clearing a space'.

In his main work on focusing-oriented psychotherapy, Gendlin (1996, p.301) stated explicitly: 'Focusing-oriented therapy is Client-Centered Therapy'. (He was, of course, referring to what we in the UK and in this present book are calling classical person-centred therapy (Chapter 2, this volume).) Today, this classical person-centred therapy has been largely incorporated into person-centred therapy and hardly exists as a separate tradition whose effectiveness could be investigated. Yet this doesn't mean that FOT and classical person-centred therapy have disappeared off the research radar. Much of the outcome research supports the effectiveness of therapies that incorporate the classical person-centred principles of active listening and reflecting and Rogers' 'receiving' of the client, and this research clearly has a bearing on FOT. There are many therapy orientations today that do not see themselves as 'focusing-oriented' yet in practice place considerable emphasis on listening, empathising and checking with the client how they are responding to the interventions the therapist is using. To a large extent, the principles of classical person-centred therapy have become part of what many counsellors would take to be central to what counselling is. The research evidence (Wampold & Imel, 2015; Cooper, 2008) seems to confirm that it is these principles that are indeed central to effective therapy, rather than specialised techniques or interventions grounded in the details of psychological theories.

I am inclined to think that there is by now sufficient evidence available to support the effectiveness of the basic principles of FOT. What would be useful in future would be: 1) studies of whether any particular mode of therapy is more effective when carried out in an FOT way, and 2) more studies of the use of FOT in specific contexts. For example, Claudia

Clark (1990) investigated what takes place when clients engage in focusing in the course of experiential therapy. Among her findings are the suggestions that focusing may be of value to unassertive clients where their inability to assert themselves comes from their difficulties in knowing what their feelings really are, and that focusing is interrupted not so much by strong emotion but by the intrusion of 'inner critics'. In more recent work, Ellis (2016) studied qualitative changes in recurrent PTSD nightmares after focusing-oriented dreamwork. And a number of studies have been made of the effectiveness of focusing in stress relief and pain control (Krycka & Ikemi, 2016).

One final line of research that may be relevant to the effectiveness of FOT is that concerning relapse rates after therapy. It is clearly important to know whether, after completing therapy, clients maintain the improvements they have made. Some randomised control studies have suggested that this is so for CBT, but less so for person-centred therapies. One explanation for this could be that CBT provides clients with techniques that they can use after therapy finishes: they can continue with *self*-therapy. However, in person-centred therapy there is little that corresponds to this aspect of CBT. Michael Barkham (Barkham et al., 2021) recently led a randomised control trial of the effectiveness of CBT for depression in comparison with person-centred experiential therapy (PCEP). This study found, as by now one would expect, that the two forms of therapy were equally effective. However, the relapse rate was higher in PCEP. It seems that the CBT clients learned something in therapy about how to continue to manage their difficulties, whereas in the PCEP group, as Barkham puts it, 'Clients leave feeling better for having told their story, but when the depression comes back, they don't have the means to process and move forward again on their own – all they can think of is going back to therapy again' (quoted in Jackson, 2021, p.22). If confirmed by subsequent studies, these findings are very relevant for focusing-oriented therapy. What they suggest is that therapy needs to include or encourage some element of self-therapy (Purton, 2022) – something the client can learn to do on their own after therapy ends. And from a person-centred perspective, what clients can learn to do is to focus.

Resources for learning

Organisations and websites

- British Focusing Association – www.focusing.org.uk
- Campbell Purton's website – www.dwelling.me.uk
- European Focusing Association – www.efa-focusing.eu
- Focusing Resources (Ann Weiser Cornell's website) – www.focusingresources.com
- The Gendlin Online Library (includes most of Gendlin's publications) – www.focusing.org/gendlin
- International Association of Focusing-Oriented Psychotherapy – www.focusingtherapy.org
- International Focusing Institute – www.focusing.org.
- London Focusing – www.londonfocusing.com
- World Association for Person-Centered and Experiential Psychotherapy and Counseling (WAPCEPC) – www.pce-world.org

Further reading

Focusing-oriented therapy

These two papers provide a good introduction to FOT:

- Gendlin, E.T. (1984). The client's client: The edge of awareness. In R. Levant & J.M. Shlien (Eds.) *Client-centered therapy and the person-centered approach* (pp.76–107). Praeger.
- Gendlin, E.T. (1990). The small steps of the therapy process: How they come and how to help them come. In G. Lietaer, J. Rombauts & R. Van Balen (Eds.), *Client-centered and experiential psychotherapy in the nineties* (pp.205–224). Leuven University Press.

This is Gendlin's major work on FOT:

- Gendlin, E.T. (1996). *Focusing-oriented psychotherapy.* Guilford Press.

A practical introduction to FOT for counsellors:

- Purton, C. (2021). *The focusing-oriented counselling primer* (2nd ed.). PCCS Books.

Focusing as a self-help procedure

Gendlin's original self-help book:

- Gendlin, E.T. (1978/2003). *Focusing.* Rider.

A new approach, 44 years on:

- Purton, C. (2022). *Self-therapy: A focusing-oriented guide.* Eurasia Publications.

Focusing theory

Gendlin's major early contribution to FOT theory:

- Gendlin, E.T. (1964). A theory of personality change. In P. Worchel & D. Byrne (Eds.), *Personality change* (pp.100–148). John Wiley. www.focusing.org/gendlin/docs/gol_2145.html

This paper relates FOT to experiential psychotherapy generally:

- Gendlin, E.T. (1968). The experiential response. In E.F. Hammer (Ed.), *Use of interpretation in treatment: Technique and art* (pp.208–227). Grune & Stratton.

This paper looks at some philosophical aspects of FOT:

- Purton, C. (2014b). Wittgenstein and the expression of feelings in psychotherapy. *Philosophical Investigations, 37*(2), 89–98. Available at www.dwelling.me.uk

Felt sense and the body

These two papers are concerned with the notion of a 'felt sense', and the role the body plays in FOT:

- Purton, C. (2014). The myth of the bodily felt sense. In G. Madison (2014). *Theory and practice of focusing-oriented psychotherapy: Beyond the talking cure* (pp.221–233). Jessica Kingsley.
- Purton, C. (2021). The role of the body in focusing. In N. Kypriotakis & J. Moore (Eds.), *Senses of focusing* (Vol. 1), (pp.221–233). Eurasia Publications.

These are two further contributions to 'felt sense' debate:

- Schoeller, D. (2021). Felt sense – a beautiful yet misleading term: Trials, errors and opportunities. In N. Kypriotakis & J. Moore (Eds.), *Senses of Focusing* (Vol. 1) (pp.203–224.) Eurasia Publications.
- Puc, J. (2022). Felt body as myth and reality: On the bodily dimension of felt sense. *Journal of Humanistic Psychology*, https://doi.org/10.1177/00221678221074185

References

Barkham, M., Saxon, D., Hardy G.E., Bradburn, M., Galloway, D., Wickramasekera, N. et al. (2021). Person-centred experiential therapy versus cognitive behavioural therapy delivered in the English Improving Access to Psychological therapies service for the treatment of moderate or severe depression (PraCTICED): A pragmatic, randomised, non-inferiority trial. *The Lancet Psychiatry, 6*(8), 487–499. https://doi.org/10.1016/S2215-0366(21)00083-3

Barrett-Lennard, G.T. (1998). *Carl Rogers' helping system: Journey and substance.* Sage.

Clark, C.A. (1990). *A comprehensive process analysis of focusing events in experiential therapy.* Doctoral dissertation. University of Toledo.

Cooper, M. (2008). *Essential research findings in counselling and psychotherapy: The facts are friendly.* Sage.

Cornell, A.W. (1996). *The power of focusing.* New Harbinger.

Elliott, R., Watson, J., Timulak, L. & Sharbanee, J. (2021). Research on humanistic-experiential psychotherapies: Updated review. In M. Barkham, W. Lutz, & L, Castonguay (Eds.), *Garfield & Bergin's handbook of psychotherapy & behavior change* (7th ed.) (pp.421–467). Wiley.

Ellis, L.A. (2016). Qualitative changes in recurrent PTSD nightmares after focusing-oriented dreamwork. *Dreaming, 26*(3), 185. doi: 10.1037/drm0000031

Freud, S. (1936). *The problem of anxiety* (H.A. Bunker, Trans.). W.W. Norton & Co.

Gendlin, E. T. (1969). Focusing. *Psychotherapy: Theory, Research and Practice, 6*(1), 4–15. www.focusing.org/gendlin/docs/gol_2048.html

Gendlin, E.T. (1978/2003). *Focusing* (Revised and updated edition). Rider.

Gendlin, E.T. (1984). The client's client: The edge of awareness. In R. Levant & J.M. Schlien (Eds.), *Client-centered therapy and the person-centered approach* (pp.76–107). Praeger. www.focusing.org/gendlin/docs/gol_2149.html

Gendlin, E.T. (1990). The small steps of the therapy process: How they come and how to help them come. In G. Lietaer, J. Rombauts & R. Van Balen (Eds.), *Client-centered and experiential psychotherapy in the nineties* (pp.205–224). Leuven University Press. www.focusing.org/gendlin/docs/gol_2110.html

Gendlin, E.T. (1993). Three assertions about the body. *The Folio, 12*(1), 21–33. https://focusing.org/gendlin/docs/gol_2064.html

Gendlin, E. T. (1996). *Focusing-oriented psychotherapy.* Guilford Press.

Gendlin, E.T. (2000). When you feel the body from inside, there is a door. In J.K. Zeig (Ed.), *The evolution of psychotherapy: A meeting of the minds.* Milton H. Erickson Foundation Press (pp.255–271). https://focusing.org/gendlin/docs/gol_2232.html

Gendlin, E.T. (2002). Foreword. In C.R. Rogers & D.E. Russell, *Carl Rogers: The quiet revolutionary. An oral history* (pp. xi-xii). Penmarin Books. www.focusing.org/gendlin/docs/gol_2155.html

Gendlin, E.T. & Lietaer, G. (1983). On client-centered and experiential psychotherapy: An interview with Gene Gendlin. In W.-R. Minsel & W. Herff (Eds.), *Research on psychotherapeutic approaches: Proceedings of the 1st European conference on psychotherapy research, Trier, 1981, Vol. 2* (pp.77-104). Verlag Peter Lang.

Gendlin, E.T. & Zimring, F. (1955/1994). The qualities or dimensions of experiencing and their change. Discussion Papers *1*(3). University of Chicago Counseling Center. Reprinted in *Person-Centered Journal, 1*(2), 55–67 (1994). https://focusing.org/gendlin/docs/gol_2139.html

Hendricks, M. (2002). Focusing-oriented/experiential psychotherapy. In D.J. Cain and J. Seeman (Eds.), *Humanistic psychotherapies: Handbook of research and practice* (pp.221–251). American Psychological Association.

Jackson, C. (2021). The big issue: What works and why. *Therapy Today, 32*(7), 22–27.

Kirtner, W.L. & Cartwright, D.S. (1958a). Success and failure in client-centered therapy as a function of client personality variables. *Journal of Consulting Psychology, 22*, 259–264.

Kirtner, W.L. & Cartwright, D.S. (1958b). Success and failure in client-centered therapy as a function of initial in-therapy behavior. *Journal of Consulting Psychology, 22*, 329–333. www.focusing.org/gendlin/docs/gol_2100.html

Korbei, L. (1994). Eugen(e) Gend(e)lin. In O. Frischenschlager (Hg.), *Wien, wo sonst! Die Entstehung der Psychoanalyse und ihrer Schulen (pp.174–181). [Vienna where else! The origin of psychoanalysis and its schools]*. Böhlau. www.focusing.org/gendlin/docs/gol_2181.html

Krycka, K.C. & Ikemi, A. (2016). Focusing-oriented-experiential psychotherapy: From research to practice. In Cain, C., Keenan, K. & Rubin, S. (Eds.), *Humanistic psychotherapies: Handbook of research and practice* (2nd ed.) (pp.251–282). American Psychological Association.

Kypriotakis, N. & Moore, J. (Eds.). (2021). *Senses of focusing, vols. 1 & 2*. Eurasia Publications.

Lietaer, G., Rombauts, J. & Van Balen, R. (Eds.). (1990). *Client-centered and experiential psychotherapy in the nineties*. Leuven University Press.

Luczaj, S. (2021). Focusing is not a 'thing'. In N. Kypriotakis & J. Moore (Eds.), *Senses of focusing, vol. 1* (pp.139–153). Eurasia Publications.

Mearns, D. & Thorne, B. (2000). *Person-centred therapy today*. Sage.

Merry, T. (2000). *Person-centred practice: The BAPCA reader*. PCCS Books.

Moore, J. (2021a) 'What is focusing and where did it come from?' In N. Kypriotakis & J. Moore (Eds.), *Senses of Focusing , vol. 2* (pp.49–71). Eurasia Publications.

Moore, J. (2021b). Eugene Gendlin's contribution to client-centred therapy. In N. Kypriotakis & J. Moore (Eds.), *Senses of Focusing , vol. 2* (pp.489–510). Eurasia Publications.

Parker, R. (2014) Focusing-oriented therapy: The message from research. In Madison, G. (Ed.), *Theory and practice of focusing-oriented psychotherapy: Beyond the talking cure* (pp.259–272). Jessica Kingsley.

Puc, J. (2022). Felt body as myth and reality: On the bodily dimension of felt sense. *Journal of Humanistic Psychology OnlineFirst*. DOI:10.1177/00221678221074185

Purton, C. (2004). *Person-centred therapy: The focusing-oriented approach*. Palgrave Macmillan.

Purton, C. (2014a). The myth of the bodily felt sense. In G. Madison (Ed.), *Theory and practice of focusing-oriented psychotherapy: Beyond the talking cure* (pp.221–233). Jessica Kingsley.

Purton, C. (2014b). Wittgenstein and the expression of feelings in psychotherapy. *Philosophical Investigations, 37(2)*, 89–98. Available at www.dwelling.me.uk

Purton, C. (2021). The role of the body in focusing. In N. Kypriotakis & J. Moore (Eds.), *Senses of Focusing , vol. 1* (pp.185–201). Eurasia Publications.

Purton, C. (2022). *Self-therapy: A focusing-oriented guide*. Eurasia Publications.

Rogers, C.R. (1954). The case of Mrs Oak: A research analysis. In C.R. Rogers & R.F. Dymond (Eds.), *Psychotherapy and personality change*. University of Chicago Press.

Rogers, C.R. (1956). *The essence of psychotherapy: Moments of movement*. Paper given at the first meeting of the American Academy of Psychotherapists, New York, 20 October.

Rogers, C.R. (1957). The necessary and sufficient conditions of therapeutic personality change. *Journal of Consulting Psychology, 21*, 95–103. Reprinted in H. Kirschenbaum & V.L. Henderson (Eds.). (1990), *The Carl Rogers reader* (pp.219–235). Constable.

Rogers, C.R. (1958/1961). A process conception of psychotherapy. *American Psychologist, 18*, 114–159. Reprinted in C.R. Rogers (1961), *On becoming a person* (pp.125–162). Constable.

Rogers, C.R. (1961). *On becoming a person*. Houghton Mifflin.

Rogers, C.R. (1986/1990). Reflection of feelings. *Person-Centered Review, 1*(4), 375–377. Reprinted in H. Kirschenbaum & V.L. Henderson (Eds.) (1990), *The Carl Rogers reader* (pp.127–129). Constable.

Slack, S. (1985). Reflections on a workshop with Carl Rogers. *Journal of Humanistic Psychology, 25*(1) 35–42.

van Woerden, R. (1990). Gendlin: The small steps of the therapy process. Questions from the audience. In G. Lietaer, J. Rombauts & R. Van Balen (Eds.), *Client-centered and experiential psychotherapy in the nineties* (pp.205–224). Leuven University Press.

Wampold, B.E. & Imel, Z.E. (2015). *The great psychotherapy debate: The evidence for what makes psychotherapy work* (2nd ed.). Routledge.

Warner, M.S. (2000). Person-centered therapy: One nation, many tribes. *The Person-Centered Journal,* 7(1), 28–39.

Watson, J.C. & Bedard, D.L. (2006). Clients' emotional processing in psychotherapy: A comparison between cognitive-behavioral and process-experiential therapies. *Journal of Consulting and Clinical Psychology 74*(1), 152–159.

Watson, J.C., Steckley, P.L. & McMullen, E.J (2014). The role of empathy in promoting change. *Psychotherapy Research, 24*, 286–298. https://doi.org/10.1080/10503307.2013.802823

5. Emotion-focused therapy

Robert Elliott

Emotion-focused therapy (EFT), previously known as process-experiential therapy, integrates active therapeutic methods from Gestalt and other humanistic therapies within the frame of a person-centred relationship (Greenberg et al., 1993; Elliott et al., 2004). In essence, EFT benefits from the creative tension between the person-centred emphasis on creating a genuinely empathic and prizing therapeutic relationship (Rogers, 1961) and the active, task-focused, process-guiding style of Gestalt therapy (Perls, 1969) and focusing (Gendlin, 1996). In addition, EFT updates these experiential, process-guiding therapies by incorporating contemporary emotion theory and affective neuroscience, along with dialectical constructivism. In this chapter, I summarise the current status of EFT, including its theory, practice and outcome evidence, and starting with its history within the person-centred-experiential approach.

A brief history

The tribes of the person-centred-experiential (PCE) nation began to divide themselves in the late 1950s when Rogers and Gendlin started to look more closely at the client side of the famous 'process equation' (Rogers, 1961). This shift in attention from the therapist-facilitating conditions to an in-depth study of the client's process led to the Client Experiencing Scale (Klein et al., 1986), and eventually to the practice of focusing (Gendlin, 1981) (see Chapter 4, this volume). This phase of the development of the PCE approach came to be called 'experiential' (Lietaer, 1998), in contrast to the approach of those therapists who continued to put the primary emphasis on the therapist-relational conditions of accurate empathy, unconditional positive regard and genuineness.

Laura Rice had been a student of Rogers in the 1950s and, after Rogers left the University of Chicago (see Chapter 1, this volume), she stayed on at the Counseling Center, which she directed for a time. While there, she and David Wexler continued the focus on client process, emphasising client information processing and drawing on early cognitive science (Wexler & Rice, 1974). In the late 1960s and early 1970s, Rice broadened the investigation of client processes to include client stylistic variables such as expressiveness and vocal quality, and also began to look at the evocative function of the therapist through the use of metaphor and vocal expressiveness.

In the meantime, beginning around 1970 and in collaboration with her then student Leslie Greenberg, Rice adapted the method of task analysis from cognitive science knowledge elicitation methods used to study 'expert systems' (Newell & Simon, 1972). This was in order to understand how clients use therapy to solve their personal, cognitive-affective problems, foreshadowing later work by Rennie (1998) and Bohart and Tallman (1999) on the client as the active agent in therapy. Using recordings from the Chicago Counseling Center, Rice first studied how clients use a process of careful re-experiencing to resolve the task of making sense out of puzzling personal over-reactions (e.g. becoming inexplicably angry at one's children for fooling around at the breakfast table). This *evocative unfolding for problematic reaction points* became the first EFT task to be mapped (Rice & Saperia, 1984).

In parallel, as proof of concept for therapeutic task analysis, Greenberg went off to learn Gestalt therapy to see what client tasks could be identified and studied there. He fastened onto the task of resolving internal conflicts using the Gestalt therapy technique of two-chair work, in which the client enacts the two conflicting aspects of self – usually a critic ('top dog') and a part that is being criticised or pressured to do something ('underdog'). This he termed *two-chair work for conflict splits*. In the late 1970s and early 1980s, Rice and Greenberg carried out a series of studies on these two tasks, which they eventually wrote up in their chapters in their co-edited book, *Patterns of Change* (1984).

In 1985, I joined them to develop an experiential therapy for depression that integrated unfolding and two-chair work within a fundamentally person-centred relationship. To their experience with person-centred therapy and Gestalt therapies, I brought my background as a therapy micro-process researcher studying therapist response modes and client in-session experiences, along with my interest in Gendlin's (1981) focusing method (see Chapter 4, this volume). The first thing we did was to develop the set of six therapeutic principles that are the basis of EFT today. These provided the starting point for everything else (see Table 5.1 for their current wording). Then, as I applied the approach to a population of clinically depressed clients, we began to develop and integrate models of additional tasks: *empty chair work for unfinished business*, *two-chair enactment for self-interruption*, *experiential focusing for an unclear felt sense*, and *empathic affirmation for vulnerability*. We named it the process-experiential (PE) approach, to distinguish it from other versions of experiential therapy (e.g. Mahrer, 1983) and because the therapy was process-oriented (Greenberg et al., 1993).

In its early years, the PE approach was controversial and its place among the tribes of the PCE nation was questioned by some. For example, John Shlien (personal communication, July 1994) once told me that he thought it would be better for the person-centred approach 'to die a noble death' than to come under the influence of 'people like you'. Even more than

Table 5.1: Basic principles of emotion-focused therapy

A.	**Relationship principles**: Facilitate a safe, productive therapy relationship
1.	*Empathic attunement*: Enter, track clients' immediate and evolving experiencing.
2.	*Therapeutic bond*: Actively offer an accepting, empathic presence to clients.
3.	*Task collaboration*: Offer and facilitate mutual involvement in the goals and tasks of therapy.
B.	**Task principles**: Facilitate work on specific therapeutic tasks
4.	*Therapist responsiveness*: Attend in a careful, differentiated manner to important client processes.
5.	*Emotional transformation through deepening*: Help clients use key therapeutic tasks to move themselves from problematic to adaptive emotions through an emotional deepening process.
6.	*Personal agency and growth*: Help clients develop new emotional meaning and a sense of personal power and forward movement in their lives.

Adapted from Elliott & Greenberg (2021).

focusing, the process-experiential approach was the object of suspicion among classical non-directive therapists (see Chapter 2, this volume) such as Brodley (1990), who felt that proposing things like two-chair work for conflict splits violated the client's autonomy and the principle of unconditional positive regard. As process-experiential therapy proponents, we argued that the traditional person-centred facilitative conditions were necessary and might be sufficient, but were not 'efficient' – an argument that we thought was clever but did not go down particularly well with many of our critics at the time.

Since its somewhat shaky emergence in the PCE world, the PE approach has evolved over the years. First, it re-branded itself as *emotion-focused therapy* (EFT). The story behind this is that, in the mid-1980s, Les Greenberg and Sue Johnson (1988) had developed an approach to working with couples that integrated experiential and systemic therapy. They named this approach 'emotionally focused therapy for couples' in order to distinguish it from the behavioural marital therapy popular at the time. Process-experiential therapy had always had a major focus on emotion and made use of important emerging work on human emotions (Greenberg & Safran, 1987). So, over the course of the 1990s and early 2000s, it began to make sense to adopt the broader term 'emotion-focused therapy'. For one thing, by this time we had elaborated the therapy's underlying emotion theory to the point where it provided a rich guiding account of psychological function, dysfunction and change, culminating in the articulation of a set of principles of emotional change (Greenberg, 2004) and models of the emotional deepening process (Elliott & Greenberg, 2021; Elliott et al., 2004; Pascual-Leone & Greenberg, 2007). These emotion-change principles and unifying models ran across the different therapeutic tasks (e.g. systematic evocative unfolding for problematic reactions, two-chair work for conflict splits, empty chair work for unfinished business) and offered an elegant integration of the many tasks and sub-processes. In addition, it became clear that 'emotion-focused therapy' was a more comprehensible and broadly appealing term than 'process-experiential therapy.'

Of course, 'emotion-focused therapy' at the same time obscured our roots and situatedness within the PCE therapy tradition and did nothing to allay the fears of folk like John Shlien, who had been inclined to distrust our intentions from the beginning. However, we took these criticisms as challenges, and during this time we developed PE/EFT formulations of relational and interpersonal processes within the approach. Thus, we articulated our understandings of therapist empathy (Greenberg & Elliott, 1997; Watson, 2002), laid out empathic exploration and relationship dialogue for alliance difficulties as therapeutic tasks (Elliott et al., 2004), and more fully described the tension or dance in EFT between relational and task processes – that is, between 'being' and 'doing' (Greenberg, 2001).

Distinctive features of emotion-focused therapy

What are the distinguishing features of emotion-focused therapy as it has developed today? A useful place to start an explication of EFT is by laying out six of its defining characteristics (Elliott et al., 2004).

EFT is a neo-humanistic therapy

It is a based on a set of key values, deriving from the tradition of humanistic psychology but reinterpreted in light of contemporary emotion theory, attachment theory and dialectical constructivism. These values include (Elliott et al., 2004):

- *emotional experiencing* – Immediate experiencing of our emotions is the basis of human perception, bodily sensation, thought, and action.
- *agency/self-determination* – Human beings are fundamentally free to choose what to do and how to construct their worlds.
- *wholeness* – People are greater than the sum of their parts and cannot be understood by attending only to single aspects.
- *pluralism/equality* – Differences within and between people should be recognised, tolerated and even prized.
- *presence/authenticity* – People function best and are best helped through authentic, person-to-person relationships.
- *growth* – People have a natural tendency toward psychological growth and development that continues throughout the life span.

EFT is based on an evolving emotion theory

As noted earlier, the major contemporary foundation of EFT is an evolving *emotion theory* (Greenberg & Safran, 1987; Greenberg & Paivio, 1997; Goldman & Greenberg, 2014). This holds that emotion is fundamentally adaptive in nature, helping the person to process complex situational information rapidly and automatically in order to produce action appropriate for meeting important organismic needs (e.g. self-protection, support). Specifically, EFT makes use of four fundamental dimensions of emotion in its theory of function and dysfunction (Elliott & Greenberg, 2021): emotion categories; aspects of emotions (emotion schemes, such as, for example, bodily experience); emotion regulation, and emotion response sequences. These will be described in more detail later in the theory section of this chapter.

EFT is person-centred but process-guiding

Essential to its practice, EFT is based on a *person-centred but process-guiding relational stance*. Therapists *follow* the track of their clients' internal experience as it evolves from moment to moment, trying to remain very empathically attuned to clients' immediate inner experiences and to communicate this. Fundamentally, EFT therapists try to follow clients' experience because they recognise that clients are human, just as therapists are – the client is another existing human being, an authentic source of experience, an active agent trying to make meaning, accomplish goals and connect with others. EFT therapists prize their clients' initiative and attempt to help them make sense of their situation or resolve problems.

At the same time, however, EFT therapists also offer active guidance on the therapeutic *process*. This does not mean lecturing clients, giving advice or controlling or manipulating them. It also does not mean doing clients' work for them, or trying to fix clients' problems, enlighten them or get them to do what we think would be good for them. EFT therapists are experiential guides who know something about the shape and feel of various experiences and also about emotional processes. EFT is often referred to as 'process directive', but 'process guiding' is actually a better phrase to describe what happens. Therapist responses continually 'offer' the client opportunities to work with experience – what Sachse (1992), referred to as 'processing proposals'.

To say that EFT therapists follow and guide at the same time sounds like a contradiction, but EFT therapists see it instead as a *dialectic* or creative tension between two vitally important aspects of therapy. Following without guiding can result in therapy getting stuck and going in circles, with clients getting lost in the same ways that they usually do. Guiding without following is ineffective and counter-productive, undermining attempts to help clients develop as empowered, self-organising persons. Thus, in EFT, therapists try to integrate following and guiding, so that the distinction disappears, analogous to a dance in which each partner responds to the other by alternately following and leading. Instead, the ideal is an easy sense of co-exploration.

EFT uses an empathic exploration response style

Most concretely, EFT is marked by a distinctive *therapist empathic exploration response style*, generally apparent simply from listening to a few minutes of the therapy. Typically, this style makes use of *exploratory reflections*, as in this short example:

> Client: I just want enough of who I used to be, so that I could live like a human being.
>
> Therapist: It's almost like, 'I don't feel like a human being right now. I feel like some kind of something else, that's not human.' Is that what it feels like?

Exploratory questions are also important, such as, 'What is it like inside right now?'; 'What are you experiencing as you say that?'; or even 'Where is the [sadness, anxiety] in your body?' Empathic exploration responses are active, engaged and often evocative or expressive, but at the same time typically tentative and sometimes even deliberately inarticulate, as they try to model and promote client self-exploration of immediate felt experiencing.

EFT is marker-guided

EFT is characterised by clear descriptions of in-session therapeutic *markers* and *tasks*. Markers are in-session behaviours that signal that a client is ready to work on a particular problem at that moment. An example is a *self-critical split* marker, in which one part of the person (a *critic*) is criticising another part (an *experiencer*). Tasks involve immediate within-session goals, such as resolving the conflict inherent in a self-critical split. EFT also describes particular therapeutic methods for helping clients resolve tasks. For example, if the therapeutic alliance is developed enough, the therapist might suggest that the client take turns speaking as the critic and the experiencer, moving back and forth between two chairs (*two-chair dialogue*). In general, EFT therapists listen for their clients to present task markers, then offer interventions to match the tasks that emerge. Using the 'following' and 'guiding' language, EFT therapists first *follow* the tasks presented by clients in the form of markers, then *guide* clients by offering them opportunities to work on these tasks in potentially productive ways.

EFT is an empirically supported psychotherapy

EFT is based on a 50-year-old programme of psychotherapy process and outcome research (see reviews by Elliott et al., 2013, 2021). As noted earlier, Rice and Greenberg (1984) first adapted the method of task analysis from research on cognitive problem-solving and used it to develop and test micro-process models of the steps clients typically go through to resolve key therapeutic tasks such as internal conflicts or puzzling personal reactions. For the past 30 years, the focus of much of this research has been on outcome research, complemented by process-outcome prediction studies, qualitative research and case studies (see Elliott et al., 2013, 2021).

Emotion-focused therapy theory

I turn now to the theory of EFT, which updates the theory of humanistic-experiential psychotherapy in the light of contemporary 'emotion theory' and 'dialectical constructivism'.

Emotion theory

Contemporary *emotion theory* (e.g. Elliott et al., 2004; Greenberg, 2015; Greenberg & Pascual-Leone, 2006; Greenberg & Watson, 2005) holds that emotion is fundamentally adaptive in nature. Emotion helps the organism to process rich incoming situational information in a rapid, automatic manner, in order to produce action appropriate for meeting important needs of the organism (e.g. self-protection, connection, exploration). As noted earlier, EFT uses a four-dimensional model of emotions (Elliott & Greenberg, 2021): emotion categories; aspects of emotion schemes; emotion intensity/regulation, and emotional productivity/adaptiveness.

First, *emotion categories* are simply the different kinds of emotion that provide us with useful information and prepare us to take useful action. Many of these emotions are unpleasant (specifically, anger, fear/anxiety, sadness, shame, guilt, disgust, emotion pain) and are particularly valuable for identifying and dealing with things that are not going right for us. Other emotions are pleasant, in the sense that they feel good or energising (interest/curiosity, happiness/joy, compassion). (Note that, in EFT, we do not find it useful to refer to *any* emotions as 'negative' or 'positive'.)

Second, *emotion schemes* provide an implicit, constantly evolving, higher-order organisation for experience but are not available to awareness until activated or reflected upon (Greenberg et al., 1993). They are idiosyncratic and highly variable, both across people and within the same person over time, requiring individualised and flexible assessment via therapist empathic attunement and client self-exploration. Although emotion schemes serve as the basis of self-organisation, they are not static entities; instead, they are continually synthesised in the person's moment-to-moment experience. Emotion schemes consist of component *aspects* linked together in a network, with the activation of single aspects spreading to other aspects. What are these emotion scheme aspects? It is useful clinically to distinguish five types of schematic component (Elliott et al., 2004):

1. The *implicit or experienced emotion* organises all of the other elements around a particular emotion and its felt quality (e.g. intense fear of being severely physically harmed). The person may be fully aware of their experienced emotion or only partially or implicitly aware of it.
2. *Situational/perceptual* elements represent the person's current or past external environments and include immediate awareness of the current situation (perceptions) and episodic memories of past situations and events. For example, a client's perception of her mother's darkened living room might remind her of a previous trauma, activating fears of being attacked again.
3. *Bodily/expressive* elements represent the emotion through the body, including both immediate sensations within the body (e.g. a round, knotted feeling in the gut, accompanied by feelings like electrical impulses in arms and legs) and bodily expression of the emotion (e.g. a fearful facial expression, nervous laughter).
4. *Symbolic/conceptual* elements are verbal or visual representations of the emotion, produced through reflective self-awareness of the other elements. Symbolic representations can be verbal ('I could be attacked again at any moment') or visual (an image of self as weak and fragile like a small, helpless animal). They can be descriptive labels or metaphors for the emotion ('The fear is like a thing'), the situation ('It's a trap'), or one's body ('shaking like a leaf').

5. *Motivational/behavioural* elements are activated by the emotion scheme and represent it in the form of associated desires, needs, wishes, intentions or actions (e.g. the wish to be safe from attack, or attempts to ignore the fear).

As Leijssen (1996) has shown, the therapeutic implication of this framework is that optimal emotional processing involves all of these schematic elements. Particular difficulties occur when the person neglects one or more types of these elements. In addition, difficulties in emotion processing can also occur when emotion schemes are activated in the wrong situations. In EFT, the therapist helps clients reflect on, understand and re-evaluate their emotion schemes through careful empathic listening and evocative or expressive work.

Third, EFT therapists attend to the client's *emotional regulation* – that is, the level of intensity of the client's emotions and whether these emotions are over-regulated (leaving the person restricted, numb or even dissociated), under-regulated (flooded or out of control), or appropriately regulated (so that they can be usefully worked with) (Greenberg, 2015). People's emotion regulation capacities include both being able to soothe their own anxiety and emotion pain and adjust the general level of emotional arousal in order to function adaptively. Effective emotion regulation requires the ability both to access and heighten emotion and also to contain or moderate it, depending on the task at hand, whether that is trying to get oneself going in the morning or psych oneself up for a presentation, or calm one's nerves before a test or unwind after a stressful day.

Fourth, emotion responses vary in their *usefulness for helping the person* deal with situations and also in their emotional depth. Four main types of emotion response have generally been recognised in the EFT literature: primary adaptive, primary maladaptive, secondary reaction and instrumental. However, over time, these have been differentiated and added to, creating the integrated emotional deepening model that is central to contemporary EFT practice. Most of these are part of the *main deepening sequence* in EFT (Elliott & Greenberg, 2021), presented below:

a. *Instrumental emotion responses* although technically outside the main deepening sequence, have to be dealt with before anything else in therapy. They are strategic displays of an emotion for their intended effect on others, such as getting others to pay attention to us, go along with something we want them to do for us, approve of us or, perhaps most often, just not disapprove of us. Common examples include 'crocodile tears' (instrumental sadness), 'crying wolf' (instrumental fear), and bullying (instrumental anger). EFT therapists try to be aware of any negative reactions they might have to such 'fake' emotions. Instead, they try to access empathy for the interpersonal intentions behind the instrumental emotion (e.g. to convince the therapist that the client needs attention).

b. *Interrupted/over-regulated emotions* are a common starting point for many clients entering psychotherapy (especially with depression or post-trauma) with a tendency to cut themselves off from or to restrict their emotions. EFT therapists help clients in these states by communicating in an empathically evocative manner and by exploring or enacting their self-restriction or self-interruption processes.

c. *Global distress* is also encountered in the earlier stages of therapy and is experienced as feeling 'bad', 'upset', 'stressed' and so forth. In EFT undifferentiated emotions are seen as a type of *secondary reactive emotion* and serve as a way of pushing away more specific painful emotions. EFT therapists help clients to specify or differentiate these emotions.

d. *Presenting symptomatic emotions* are another form of secondary reactive emotion and include in particular depressive and anxiety symptoms, but also reactive anger and unwanted nervous laughter. Here, the person reacts to their initial, direct response to a situation, replacing it with a secondary emotion. Note that *secondary* simply means 'second' – a different emotion occurred first. For example, a client who encounters danger and begins to feel fear may become angry with herself for being afraid or may become angry at the danger, even when angry behaviour increases the danger. EFT therapists help clients explore these emotions but don't dwell on them, listening instead for the emotions that came before or are underneath them.

e. *Primary maladaptive* emotion responses are initial, direct (that is, *first*) reactions to situations. However, they involve overlearned responses based on previous, often traumatic experiences. Here, 'maladaptive' simply means the response is no longer useful because it does not fit the current situation and instead feels stuck, like 'this is the story of my life'. For example, a client with 'fragile processes' may have learned when she was growing up that an offer of caring was usually followed by physical or sexual abuse. As a result, the therapist's empathy and caring are responded to with anger, as a potential violation. The client's angry response is understandable and needs to be met with empathy and compassion but is not useful to the client in their immediate situation. EFT therapists respond to these emotions with empathy and curiosity, in order to help clients fully arrive at and accept them, before exploring what is most painful or difficult about them.

f. *Core pain* is the deepest, most painful aspect of a one's primary maladaptive emotions – 'What hurts the most'. For example, deep, stuck shame about one's basic defectiveness might have at its core a feeling of being unfixably broken, utterly alone and abandoned or terrifyingly exposed and vulnerable. EFT therapists meet core pain with genuine compassion and gently ask this pain what it needs. Doing this taps universal, existential human needs (see Chapter 8, this volume), which in turn activates primary adaptive emotions.

g. *Primary adaptive* emotion responses are the ones most likely to have helped our evolutionary ancestors deal usefully with a given situation. They are thus our first, natural reactions to the current situation that would help us take appropriate action. (Here the word 'primary' again simply means 'first'.) For example, if a person is being violated by someone, anger is an adaptive response, because it helps the person to take assertive action to end the violation; fear signals immediate, overwhelming danger that needs to be avoided or escaped; sadness indicates loss and motivates the need for connection, and so on. EFT therapists help clients dwell on these emotions in order to fully receive the useful information they contain. In the emotional transformation process we've been describing, three key primary adaptive emotions are connecting sadness (which fuels a hunger for connection with others), assertive anger (which helps us set effective boundaries in the face of violation), and self-compassion (which helps heal emotional injuries).

Assessing these various types of emotion response requires close empathic attunement to the nuances of clients' expressions of the emotion and the perceived situation in which the emotion emerged and is worked out collaboratively with clients in session.

Dialectical constructivism

EFT is based on a *dialectical constructivist* theory of knowledge, self and the change process. This is a pluralist, neo-Piagetian perspective, in which the process of knowing changes both the knower and the known. The self is viewed as a process made up of various elements continuously interacting to produce experience and action, and therapy changes both the client and the therapist (Greenberg & Pascual-Leone, 1995). The multiple interacting self-processes are often organised around emotion schemes, which parallels the related person-centred concept of 'configurations of self' (Mearns et al., 2013). For EFT, the 'I' is an agent self-aspect or self-narrating voice that constructs a coherent story of the self by integrating different aspects of experience in a given situation. However, this voice has no special status as an executive self.

A dialectically constructive change process starts with clear separation between the different self-processes, emotion schemes or configurations, and especially between the internal or experiential and the external or conceptual processes, some dominant or salient, others implicit or unacknowledged. Next, the therapist helps the client to bring the different aspects into direct contact with each other so that discords and harmonies can be heard. By accessing emerging or implicit inner aspects and helping these interact with the more obvious aspects, an internal dialogue is created. If this dialogue is successful, some form of newness will be generated, in the form of new experiences and restructuring of existing emotion schemes. This dialectic process can be seen most clearly in EFT's use of two-chair dialogue for conflict splits. However, interaction between different aspects of the client runs through most EFT tasks and is a general change process in EFT (Elliott et al., 2004). When successful, this process leads to change in both aspects, or voices. Importantly, the therapist can only facilitate such a process but cannot know or direct the specific nature of the change that takes place as a result.

The practice of emotion-focused therapy

The basis of EFT practice is the set of six therapeutic principles mentioned here (see Table 5.1). Practice in EFT can be further described using two complementary sets of concepts: *therapist EFT response modes*, which occur at the level of individual therapist responses, and *therapeutic tasks*, which encompass substantial portions of therapy sessions centred on a particular kind of therapeutic work, such as two-chair work for conflict splits.

Therapist EFT response modes

It is useful to describe what therapists do in EFT in terms of four sets of therapist response modes or 'speech acts' (Elliott et al., 2004):

1. *Empathic understanding*

Consistent with its person-centred heritage, the bedrock of therapist responding in EFT is empathic reflection and following, using responses that try to communicate understanding of the client's message, including simple reflections and brief acknowledgements or minimal encouragers ('Uh-huhs') (see Chapter 2, this volume, in particular). For example, Beth, a client with severe crime-related post-trauma difficulties, talked about her inability to do things on her own:

Beth: I mean that's the biggest grief, that's my biggest sadness.

[Her therapist reflects with:]

Therapist: That's what you grieve for, the loss of independence.

2. *Empathic exploration responses*

The most characteristic kind of EFT response is empathic exploration (Elliott et al., 2004). This set of responses simultaneously communicates understanding and helps clients move toward the unclear or emerging edges of their experience. Empathic exploration responses take many different forms, including evocative reflections, exploratory questions, 'fit' questions (to check understanding), empathic conjectures, empathic formulations and empathic refocusing responses. Here is a brief excerpt illustrating empathic exploration responses, taken from a two-chair self-soothing exchange between Beth's strong pre-victimisation self and her weak post-victimisation self:

Beth: I just want enough of who I used to be, so that I could live like a human being.

Therapist: 'I don't feel like a human being right now. I feel like some kind of something else that's not human.' [First-person *evocative reflection* spoken as the post-victimisation self]

Beth: Just like a paranoid little, girl, ya' know.

Therapist: It's like what you want from that part is some of the courage. Is that right? [*Empathic conjecture*, intended to offer Beth a chance to turn her attention back to her current, post-victimisation self; followed by a *'fit' question* to assess accuracy]

[A little later, the therapist offers a response with two exploratory questions addressed to the lost, pre-victimisation self, in order to help Beth access this part of herself:]

Therapist: What's that like? What do you feel in that part?

Beth: Happy. [*Laughs softly*]

3. *Process guiding*

The difference between classical person-centred therapy (see Chapter 2, this volume) and EFT is most apparent in the use of process guiding responses in EFT to facilitate productive client experiencing. Although EFT therapists do not give advice about possible solutions to client life problems, they do offer process suggestions, proposing in a non-imposing way that the client try engaging in particular in-session activities, such as turning attention inside or saying something to an imagined person or self-aspect in the other chair. EFT therapists also sometimes provide experiential teaching, giving orienting information about the nature of therapy or of emotional experience, or they offer gentle support, orienting suggestions or encouragement to work on the task at hand. Finally, at the end of the session, EFT therapists may offer awareness homework, encouraging the client to continue work from the session on their own. Many of these are illustrated in this example of process-guiding responses used to help Beth to grieve and re-access her lost, pre-victimisation 'strong self':

Therapist: [Early in session, *process suggestion* about Beth's discouragement at not overcoming her fears] Can you stay with that hurt and sadness for a minute, and just feel what that's about and what that's like?

Therapist: [Later in session, *experiential teaching* about a potentially useful therapeutic strategy] One way to try to work with the grief is to put that part of you that you've lost in the chair and talk to her. There are other ways but that is one way that occurs to me.

[Finally, near the end of the session, the therapist helps Beth reintegrate her lost, pre-victimisation self, using a couple of *process suggestions*:]

Therapist: [*Gently*] Can you go over and *be* the strong part?

Beth: I would but I wouldn't know how.

Therapist: Tell her, 'I'd like you to have that strength.'

Beth: I'd like you to have my strength.

Therapist: What's that feel like? [*Exploratory question*]

Beth: Like a – like a mom.

4. *Experiential presence*

In EFT, therapist empathic attunement, prizing, genuineness and collaboration are largely communicated through the therapist's genuine presence or manner of being with the client. Although the specific configuration of therapist paralinguistic and non-verbal behaviours, including silence, vocal quality, posture and expression, varies among therapists, there is a distinctive, easily recognised EFT style. For example, when offering process guiding, the therapist typically uses a gentle, affirming voice (and sometimes humour), while empathic exploration responses often have a tentative, pondering quality. Presence is also indicated by direct eye contact at moments of connection between client and therapist.

Therapist *process* and *personal disclosures* are actually explicit forms of experiential presence, in that they are commonly used to communicate relationship attitudes. For example, the therapist begins the first session of Beth's therapy with a process disclosure of excitement:

> Therapist: ... So I'm excited about giving it [the therapy] a try.

In the fifth session, he uses another process disclosure to frame an empathic conjecture in helping Beth explore her crime-related fear:

> Therapist: You know it reminds me of, you know, those creepy old science fiction horror movies about things that take possession of people.

EFT tasks

EFT integrates a variety of different experiential *tasks*, drawn from person-centred, experiential, Gestalt and existential therapy traditions. These tasks all include three main elements:

- a *marker* of a client problem state signalling the client's wish to work on a particular experiential task (e.g. an unclear feeling)
- the *general thing* the therapist does to facilitate the task (e.g. help the client slow down and turn their attention inward to what they feel in their body)
- the *key change point*, in which the client begins to resolve the task (e.g. experience a bodily shift or release) (Elliott & Greenberg, 2021).

We find it useful to divide EFT tasks into four *task families* based on their most distinctive change processes: therapeutic relationship; experiencing; reprocessing, and enactment (see Table 5.2 for the current list of EFT tasks; for more detail see Elliott et al., 2004; Elliott & Greenberg, 2021).

1. Relational tasks

These emphasise the relational strand of the PCE therapy tradition and involve the development and repair of a safe working relationship between client and therapist. Change is believed to emerge directly from a therapeutic relationship characterised by empathic attunement, prizing (valuing), genuineness and collaboration. These tasks take priority because they provide the relational foundation for other kinds of work. (See also Chapters 2, 5 and 6, this volume.)

- *Alliance formation* is the first task of therapy, working with the client to establish mutual trust and a safe environment so that clients can engage in experiencing and exploring more painful experiences (Elliott et al., 2004). Alliance formation unfolds through several successive stages, culminating in the achievement of a productive

Table 5.2: Emotion-focused therapy tasks: Markers, interventions and end states (2021)

TASK MARKER	PROCESS	END STATE
1. Relational tasks		
Beginning of therapy	**Alliance formation**	Productive working environment
Therapy complaint or withdrawal difficulty (questioning goals or tasks; persistent avoidance of relationship or work)	**Alliance dialogue** (each explores own role in difficulty)	Alliance repair (stronger therapeutic bond or investment in therapy; greater self-understanding)
Vulnerability (painful emotion related to self, more based in the present)	**Empathic affirmation**	Self-affirmation (feels understood, hopeful, stronger)
Loss of psychological contact (psychotic, dissociative, or panic states)	**Pre-therapy contact work** (concrete reflections of present situation)	Restoration of psychological contact between client and therapist
2. Experiencing tasks		
Attentional focus difficulty (e.g. confused, overwhelmed, blank)	**Clearing a space**	Therapeutic focus; ability to work productively with experiencing (working distance)
Unclear feeling (vague, external or abstract)	**Experiential focusing**	Symbolisation of felt sense; sense of easing (feeling shift); readiness to apply outside of therapy (carrying forward)
3. Reprocessing tasks		
Narrative pressure (to tell painful life stories)	**Narrative retelling**	Relief, validation, restoration of narrative gaps, understanding of broader meaning
Problematic reaction point (puzzling over-reaction to specific situation)	**Systematic evocative unfolding**	New view of self in-the-world-functioning
Meaning protest (life event violates cherished belief)	**Meaning re-creation**	Revision of cherished belief
4. Enactment tasks		
Negative treatment of self (especially self-criticism, self-coercion, self-interruption; also attribution split)	**Two-chair work**	Softening of negative treatment of self; self-acceptance, integration
Unfinished business (Lingering bad feeling re: significant other)	**Empty chair work**	Let go of resentments, unmet needs re: other; affirm self; understand or hold other accountable
Stuck, dysregulated anguish (more about past than present)	**Compassionate self-soothing**	Emotional/bodily relief, self-empowerment

working relationship. EFT therapists begin therapy by being emotionally present and highly empathically attuned, which helps the client experience safety and feel safe within the therapeutic environment. Next, the therapist works actively with the client to establish a specific focus for therapy (Watson & Greenberg, 1996). In particular, the therapist uses their client's emotional responses as a compass to direct them where to focus attention and to establish shared agreement on therapeutic goals (what to work on) and tasks (how to go about working).

- *Alliance dialogue*, the next task, takes place when the client expresses some form of *complaint or difficulty* about therapy. For example, they might say: 'I feel stuck, like I'm not progressing anymore, or maybe even going backwards' or, 'I have the feeling that you are getting tired of me complaining all the time' or, 'I know you're not supposed to give advice, but I really think I need someone to tell me what to do about these fear attacks I keep having.' Therapeutic errors, empathic failures and mismatches between client expectations and treatment are inevitable in any therapy. These result in disappointment and sometimes anger on the part of the client and warrant immediate attention and the suspension of other therapeutic tasks. The therapist begins alliance dialogue work by offering solid empathic reflection of the potential difficulty, trying to capture it as accurately and thoroughly as possible. The difficulty is presented as a shared responsibility for client and therapist to work on together. The therapist models and fosters this process by genuinely considering and disclosing their own possible role in it, and client and therapist explore what is at stake for the client in the difficulty, as well as how it might be resolved between them.

- *Empathic affirmation* is offered when clients present a *vulnerability marker*, indicating the emergence of general, self-related emotional pain primarily based in the present. The client confesses to the therapist that they are struggling with strong feelings of vulnerability, despair or hopelessness. In emotional vulnerability, the client's need is to face and admit to another person an intense, feared aspect of self that had previously been kept hidden. The therapist's task is to offer a non-intrusive empathic presence, accepting and prizing whatever the client is experiencing, allowing the client to descend into their pain or despair as far as they care to go. The therapist does not push for inner exploration; indeed, they do not try to 'do' anything with the client's experience except understand and accept it. When the therapist follows and affirms the client's experience in this way, it helps to heighten the vulnerability to the point where the client hits bottom before beginning spontaneously to turn back toward hope. It can be challenging for therapists to maintain faith that the client's innate growth tendencies will enable them to come back from this process. Resolution consists of enhanced client self-acceptance and wholeness, together with decreased sense of isolation and increased self-agency.

- *Pre-therapy contact work* is another of the tasks. Although it did not emerge from the EFT tradition, Prouty's pre-therapy work (see Sanders, 2007, for an accessible account;

also Chapter 11, this volume) has the same structure as the other EFT tasks and is therefore very easy to assimilate into EFT. The marker is in-session loss of psychological contact in the form of immediate psychotic state, dissociation or panic. The general thing the therapist does is offer concrete contact reflections, such as: '[Client's name] is looking away but listening to the sound of [therapist's name] voice.' These contact responses allow the client to gradually recover psychological contact in the session.

2. Experiencing tasks

Experiencing tasks are derived from the work of focusing-oriented therapists (see Chapter 4, this volume).

- *Experiential focusing* has been described by Gendlin (1981) and Cornell (1996) as a general task for deepening client experiencing (see Chapter 4, this volume). For example, the client may be experiencing emotional distancing in the session, in the form of speaking in an intellectual or externalising manner or talking around in circles without getting to what is important to them. When this occurs, the therapist can gently interrupt the client, as in this hypothetical but typical example:

  Therapist: I wonder, as you are talking, what are you experiencing?

  Client: I'm not sure, I'm just going on [talking].

  Therapist: I wonder if we could try something here?

  Client: (*Nods*)

  Therapist: Can you take a minute, maybe slow down... and see if you can look inside... Ask yourself, 'What's going on with me right now?' and see what comes to you?

  As focusing progresses the client shifts to internal self-exploration. Resolution involves developing an accurately labelled felt sense, accompanied by an experienced sense of easing or relief and a direction for carrying this 'felt shift' into life outside the therapy session.

- Another of these experiencing tasks is *clearing a space*. If the client feels overwhelmed by multiple worries or by strongly painful experience (e.g. trauma memories), the therapist can help the client by using the clearing-a-space process from focusing (Gendlin, 1996). That is, the therapist helps the client mentally set side aside each of their problems to establish a safe, clear internal space. Here, resolution involves the attainment and full appreciation of the imagined safe space. Resolution occurs when the client attains a sense of an internal, clear safe space.

3. Reprocessing tasks

These are tasks in which clients present some form of problematic experience that has happened to them outside of therapy. They reflect the person-centred and existential heritage of EFT. The therapist helps the client examine the experience closely in order to make sense of it and to create new meaning about it in the broader context of their life.

- *Narrative retelling of difficult or traumatic experiences* is common in EFT for post-trauma difficulties. While telling stories of difficult or traumatic experiences is usually painful, people typically have a strong need to tell others about such experiences. The *narrative pressure* marker is an indication that the client is experiencing some internal pressure to tell their story (e.g. 'When I was robbed, there was nothing I could do to stop them!'). Often, it is useful for the therapist to encourage the client, by saying: 'Tell me the story of _______ in as much detail as you feel comfortable giving.' This also signals the therapist's willingness to 'hear the client through their pain' (Egendorf, 1995). A resolved retelling is a relatively complete narrative experienced by the client as making sense, with an overall meaning in the broad context of their life, typically accompanied by a sense of relief.

- *Systematic evocative unfolding* is used for *problematic reaction points*, or instances in which the client is puzzled by an overreaction they had to a specific situation. This task is particularly relevant to clients who experience sudden episodes of unwanted emotion, including post-traumatic flashbacks, panic or anxiety attacks, anger outbursts, impulsive acts, or episodes of strong emotion dysregulation. Unfolding tasks resemble retelling tasks in that both involve helping the client elaborate narratives with immediacy and vividness, but unfoldings are driven by curiosity or puzzlement (they are like a mystery story), while retellings are driven by the need to share distress or emotional pain (they are like a painful history). In unfolding, the therapist suggests that the client take them through the puzzling episode, including exactly what it was that the client reacted to. As the client re-enters the situation in imagination, they commonly re-experience what they felt at the time. The key change point involves the client reaching an understanding of the reason for the puzzling reaction (the *meaning bridge*), and typically leads to further exploration.

- *Meaning re-creation* work involves a *meaning protest* against a life event – usually some kind of trauma. Clarke (1989) described the meaning protest marker as the expression of strong emotion and confusion or puzzlement about a painful life event, in conjunction with description of a challenged cherished belief. This task is probably the most existential of EFT tasks (see Chapter 8, this volume) and involves helping clients in states of high emotional arousal to capture their experience in words and images that symbolise and begin to contain their emotional experience. Therapist interventions that facilitate this task attempt to help the client clarify and symbolise the cherished belief (e.g. bad things don't happen to good people) and the discrepant experience (a trauma or other painful life event). As this work progresses, client and therapist explore the basis and continued tenability of the cherished belief. However, the therapist does not challenge the cherished belief, or call it 'dysfunctional'; instead, the belief is accepted and understood, while being held up for reflection. In full resolution, the client modifies some aspect of the cherished belief, symbolises this change and considers new behaviour. For example, Labott and colleagues (1992) describe how a depressed client wept intensely as she accessed her disappointment and anger with her alcoholic father for beating her as a child. When exploring her reaction, she discovered that his behaviour had violated her cherished belief that 'If you love someone, you don't hurt them.' Through examining this belief and her experience, she concluded that her father hadn't really loved her and that his behaviour was not really her fault.

4. Active expression tasks

The last family of EFT tasks comes out of Gestalt and psychodrama traditions. Active expression tasks ask the client to enact a conversation between aspects of self or between self and others. These active, highly evocative tasks generally require a strong therapeutic alliance and a fair amount of therapist skill. They are rarely attempted before session three or four.

- *Two-chair dialogues* are used when the client presents some form of *negative treatment of self* (Elliott & Greenberg, 2021). There are three main forms of negative treatment of self:
    - *self-criticism split*, where the client criticises self. This is seen as a conflict between critic and self-aspects
    - *self-coercion split*, where the client tries to force self to do or feel something. Here, the conflict is between coercive and self-aspects of the person
    - *self-interruption split*, where the client tries to stop or block self from saying, doing or feeling something (e.g. anger).

Some other forms of conflict split include:

- *decisional conflict*, where the client feels torn between two alternative courses of action (e.g. to end a relationship or not)
- *attribution split*, where the client describes what they perceive as an overreaction to a perceived critical or controlling another person or situation. This is understood as a conflict between the self-aspect and the client's own negative treatment of self, projected onto the other person or situation.

Anxiety splits and *depressive splits* are common forms of split found in anxious or depressed clients, while *motivational splits* involve self-damaging activities such as problem drinking (see also Chapter 7, this volume). The conflict split marker is the broadest, most complex of all the EFT task markers.

The therapist initiates the two-chair dialogue by suggesting that the client move back and forth between two chairs, each representing one self-aspect, in order to enact the internal conversation between the two parts. In the case of an attributional split, the client is asked to enact the other or the external situation. For example, a traumatised client with a fear of driving on the motorway might be asked to 'be' the motorway and 'show how you scare (client).' This gives the client the opportunity to identify with and re-own the powerful, fear-inducing parts of the self. This re-owning provides a partial resolution, while a full resolution would require some kind of mutual understanding and accommodation between the fearful self and the fear-inducing coercive/critical aspect, with the fearful aspect asserting its needs, and the fear-inducing aspect softening its stance toward the self.

- *Empty chair work* is based specifically on the idea that attachment injuries, such as childhood mistreatment or emotional neglect, lead to unresolved issues with important others, including lingering bad feelings (usually sadness and anger) and unmet needs (e.g. for validation). The marker, referred to as *unfinished business*, involves interrupted expression of the negative feelings, often in the form of complaining or blaming. Empty chair work is used extensively with clients with depression and post-trauma difficulties. In this task, the therapist suggests that the client imagine the other in the empty chair and express unexpressed or unresolved feelings toward them. Although not necessary, the therapist sometimes suggests that the client also takes the role of the other and speaks to the self. The key change point consists of moderately strong emotional expression toward the other. Empty chair work is highly evocative and emotionally arousing. If the client is already in a highly emotional state, they are likely to feel overwhelmed even by the suggestion to speak to the other in the empty chair. Therefore, it is best to follow Clarke's (1993) suggestion that, when emotional arousal is high to start with, it is preferable to use the meaning re-creation task described above, because it helps the client to symbolise and contain painful emotion. In empty chair work, it is important for the therapist to maintain constant empathic attunement to the client's level of emotional arousal and whether the client feels safe enough with the therapist to undertake or continue with the work.

- *Compassionate self-soothing* is the most recently developed EFT task (Goldman & Fox, 2010; Sutherland et al., 2014) and is used when the client experiences a familiar stuck *anguish*, typically in the face of a powerful unmet existential need (e.g. for love or validation) that has not been or cannot be met by others. Compassion is the opposite of self-criticism, and expressing compassion toward oneself is a way of changing painful emotions (e.g. shame, fear, sadness) by internally confronting them with a different emotion. In this task, the therapist first helps the client deepen their sense of anguish so that they can access their core existential pain and express the unmet needs associated with it. Then, the therapist offers a two-chair process to the client in which they enact providing what is needed (e.g. validation, support, protection) to themselves. This can be done either directly or with the needy part symbolised as child or close friend experiencing the same things that the client is experiencing. The comforting aspect is represented either as a strong, nurturing aspect of self or as an idealised parental figure. Working this task is typically an intense, powerful experience that needs to be carefully and patiently held by a deep empathic, prizing connection between client and therapist.

Practical implementation of EFT

Modality

EFT is generally carried out in an individual format. However, under different names ('focused expressive therapy,' 'emotionally focused therapy') and with somewhat different emphases, EFT has been used extensively in a conjoint format (e.g. Greenberg & Johnson, 1988) as well as in groups (e.g., Thompson & Girz, 2020), and more recently as a family-based approach for working with caregivers and children/young people (Foroughe, 2018).

Appropriate clients

EFT is most appropriate for use in outpatient settings with clients experiencing mild-to-moderate levels of clinical distress and symptoms. Some clients seem to enter therapy with processing styles that allow them to engage almost immediately in the mindful attending, experiential search and active expression modes of engagement so critical to this approach. Such clients may have a variety of diagnoses and problems, including adjustment reactions, depression, post-trauma difficulties, anxiety, low self-esteem, internal conflicts and emotional injuries and difficulties with others.

In our experience, however, not all clients enter therapy with this inclination to explore the 'edges' of their own experience. In fact, much of the challenge and art of EFT comes in adapting it to meet the needs of clients with various processing styles. For instance, some clients seem to be persistently focused on external factors, such as unsupportive others and financial or medical problems, to which they return repeatedly in the face of the therapist's best efforts to help them look inside. Other clients enter therapy seeking expert guidance or advice. For clients whose styles are generally external or interpersonally dependent, the therapist needs to help the client gradually increase their ability to turn their attention inward. This is done through consistent empathic exploration of inner experience and by providing a rationale for this sort of work. In addition, with these clients, therapy may emphasise the use of the more process guiding tasks, such as focusing and empty chair work. Furthermore, with such clients, the therapist is always ready to engage in relationship dialogue regarding therapy tasks and activities.

Session length and frequency

In EFT the standard session length and frequency of 50–60 minutes once a week is typical. In order to maintain continuity, sessions generally occur on a weekly basis, particularly in the main working phase. Nevertheless, the therapist is flexible and allows for client self-determination within the limits imposed by scheduling. Particularly as therapy progresses, it makes sense to offer the client the option of less frequent sessions, including monthly maintenance sessions after the main work of therapy has been completed.

Length of therapy

EFT is appropriate as either a brief or long-term therapy, although relationship elements appear to play a larger role in the longer therapies needed for clients suffering from chronic interpersonal difficulties. As a brief therapy, EFT emphasises task interventions, and there are standard protocols for clients presenting with depression (Greenberg & Watson, 2005), complex trauma (Paivio & Pascual-Leone, 2023), and social and generalised anxiety (e.g. Elliott & Shahar, 2017; Timulak & McElvaney, 2017). In open-ended work, it is good practice to ask clients at the beginning of therapy how many sessions they feel are needed, and to review progress and goals every 10 sessions or so. As much as external constraints allow, clients are encouraged to judge when they are ready to end therapy.

Training, supervision and accreditation

Learning EFT presents trainees with substantial demands in that they are asked to learn general theories of function, dysfunction and the change process, along with sets of therapy principles, therapist response modes and therapy tasks and their variations (Elliott et al., 2004). Elliott and colleagues (2004) have devised a multi-faceted training programme to promote the development of these therapist capacities. The training consists of the following components:

- trainee selection and self-selection for basic experiential capacities and interests
- safe, supportive but stimulating training context
- didactic learning, including lectures and readings
- observation of recorded examples/modelling
- supervised practice in therapist role, including focus on both technique and personal development
- direct experience in client role, in order to experience the effects of task interventions
- reflexivity, supported by self-observation/evaluation, client feedback and participation in continuing treatment development.

Ideally, therapists learning EFT will have previously learned some form of humanistic-experiential therapy or counselling (e.g. person-centred). Alternatively, the initial phase of EFT training needs to focus on the person-centred facilitative skills of accurate empathy, unconditional positive regard and genuineness/transparency. Without this, training in the more active tasks, such as the various kinds of chair work, will be hampered, as these rely heavily on PCT skills. EFT training often begins with the less process-guiding tasks of focusing, evocative unfolding and meaning re-creation, and then shifts increasingly to the different forms of chair work. After this, trainees are closely supervised with actual clients. In order to be certified as an EFT therapist, they must complete about 80 hours of formal training and supervision in EFT tasks and then successfully apply a range of

EFT tasks in at least 60 sessions involving two or more clients. Accreditation as an EFT therapist (via the International Society for Emotion-Focused Therapy (ISEFT)) is carried out by a supervisor-level EFT therapist using the Person-Centred and Experiential Process Scale – EFT Addendum (PCEPS-EFT-5) (see appendix to Elliott & Greenberg, 2021). A competency framework and training curricula for EFT therapists, supervisors and trainers are available from EFT@EU.[1]

After reading this chapter, you might be wondering whether it would be okay for you to try chair work without specialised EFT training. This answer is, it depends: Do you have well-developed empathy skills? Have you read the more detailed coverage of these tasks in books like Elliott & Greenberg (2021)? Have you discussed it with your supervisor, and are they willing to support you in trying out chair work? Are you working with a client who is resilient and adventurous? Has this client presented a clear conflict split or unfinished business marker? Have you already tried other more person-centred ways of working with this marker, such as 'configuration work' (if it was a conflict split, Mearns et al., 2013) or 'speaking your truth' (if it was unfinished business, Elliott & Greenberg, 2021)? And, finally, is your client's wellbeing more important to you than trying out a cool new therapy technique? If the answer to all these questions is 'yes', then it might be okay for you to begin trying out chair work.

Research

Based on data from meta-analyses of humanistic-experiential psychotherapy outcome by Elliott and colleagues (2013, 2021), the outcomes of individual EFT have been the subject of at least 27 separate studies. Four client populations have been studied:

- major depression (e.g. Goldman et al, 2006)
- abuse, trauma and other unresolved interpersonal relationships (e.g. Paivio & Greenberg, 1995)
- anxiety presentations (e.g. Shahar et al., 2017)
- mixed or other problems (e.g. Klein & Elliott, 2006).

The overall uncontrolled pre-post weighted mean effect size (Hedges' g) for these studies is 1.23 standard deviation units, with a 95% confidence interval of 1.03 to 1.42 (i.e. there is a 95% probability that the actual value for this effect falls between these two values). This is a very large effect size.

Six of these were controlled studies – that is, they compared clients in EFT with clients not receiving therapy (e.g. Paivio & Nieuwenhuis, 2001), with a very large weighted controlled effect size of 0.90 sd. Eleven comparative outcome studies compared EFT with some other non-humanistic-experiential therapy, either CBT (e.g. Watson et al., 2003) or psychoeducation (Paivio & Greenberg, 1995). The comparative effect size overall was 0.46

1. Empowering Emotion-Focused Practice in Europe – https://emotionfocusedtherapy.eu

in favour of EFT, pointing to a substantial and clinically significant advantage. However, these studies were almost all carried out by EFT researchers, so they are probably subject to researcher allegiance effects. Finally, two studies (e.g. Goldman et al., 2006) have addressed the issue of the comparative effectiveness of EFT vs PCT (essentially PCE therapy for depression; see Chapter 6, this volume), yielding a statistically and clinically significant effect size of .49 in favour of EFT. While the results of these studies could have been influenced by researcher allegiance, the therapists were carefully trained and supervised in both PCE therapy and EFT, and were also monitored for treatment adherence, including empathy.

EFT thus appears to be a promising approach to therapy, especially for depression, anxiety and trauma/relational/interpersonal problems. However, more research is needed to document its effects with these and other clinical populations.

Conclusions

Since its roots in the 1970s task analytic research of Rice and Greenberg (1984), EFT has developed into an integrated approach with a theory of human function and dysfunction, a detailed theory of practice and the change process, and a set of therapeutic tasks and appropriate interventions, accompanied by a large practice literature (see key books and web resources below). As I have tried to show in this chapter, EFT continues to develop, adding new therapeutic tasks (e.g. meaning re-creation, relationship dialogue, compassionate self-soothing), developing applications to new clinical populations (e.g. complex PTSD, anxiety difficulties), refining training methods (Elliott et al., 2004), continuing outcome and process research (for reviews, see Elliott et al., 2013, 2021), and generating a thriving international EFT community, with conferences every two years and numerous trainings in many countries, including the UK.

EFT seems to appeal to person-centred and humanistic therapists who are interested in the transformative power of emotion or who share humanistic values of focusing on people's internal resources and strengths. At the same time, it offers a bridge into person-centred and humanistic therapy for CBT and psychodynamic practitioners. CBT therapists like EFT's systematic formulations and effectiveness data, while psychodynamic therapists like its depth and focus on emotion.

In an era of increasing demands for brief, effective treatments and criticism of person-centred and humanistic therapies for lack of theory and empirical support, EFT appears to offer a viable development of the humanistic and person-centred traditions, while at the same time appealing to therapists from other approaches. The continuing efforts described here in the areas of theory development, research, training and extension to new clinical populations are all part of a larger effort to help re-establish person-centred and humanistic therapies as empirically supported and generally respected psychotherapies for the 21st century.

Resources

Key books

User-friendly introduction to EFT for counselling students:

- Elliott, R. & Greenberg, L.S. (2021). *Emotion-focused counselling in action.* Sage.

The latest word from the primary developer of EFT; emphasises change processes over tasks:

- Greenberg, L.S. (2021). *Changing emotion with emotion.* APA.

Up-to-date coverage of key topics in EFT from a wide range of contributors; for EFT 'nerds':

- Greenberg, L.S. & Goldman, R.N. (Eds.) (2019). *Clinical handbook of emotion-focused therapy*. APA.

Masterful description of EFT as applied to a challenging, fragile client population:

- Paivio, S.C. & Pascual-Leone, A. (2023). *Emotion-focused therapy for complex trauma* (2nd ed.). APA.

Another user-friendly introduction to EFT, organised around the emotional deepening process:

- Timulak, L. (2015). *Transforming emotional pain in psychotherapy: An emotion-focused approach.* Routledge.

Key web resources

- Empowering Emotion-Focused Practice in Europe: https://emotionfocusedtherapy.eu/

Contains outputs from an Erasmus project to develop training opportunities and good practice guides for EFT trainers and clinical supervisors and a digital platform to support EFT training, supervision and practice in different countries.

- International Society for Emotion-Focused Therapy: www.iseft.org

Website with information about books, conferences, trainings and so forth.

- Emotion-Focused Podcast: www.emotionfocused.com

Hosted by Lou Cooper, of engaging interviews with well-known EFT therapists.

References

Bohart, A.C. & Tallman, K. (1999). *How clients make therapy work: The process of active self-healing*. American Psychological Association.

Brodley, B.T. (1990). Client-centered and experiential: Two different therapies. In G. Lietaer, J. Rombauts & R. Van Balen (Eds.), *Client-centered and experiential psychotherapy towards the nineties* (pp.87–107). Leuven University Press.

Clarke, K.M. (1989). Creation of meaning: An emotional processing task in psychotherapy. *Psychotherapy*, *26*, 139-148.

Clarke, K.M. (1993). Creation of meaning in incest survivors. *Journal of Cognitive Psychotherapy*, *7*, 195–203.

Cornell, A.W. (1996). *The power of focusing*. New Harbinger.

Egendorf, A. (1995). Hearing people through their pain. *Journal of Traumatic Stress, 8*, 5–28.

Elliott, R. & Greenberg, L.S. (2021). *Emotion-focused counselling in action*. Sage.

Elliott, R. & Shahar, B. (2017). Emotion-focused therapy for social anxiety. *Person-Centered & Experiential Psychotherapies, 16*, 140–158. doi: 10.1080/14779757.2017.1330701

Elliott, R., Watson, J.C., Goldman, R.N. & Greenberg, L.S. (2004). *Learning emotion-focused therapy: The process-experiential approach to change*. APA.

Elliott, R., Watson, J., Greenberg, L.S., Timulak, L. & Freire, E. (2013). Research on humanistic-experiential psychotherapies. In M.J. Lambert (Ed.), *Bergin & Garfield's handbook of psychotherapy and behavior change* (6th ed.) (pp.495–538). Wiley.

Elliott, R., Watson, J., Timulak, L. & Sharbanee, J. (2021). Research on humanistic-experiential psychotherapies. In M. Barkham, W. Lutz, & L. Castonguay (Eds.), *Garfield & Bergin's handbook of psychotherapy & behavior change* (7th ed.) (pp.425–472). Wiley.

Foroughe, M. (Ed.). (2018). *Emotion-focused family therapy with children and caregivers: A trauma-informed approach*. Routledge.

Gendlin, E.T. (1981). *Focusing* (2nd ed.). Bantam Books.

Gendlin, E.T. (1996). *Focusing-oriented psychotherapy: A manual of the experiential method*. Guilford Press.

Goldman, R., & Fox, A. (May, 2010). *Self-soothing in emotion-focused therapy: Findings from a task analysis*. Paper presented at conference of Society for the Exploration of Psychotherapy Integration, Florence, Italy.

Goldman, R. & Greenberg, L.S. (2014). *Case formulation in emotion-focused therapy*. APA.

Goldman, R.N., Greenberg, L.S. & Angus, L. (2006). The effects of adding emotion-focused interventions to the client-centered relationship conditions in the treatment of depression. *Psychotherapy Research, 16*, 537–549.

Greenberg, L.S. (2004). Being and doing: Person-centeredness, process guidance and differential treatment. *Person-Centered & Experiential Psychotherapies, 3*, 52–64. doi: 10.1080/14779757.2004.9688329

Greenberg, L.S. (2015). *Emotion-focused therapy: Coaching clients to work through their feelings* (2nd ed.). APA.

Greenberg, L.S. & Elliott, R. (1997). Varieties of empathic responding. In A. Bohart & L.S. Greenberg (Eds.), *Empathy reconsidered: New directions in psychotherapy* (pp.167–186). American Psychological Association Press.

Greenberg, L.S. & Johnson, S.M (1988). *Emotionally focused therapy for couples*. Guilford Press.

Greenberg, L.S. & Paivio, S. (1997). *Working with emotions in psychotherapy*. Guilford Press.

Greenberg, L.S. & Pascual-Leone, J. (1995). A dialectical constructivist approach to experiential change. In R. Neimeyer & M. Mahoney (Eds.), *Constructivism in psychotherapy* (pp.169–191). American Psychological Association.

Greenberg, L.S. & Pascual-Leone, A. (2006). Emotion in psychotherapy: A practice-friendly research review. *Journal of Clinical Psychology*, 62, 611–630. DOI: 10.1002/jclp.20252

Greenberg, L.S., Rice, L.N. & Elliott, R. (1993). *Facilitating emotional change: The moment-by-moment process.* Guilford Press.

Greenberg, L.S. & Safran, J.D. (1987). *Emotion in psychotherapy.* Guilford Press.

Greenberg, L.S. & Watson, J.C. (2005). *Emotion-focused therapy for depression.* American Psychological Association Press.

Klein, M.H., Mathieu-Coughlan, P. & Kiesler, D.J. (1986). The experiencing scales. In L. Greenberg & W. Pinsof (Eds.), *The psychotherapeutic process* (pp.21–71). Guilford Press.

Klein, M.J. & Elliott, J. (2006). Client accounts of personal change in process-experiential psychotherapy: A methodologically pluralistic approach. *Psychotherapy Research, 16,* 91–105.

Labott, S., Elliott, R. & Eason, P. (1992). 'If you love someone, you don't hurt them': A comprehensive process analysis of a weeping event in psychotherapy. *Psychiatry, 55*, 49–62.

Leijssen, M. (1996). Characteristics of a healing inner relationship. In R. Hutterer, G. Pawlowsky, P.F. Schmid & R. Stipsits (Eds.), *Client-centered and experiential psychotherapy: A paradigm in motion* (pp.427–438). Peter Lang.

Lietaer, G. (1998), From non-directive to experiential: A paradigm unfolding. In B. Thorne & E. Lambers (Eds.), *Person-centred therapy: European perspectives* (pp.62–73). Sage.

Mahrer, A.R. (1983). *Experiential psychotherapy: Basic practices.* Brunner/Mazel.

Mearns, D., Thorne, B. & McLeod, J. (2013). *Person-centred counselling in action* (4th ed.) Sage.

Newell, A. & Simon, H. (1972). *Human problem solving.* Prentice-Hall.

Paivio, S.C. & Greenberg, L.S. (1995). Resolving 'unfinished business': Efficacy of experiential therapy using empty chair dialogue. *Journal of Consulting and Clinical Psychology, 63*, 419–425.

Paivio, S.C. & Nieuwenhuis, J.A. (2001). Efficacy of emotion-focused therapy for adult survivors of child abuse: A preliminary study. *Journal of Traumatic Stress, 14*, 115–134.

Paivio, S.C. & Pascual-Leone, A. (2023). *Emotion-focused therapy for complex trauma* (2nd ed.). APA.

Pascual-Leone, A. & Greenberg, L.S. (2007). Emotional processing in experiential therapy: Why 'the only way out is through.' *Journal of Consulting & Clinical Psychology, 75*, 875–887. doi: 10.1037/0022-006X.75.6.875

Perls, F.S. (1969). *Gestalt therapy verbatim.* Real People Press.

Rennie, D. (1998). *Person-centred counselling: An experiential approach.* Sage.

Rice, L.N. & Greenberg, L. (Eds.) (1984). *Patterns of change.* Guilford Press.

Rice, L.N. & Saperia, E.P. (1984). Task analysis and the resolution of problematic reactions. In L.N. Rice & L.S. Greenberg (Eds.), *Patterns of change* (pp. 29-66). Guilford.

Rogers, C.R. (1961). *On becoming a person.* Boston: Houghton Mifflin.

Sachse, R. (1992). Differential effects of processing proposals and content references on the explication process of clients with different starting conditions. *Psychotherapy Research, 2,* 235–251.

Sanders, P. (ed.) (2007). *The contact work primer: A concise, accessible and comprehensive introduction to pre-therapy and the work of Garry Prouty.* PCCS Books.

Shahar, B., Bar-Kalifa, E. & Alon, E. (2017). Emotion-focused therapy for social anxiety disorder: Results from a multiple-baseline study. *Journal of Consulting & Clinical Psychology, 85*(3), 238–249. doi: 10.1037/ccp0000166

Sutherland [Smoliak], O., Peräkylä, A. & Elliott, R. (2014). Conversation analysis of the two-chair self-soothing task in emotion-focused therapy. *Psychotherapy Research, 24,* 738–751. doi: 10.1080/10503307.2014.885146

Thompson, S. & Girz, L. (2020). Overcoming shame and aloneness: Emotion-focused group therapy for self-criticism. *Person-Centered & Experiential Psychotherapies, 19*(1), 1–11. doi:10.1080/14779757.2019.1618370

Timulak, L. & McElvaney, J. (2017). *Transforming generalized anxiety: An emotion-focused approach.* Routledge.

Watson, J.C. (2002). Re-visioning empathy. In D. Cain & J. Seeman (Eds.), *Humanistic psychotherapies: Handbook of research and practice* (pp.445–471). APA.

Watson, J.C., & Greenberg, L.S. (1996). Pathways to change in the psychotherapy of depression: Relating process to session change and outcome. *Psychotherapy, 33,* 262–274.

Watson, J.C., Gordon, L.B., Stermac, L., Kalogerakos, F. & Steckley, P. (2003). Comparing the effectiveness of process-experiential with cognitive-behavioral psychotherapy in the treatment of depression. *Journal of Consulting and Clinical Psychology, 71*(4), 773–781. doi: 10.1037/0022-006X.71.4.773

Wexler, D.A. & Rice, L.N. (1974). *Innovations in client-centered therapy.* Wiley.

6. Person-centred experiential counselling for depression

Richard Doyle and David Murphy

In this chapter we will explore person-centred experiential counselling for depression (PCE-CfD), a counselling modality most commonly offered in NHS primary care in England. People can access PCE-CfD through their local NHS Talking Therapies services, previously known as Improving Access to Psychological Therapies (IAPT) services.

The presence of 'depression' in the name of the therapy indicates a medicalised model of psychological distress and diagnostic constructs commonly used throughout the Western world and specifically in the UK's National Health Service (NHS). Various criticisms of the medical model challenge the validity of mental health diagnoses and highlight the risks of over-medicalising human experience (Sanders, 2017; Levitt, 2019). Articulating the person-centred approach with the medical model naturally creates a tension. Some readers may question such engagement, as the person-centred approach is based on a growth model that values unique human experience above labels and treatment plans. Others, on the other hand, may feel this is part of a necessary dialogue between paradigms, giving person-centred experiential therapies a foothold within the medical world, and is therefore a justifiable compromise. It is hoped that this chapter will help to inform and contribute to the debate.

We use the term *person-centred experiential* (PCE) therapy in this chapter to refer to the contemporary practice, grounded in person-centred therapy, in which the experiential is inherent (Murphy, 2017, 2019). As an expression of this approach, PCE-CfD originated through a drive to secure and maintain humanistic, person-centred counselling provision within England's NHS. It is within this context that we will review the genesis and current status of PCE-CfD.

IAPT emerged in NHS primary care services from 2006, following the publication of *The Depression Report* (CEPMHPG, 2006; also known as *The Layard Report*, after its lead author, the economist Professor Sir Richard Layard), which advocated for talking therapies services to be available in NHS primary care as a means to reduce the numbers of people claiming sickness benefits due to mental health issues. This, and subsequent lobbying, resulted in substantial government funding to roll out IAPT across England, to deliver therapies recommended by the National Institute for Health and Care Excellence (NICE) guidelines (2004, 2009, 2022) for the treatment of 'common' mental health problems, and specifically anxiety and depression.

From the start, there was an economic justification for increased public funding for talking therapies, with the report arguing that such a service would 'pay for itself,' due to reduced expenditure on incapacity benefits through people being helped to return to work sooner (CEPMHPG, 2006, p.7).

The IAPT programme was implemented via a top-down, managerialist agenda that significantly disrupted the existing provision of psychological therapies through the employment of counsellors based in GP surgeries. With the concomitant move towards the 'evidence-based practice' paradigm, spearheaded by NICE, priority was given to cognitive-behavioural therapies (CBT), which benefitted from a wealth of randomised controlled trial (RCT) data in support of their effectiveness. As a result, counsellors and therapists in primary care services who offered modalities other than CBT found themselves sidelined and, in many cases, out of a job.

A related development at this time was the introduction of the therapeutic competences agenda, and the 'manualisation' of therapies, in alignment with the dominant approach to research (Sanders & Hill, 2014). The idea here was to attempt to establish some consistency and fidelity in the delivery of therapies in trials and in practice, these things being valued by NICE and IAPT. A 'competence framework' for humanistic therapies was developed by a team of experts, including academics and representatives from the British Association for the Person-Centred Approach (BAPCA) and the British Association for Counselling and Psychotherapy (BACP) (Roth et al., 2009).

Following an update of the NICE guidelines for depression in 2009, it was decided to include a number of other therapies, including counselling, alongside CBT. The intention was to build capacity and offer broader choice within IAPT. BACP was commissioned to develop a new competence framework and training curriculum specifically for what came to be called Counselling for Depression (CfD) (Hill, 2011a; 2011b). This was based on person-centred therapy principles and over time developed further into PCE-CfD (Murphy, 2019).

Murphy (2019) describes the history of the emergence of PCE-CfD. PCE, he points out, evolved from Carl Rogers' work in the late 1950s, as influenced by Gendlin's research into 'experiencing' (see Chapter 4, this volume), and following Lietaer's explorations of the experiential nature of person-centred therapy (see Chapter 5, this volume). Baker (2012) coined the term 'experiential person-centred' to describe a specific tribe within the person-centred approach, and phrasing this as 'person-centred experiential' intentionally gives primacy to the concept of the person. The addition of CfD simply indicated its focus on depression in the context of NHS Talking Therapies. Murphy (2019) argues: 'PCE-CfD is not… an integration of disparate approaches… PCE therapy can be defined as a contemporary evolution of a radical paradigm for therapy' (p.3).

Creating the competence framework and training curriculum was a challenging proposition, as PCE therapy had not traditionally used diagnostic terms as a basis for describing its practice. To support the endeavour, a number of published RCT studies were identified that included ('classical') person-centred counselling (see Chapter 2, this volume) as well as emotion-focused therapy (EFT) (see Chapter 5, this volume). Together, these provided sufficient evidence of effectiveness to meet the NICE requirements for evidence-based practice. The competency framework that emerged was thus informed by practices and theory from classical person-centred and emotion-focused approaches to person-centred therapy. Trainers' and practitioners' manuals were produced that provided a detailed description of the approach, highlighting how it might be practiced in the NHS and IAPT settings (Hill, 2011a). The approach had to be presented as a manual that identified key skills and competences. The framework was accepted by NICE and, since then, PCE-CfD training courses have been established at various sites across England. Principally taken by qualified and experienced person-centred counsellors employed in an NHS Talking Therapy service, the trainings have also been taken by counsellors working in private practice.

The approach has gradually grown to become a significant element of therapeutic provision within NHS England, with 84% of NHS Talking Therapies providers offering it as of March 2022 (Health Education England, 2023). As such, PCE-CfD enables routes to employment in the NHS for counsellors trained in the person-centred approach and offers a publicly funded form of person-centred experiential therapy. Research into the approach has gradually been building, some of which is described later in this chapter. NHS England is now (as of March 2024) funding a pilot programme in which trainee counsellors are paid a full-time salary to work in an NHS Talking Therapies service for two to three days per week while they complete a training in psychotherapeutic counselling, including PCE-CfD (see further below, in the section on 'Training').

Depression and the medical model

Given that we are covering an approach to counselling that is labelled 'for depression', it seems important to consider what might be meant by this term. In this section we will do this briefly in terms of the medical model, and in the next section we will consider how depression may be conceptualised differently from a person-centred experiential viewpoint.

From a medical perspective, depression may be considered as a 'disorder' – something abnormal that negatively affects human functioning. Such conditions are associated with specific signs and symptoms, and we can refer to manuals for criteria used by those vested with the power to diagnose medical disorders. The American Psychiatric Association's *Diagnostic and Statistical Manual of Mental Disorders* (DSM), currently in its fifth edition (APA, 2013), lists a range of different 'depressive disorders' that are considered to be specific and differentiable conditions while sharing some characteristics. These include major depressive disorder (including major depressive episode), persistent depressive disorder (dysthymia), premenstrual dysphoric disorder and substance/medication-induced depressive disorder, among others. The diagnostic criteria for major depressive disorder are described in terms of five or more symptoms (out of nine listed) being present over a two-week period. The symptoms are described in some detail: depressed mood, consistent lack of pleasure in most activities, changes in weight/appetite, insomnia or hypersomnia, psychomotor agitation or retardation, fatigue, feelings of worthlessness, indecisiveness, recurrent thoughts of death, and so forth, with many clarifying notes and caveats. In further criteria, the symptoms must cause 'clinically significant distress or impairment in social, occupational, or other important areas of functioning' and not be attributable to various alternative causes (APA, 2013, pp. 160–161). A diagnosis, then, requires an objective assessment and identification of highly specific and detailed criteria.

In the medical model, disorders are associated with specific treatments that are intended to help restore the affected individual towards good health. In the NHS, treatment for depression is governed by the relevant NICE guidelines (in this instance, the revised guidelines on *Depression in Adults: Treatment and management* (NICE, 2022). Various talking therapies are listed as treatment options, as well as medications such as selective serotonin reuptake inhibitors (SSRIs) and the antidepressant mirtazapine. It's worth noting that, while such drugs may 'work' in the sense of helping the client, or patient, to manage their symptoms, the evidence does not support there being an association between levels of serotonin and depression (Moncrieff et al., 2022). Various side effects are also reported for such drugs (see, for example, Morriss et al., 2021).

In NHS Talking Therapies services, the severity of depression is routinely monitored using a questionnaire known as the Patient Health Questionnaire (PHQ-9). This forms part of the National Minimum Data Set, a collection of scales used in almost all NHS Talking Therapies services in the UK. In the current NICE guidelines (2022), someone scoring below 16 on the PHQ-9 is identified as having 'less severe depression', while scores of 16 or above are classified as 'more severe depression'.

Another widely used scale in the Minimum Data Set is the Generalised Anxiety Disorder measure (GAD-7), which aims to quantify symptoms of anxiety. The GAD-7 and the PHQ-9 were developed by Spitzer and colleagues (2006) for use in clinical trials for antidepressants and other prescribed psychiatric drugs. They are available online courtesy of the drug manufacturer Pfizer.[1] Data from such scales are used within NHS Talking Therapy services to monitor performance against targets for reliable improvement and recovery.

Depression and the person-centred approach

At this point, it is worth remembering just how different the person-centred approach is from the medical model of assessment, diagnosis of symptoms of ill health or malfunctioning, and treatment. In an interview, Carl Rogers said (1976):

> We regard the medical model as an extremely inappropriate model for dealing with psychological disturbances. The model that makes more sense is a growth model

1. See Patient Health Questionnaire (PHQ) Screeners: https://www.phqscreeners.com

> or a developmental model. In other words, we see people as having a potential for growth and development, and that can be released under the right psychological climate. We don't see them as sick and needing a diagnosis, prescription and a cure. And that is a fundamental difference with a good many implications.

This neatly captures the opposing philosophical outlooks of the two approaches. The reference to a 'growth' or 'developmental' model relates to a fundamental person-centred postulate: the 'actualising tendency' towards maintenance, growth and development of potentials that is considered to be the sole source of motivation for living organisms (Rogers, 1963). Rogers (1957a) wrote of humans as being essentially trustworthy and having a tendency:

> towards development, differentiation, cooperative relationships; whose life tends to move from dependence to independence; whose impulses tend naturally to harmonise into a complex and changing pattern of self-regulation; whose total character is such as to tend to preserve himself and his species, and perhaps to move towards its further evolution. (p.201)

This speaks to the ontology of PCE theory in relation to the nature of humans: namely, humans are viewed as being pro-social, essentially trustworthy and tending towards growth and development. While in this theory the unidirectional nature of actualisation is always growthful and towards greater differentiation and complexity of the organism, this directional tendency is also non-specific. The actualising tendency can and will be lived out differently for each person. In this way, PCE theory offers a non-pathologising way to comprehend the diversity of human experiencing, including a wide variety of expressions of distress, some of which may be described as depression.

Generic diagnostic labels such as 'depression' have long been controversial within the PCE community, largely because of their homogenising effect, whereby many subtleties of individual experience are at risk of being airbrushed away behind a simple label. Having said this, commonalities and patterns can be observed, and it makes sense to talk of a phenomenology of depression, while recognising that this will be felt in different ways by each person who identifies with this.

In order to account for the phenomenology of depression from a PCE viewpoint, we will discuss 10 hypotheses, which were originally presented by Sanders and Hill (2014) and updated by Murphy (2019). In doing so, we will touch on key aspects of personality theory that are relevant to PCE-CfD. The practice of this approach is grounded in Rogers' original theory of personality and behaviour (1951) (see Chapter 2, this volume) and incorporates the evolution in focus of the central role of *experiencing* (Rogers, 1959, 1961) as well as the emotion theory developed initially by Greenberg (1984) and Greenberg and Safran (1989).

Hypothesis 1: The phenomenology of depression can result from rigidity within the self-structure arising as a result of threat to the integrity of the self-concept.

In this model, we consider the self-concept (Rogers, 1959) as a construct related to experiences that individuals associate with a sense of who they are. The idea of a self-structure relates to the multiplicity that exists within the human organism and how we might have numerous self-configurations in constant interaction with one another. Rogers (1959), and others since (e.g. Mearns, 1999), considered the self-concept as a process. Someone's sense of who they are can adapt over time, to the extent that shifting experiences are accurately symbolised in awareness. A well-functioning self is therefore a fluid process. Rigidity in processing will restrict the potential range of experiences and consequent responses to the world. The structure of the self may become rigid due to threats, such as negative judgements from others, or abuse or trauma. Threats may also be experienced internally, such as intrusive thoughts or self-criticisms. At a quite simple and straightforward level, these threats can result in patterned restrictions of perception and response that become configured and experienced as depression.

Hypothesis 2: Some aspects of depression can result from the embodied self.

In PCE-CfD, individuals are considered as integrated organisms, and as such, psychological tension can be embodied. Experiences associated with the self-structure can often include things felt in the body. Feeling physically weak or in pain or having a sense of heaviness in the body (to offer just a few examples) can contribute to what might be called depression. Rogers also described the self-concept in terms of the organism. Indeed, Tudor and Worrall (2006) assert that the concepts of self and organism are conflated in Rogers' theory. Physical sensations are therefore important elements of experience that are available for work in therapy. There is no formula or taxonomy of embodied feelings in PCE-CfD. Each is unique and is liable to change from moment to moment.

Hypothesis 3: Symptoms of depression can result from problematic dialogue between parts of the self.

In PCE theory, communication within the self-structure and between its constituent self-configurations is crucial for development. A trajectory of healthy organismic maintenance and growth will likely be indicated by free and uninhibited communication between the different systems within us, including the accurate symbolisation of thoughts and emotions and, crucially, the expression of these through behaviours that are felt as consistent. Psychological distress is indicated by problematic communication within the self-structure.

Hypothesis 4: Symptoms of depression can uniquely result from the discrepancy between a person's real or actual self and their introjected ideal self.

Self-discrepancy theory (Higgins, 1987) provides a way of considering aspects of the self and how these may be viewed from your own standpoint or that of others. The theory posits three domains of self:

- *the actual self* – representations or experiences of the attributes you (or someone else, another) thinks that you possess

- *the ideal self* – experiences of the attributes that you (or another) would like you, ideally, to possess (hopes and aspirations for you)
- *the ought self* – experiences of the attributes that you (or another) believe you ought to possess (a representation of your duty and responsibilities).

While this theory is not required in order to grasp the PCE-CfD conceptualisation, it can be helpful to consider how a mismatch between the actual self (from your standpoint) and the ideal self (from either standpoint) could relate to depression. Various discrepancies within the model have been measured and validated in a range of studies (Watson et al., 2010).

Hypothesis 5: Symptoms of depression can result from conflicts between parts of the self that result in shutting down of experiencing, withdrawal and feelings of guilt, unworthiness, hopelessness, helplessness, blame and so on.

A concept adapted from emotion-focused therapy (EFT) (see Chapter 5, this volume), conflict-splits occur when one part of the self treats another part negatively (Elliott & Greenberg, 2021). For example, one part (a 'critic') may display aggression or harshness towards a second (the 'experiencing' part). When the critic dominates, this can lead to the client shutting down experiencing, or feeling guilty, blameworthy, unworthy, helpless and so forth, and this can be associated with the phenomenology of depression. Such inner conflict can often be on the edge or outside of people's awareness. Process-facilitative work can help encourage awareness of and therapeutic dialogue between such splits, as touched on in the next section.

Hypothesis 6: Depression can be the result of, or exacerbated by, emotions that are too overwhelming to be faced or worked with in therapy.

Sometimes people can be overwhelmed by an intense emotional experience that might, for example, be associated with trauma or grief, and can also feed into the phenomenology of depression. When feelings are so powerful that it's hard to step back and begin to process the experience, it can feel like you are stuck – in life and/or therapy. The concept of emotion regulation – that is, ways by which we can moderate our emotions (or, alternatively, tune into weaker emotions) in order that we can begin to work with them therapeutically – is important in this approach. We will return to this in the next section.

Hypothesis 7: Some aspects of depression can be the result of, or exacerbated by, puzzling, unexplained experiences that feel exaggerated or out of character.

At times, clients describe feelings of confusion following experiences in which they struggle to understand why they did what they did, or why they reacted (or didn't react) in a certain way. Examples could include not feeling sad following news of the death of a close family member or engaging in risky behaviour when 'that's not me'. The reaction can seem so out of character that it doesn't seem to belong to them and can relate to depression. A term from EFT, 'problematic reaction points', is used to refer to such puzzling experiences. In person-centred theory, these might be considered as bodily needs and experiences that haven't yet been symbolised in awareness (Rogers, 1951).

Hypothesis 8: Some aspects of depression can be the result of having a cherished belief about the world destroyed.

An athletic client in their 20s prides themselves on being strong and healthy, with many decades of life to live, until they receive a diagnosis of a life-threatening illness. 'But marriage is forever,' protests a client whose partner has, without any warning, just asked them for a divorce. When firm beliefs that have become central to the self-structure are crushed, feelings of shock, outrage, anger, injustice and so on often result. The term 'meaning protest' refers to this, and such traumatic events can relate to aspects of depression.

Hypothesis 9: Some aspects of depression can be the result of particular types of incompletely processed life events.

Clients can describe themselves as being depressed following unresolved distressing life events, often involving another person (e.g. bullying, abuse, neglect, loss, unfair accusations and so on). The term 'unfinished business' is used to refer to such insufficiently processed issues and the emotions surrounding them.

Hypothesis 10: Some aspects of depression can be the result of inappropriate and unhelpful learned emotions.

Within PCE-CfD, depression is conceptualised as resulting from certain emotional and emotional experience processes. Greater openness to feelings is associated with greater psychological health and less likelihood of experiences associated with depression. While being emotional in itself does not necessarily have therapeutic benefit, a focus on feelings and emotions can help clients to process their emotional responses, perhaps by identifying unhelpful patterns and seeking more congruent expressions.

This section has presented a brief overview of how depression may be considered from a PCE viewpoint. The processes summarised above involving the self-structure and emotions can help us conceptualise the phenomenon. Having said this, in PCE-CfD, the client's unique subjective experience is key; we seek to understand them as an individual, irrespective of any diagnostic labels.

PCE-CfD theory

PCE therapy represents a modern evolution of the person-centred approach. Rooted in Rogers' (1951) 'client-centered therapy' (what we in the UK would call 'person-centred therapy'; see Chapter 2, this volume), the approach also draws on developments relating to experiencing presented by Gendlin (1962) (see Chapter 4, this volume) and emotion theory associated with EFT (Elliott & Greenberg, 2021; see Chapter 5, this volume). PCE-CfD might be considered as an application of PCE therapy, rather than a separate 'tribe' or 'branch'. In this section, we provide a brief overview of relevant theory, noting that some aspects were touched on in the previous section and are also described in other chapters of this book, hence the very concise treatment here.

Theory of personality

The previous section made reference to the phenomenology of depression and how this links to clients' subjective experience, emotional processes and self-structure. The phenomenological nature of PCE theory is represented within Rogers' 19 propositions in his original theory of personality and behaviour (1951). Any shifts in perception or experiencing indicate changes within the person and their individual reality. As clients make use of therapy and begin to see the world differently, they will inevitably behave differently.

In PCE-CfD, the concept of experiencing is important in considering personality and how the body has a role in processing individual experience. Drawing from Gendlin's (1962) theorising, as well as the theory of emotion processing (Elliott et al., 2004), it is recognised that clients can gain new meanings by attending to an implicit felt sense that may arise from bodily sensations, emotions, memories, thoughts, beliefs, feelings and so forth. New understandings can arise from these, whether they are clear in awareness or undifferentiated and murky.

In terms of human motivation, the concept of the actualising tendency (Rogers, 1959) discussed in the previous section (see also Chapter 2, this volume) indicates the constant organismic striving for maintenance and growth that underpins the philosophy of this approach. In PCE-CfD, emotions are seen as related to motivation in that they provide information that can point to our needs and prompt goal-directed behaviour. Emotion schemes (Elliott & Greenberg, 2021) can be considered as interlinked networks of experience relating to emotions, including perception, bodily sensations and expression, meaning and motivation.

Also described in the previous section was the self-concept, which in Rogers' theory (1959) comprises the fluid and changing, yet organised and consistent Gestalt of experiences associated with 'I' or 'me'. People are considered to have a need for positive regard from others around them. If this regard is only given conditionally, then *conditions of worth* may become assimilated into the self-structure. When situations arise where an accurate representation of experience would clash with someone's self-concept, including any introjected conditions of worth, this can lead to distortion or denial of experience in awareness, such is the power of the need for positive regard. In these states, there is an *incongruence* between experience and self. If experiences aren't accurately represented in awareness, this can hamper the organismic process by which we value experiences as growthful or not. Rather than acknowledging, processing and learning from emotions in a healthy way, for example, we might bury them and become stuck. Incongruence is thus, in Rogers' theory, at the root of psychological distress or maladjustment.

Therapeutic conditions

The *necessary* and *sufficient* conditions for therapeutic change (Rogers, 1957b) will be familiar to most readers:

1. That two persons are in psychological contact.
2. That the first person, whom we shall term 'the client', is in a state of incongruence, being vulnerable, or anxious.
3. That the second person, whom we shall term 'the therapist', is congruent or integrated in the relationship.
4. That the therapist is experiencing unconditional positive regard toward the client.
5. That the therapist is experiencing an empathic understanding of the client's internal frame of reference and endeavours to communicate this to the client.
6. That the client perceives, at least to a minimal degree, conditions 4 and 5, the unconditional positive regard of the therapist for him [sic], and the empathic understanding of the therapist. The communication to the client of the therapist's empathic understanding and unconditional positive regard is to a minimal degree achieved.

According to the theory, if these conditions are present, then the client will become more open to their experience, less rigid in their thinking, and more able to make their own choices and judgements (rather than seeking an external source of authority), and will experience other changes associated with greater congruence.

It is important therefore for the PCE-CfD therapist to attempt to establish a relationship with their client that exhibits the above characteristics. They will endeavour to hold the apposite attitudinal qualities and work collaboratively with the client to foster change and growth. If they allow themselves to be touched by the client's inner world and seek to experience this as if they were the client, they can communicate through empathic responses. At the same time, they will strive to accept and prize all aspects of the client's experience unconditionally, and be more genuinely and authentically themselves in the relationship. Clients are considered to be the experts on their experience and their autonomy is respected; attempts to direct their content through interpretation or advising a course of action, or by other means, are avoided. Such real relationships are often deeply enriching for both the client and therapist.

Process-facilitation responses

Integral to PCE-CfD is that a number of insights and practices originating from focusing and EFT are called on sensitively, in response to the client's self-direction, to help facilitate experiential processing. This is done without compromising the core relationship conditions (Murphy, 2017) (see Chapters 4 and 5, this volume, respectively). These can help support the expression and processing of emotions and aid clients in developing greater understanding of self-experiences and their implicit meanings. Any such engagement will be offered as an invitation appropriate to the moment, often emerging from the natural flow of therapeutic dialogue. Several such *process facilitation* responses are recognised as being part of PCE-CfD.

- *Systematic evocative unfolding* refers to a close empathic following, aiding the re-exploration of an experience using evocative empathic responses. Through this, clients are often able to unpack and clarify confusing or problematic reactions, leading to new meanings and understandings about experiences and the self.

- *Emotion regulation* relates to the idea that, if emotions are felt too intensely and overwhelmingly, or too subtly or flatly, it can be hard for clients to observe and process their experience. Clients may already be aware of ways they might manage over-intense emotional arousal, by using breathing techniques, for example. Empathic responses that pick up on subtle emotions (perhaps expressed by the client non-verbally) can help clients bring these more clearly into awareness. 'Clearing a space' can help in either direction: managing overwhelm or tuning into weak emotions.

- *Clearing a space*, originally derived from focusing (Gendlin, 1978), refers to ways by which clients draw their attention inward and name their main concerns or worries – things that are getting in the way of them feeling okay right now. One by one, the client can place these aside, perhaps metaphorically using containers or safe spaces, in order to get some distance from them, until they run out of things to mention. This exercise can help the client who feels overwhelmed by many worries, as well as someone who is struggling to find something to bring to the session.

- *Processing problematic dialogue between self-configurations* describes those times when clients experience inner dialogue in which there is a harshness, perhaps conceptualised as one part being overly self-critical: for example, 'I can hear myself sounding really stupid.' The different self-configurations can be brought into empathic responses to help clients identify and become more aware of them and differentiate and explore their thoughts and feelings. An invitation to respond and dialogue with and between parts can sometimes lead to changes, softening of harshness, internal forgiveness and suchlike.

- *Unfinished business* involves a sense of unresolved interpersonal concerns. Examples are hurt and resentment from bullying or abuse, feelings of being deceived or manipulated, or not having expressed something to someone who has since died. The counsellor can be alongside the client as they explore these feelings. Similar to exploring dialogue between self-configurations, clients sometimes find it helpful to dialogue with an imagined third other, metaphorically brought into the session.

- *Meaning creation* relates to traumatic situations in which firm and cherished beliefs are destroyed. By helping to sensitively explore what happened and identify the belief and related feelings, clients can be supported in their process of changing or revising the belief to adapt to their new circumstances.

Theory of change

Patterns of change generally observed throughout counselling were described by Rogers in terms of a continuous process (1961). People tend to move in a direction from relative rigidity towards fluidity, from fixity to flow. This was described using an arbitrary array of seven pointers or 'stages of process' on a continuum. The first stage can be described as when someone's process is so stuck that they are unlikely to come for therapy (they think everyone else has a problem). Stage seven can be described as when someone's process is so spontaneous and fluid that almost continuous change happens outside and inside sessions. Between these extremes, predictable changes are described in terms of feelings, expression, personal constructs, perception of problems, differentiation and elaboration of experience, and attitude to change, as well as bodily changes. It should be noted that everyone's change process is unique; it may follow an irregular or non-linear pattern, proceeding at different rates in different areas of their life. The 'stages' don't exist beyond providing a possible description of arbitrary points on a continuous process.

PCE counsellors working in NHS Talking Therapy services often find themselves being asked to make initial assessments of potential new clients, to help determine the appropriate therapeutic offer. The above therapeutic conditions and stages of process can be used as criteria to inform such assessment (Wilkins, 2019). By asking yourself whether you and the potential client may be capable of forming a relationship characterised by the six necessary and sufficient conditions, a sense can be developed of whether PCE-CfD could be helpful. Similarly, a sense of whereabouts in the stages of process a client is can also contribute to such an assessment.

Working briefly

The PCE therapist will attend to the relationship and therapeutic conditions together with the client, who is trusted to determine the content of sessions, direction and pace and, in some settings, may be able to decide when to end therapy. While it need not necessarily be the case (a therapist may offer it in private practice, for example), PCE-CfD is mainly practised in NHS settings, where therapy will be time-limited due to the way services are managed and limitations on resources. The number of sessions is therefore determined by external factors before therapy starts and forms part of contracting, and may be revisited if necessary, over the course of therapy. The therapist holds the frame and boundaries delineated in the contract, including, in these circumstances, the number of sessions.

Communicating the ethos of PCE-CfD, setting the scene, establishing expectations and parameters within the service, the contracting and so forth all contribute to what might be described as 'structuring the relationship'. You may want to consider your attitude to working briefly and how this may impact on the client. The client themself may already have preconceptions around what they want or think would be helpful in relation to the number of sessions. A lot can happen in the opening minutes of the first session, so it's worth reflecting on how what you say, and how you say it, may be received.

PCE counselling involves a collaboration between therapist and client. The client may identify aims, goals or a focus for the work, and if so, then these can be discussed and clarified in sessions. When reviewing the work, it can help if clients reflect on any goals they have previously identified and how they now feel about them, and exchange feedback with the therapist.

How brief is brief? The NICE guidelines for depression suggest eight regularly spaced sessions for a new episode of less severe depression, and 12–16 sessions for a new episode of more severe depression, 'although additional sessions may be needed for people with comorbid mental or physical health problems or complex social needs, or to address residual symptoms' (NICE, 2022, p.55). The IAPT manual states (National Collaborating Centre for Mental Health, 2023):

> In general, patients should be offered up to the NICE-recommended number of sessions for the relevant clinical condition. For high-intensity work this would generally be in the range of 12 to 20 sessions, depending on the problem descriptor and severity. It is good practice to offer an initial number of sessions (around six) followed by a review to decide whether treatment should continue, whether there should be a change of approach (such as stepping up), or whether a reformulation would be appropriate. (p.51)

How each NHS Talking Therapies service delivers this will, in reality, also be influenced by the need to manage waiting lists and pressures to reach 'reliable improvement' or 'recovery' targets. It is important to consider how clients might feel about having a set number of sessions, or even the possibility of having to end when they don't feel ready to. If appropriate, it may be possible to make a case for additional sessions within the service, or to signpost to other potential suitable sources of support.

Case studies

Here we present two short illustrative examples of extracts from PCE-CfD sessions. All people and incidents portrayed here are fictional but representative of themes and approaches in PCE-CfD work.

Jane and Amina

Jane is a 45-year-old white woman who grew up in the North of England and has struggled with some serious setbacks and losses throughout her life. Her father died in a road traffic accident when Jane was 12, and her mother then had a series of relationships, each of which seemed to end shortly after Jane and her younger sister had begun to trust the new father figure.

On leaving school, Jane trained as an accountant and has since worked in a number of local firms. In her late 20s, she married and felt happy and settled for some years before the couple found they were unable to have children. Following other difficulties, they divorced when Jane was 38, and she is currently living alone. Last year, her sister was diagnosed with ovarian cancer.

Struggling to focus at work and feeling socially withdrawn, Jane consulted her GP, who suggested she might benefit from counselling (PCE-CfD) with her local NHS Talking Therapies service. She has now started sessions with Amina, a qualified PCE-CfD therapist with more than five years' experience. In the first two sessions Jane talked about her various life experiences but found it hard to go into much depth. Amina followed her empathically and with an accepting presence, paying attention to the glimpses of emotion that were present. The following dialogue starts at the beginning of the third session. The accompanying commentary is in italics.

Amina: Hello Jane, thank you for completing the forms. Where would you like to start today?

Jane: Yeah, uh… [*Pause 9 seconds*] I'm actually not sure. I haven't really thought about it much. Things have been pretty much the same. I did go to work on Friday. Everyone seems okay. They were glad to see me back.

A: So things feel the same, more or less, although you did go back to the office and felt welcomed there.

J: Yeah. And my colleague Caroline asked if I wanted to go for a drink on Friday, but I didn't want to go, what with everything.

A: When you say everything…

J: Oh you know, just, er, everything I've talked about the last couple of weeks. It's a lot.

A: So all those things are weighing on you, and because of that you don't feel ready to socialise with Caroline.

J: That's right, yeah. That's right. [*Pause 8 seconds*]

A: You sounded quite calm, Jane, as you said that. But I'm wondering if perhaps I'm picking up some sadness as well?

Jane has been coming across as quite flat emotionally. As Amina focuses on the hint of sadness perceived in her voice, it's possible that Jane may become more aware of her emotional process.

J: Oh, I don't know, I guess, what with everything, I guess. I don't really know. It's hard to say.

Jane seems to be too distant from her emotions to be able to clearly acknowledge and work with them.

A: It's hard to talk about it when you don't really know what you're feeling. Is that right?

J: Yeah.

A: Can I make a suggestion? I want to ask you to try something. You can let me know if you'd rather not.

Amina decides to offer Jane a possible way to get closer to her emotions, using the process facilitation response known as clearing a space.

J: Okay. That's okay, go ahead.

A: First, if you could try to bring your awareness inside yourself. Take your time. Perhaps close your eyes if you wish.

J: Alright, I'm doing that.

A: So, try asking yourself if there's something getting in the way of you feeling okay right now. Let me know what comes up, if anything.

J: [*Pause 11 seconds*] Oh, I just thought of my sister.

A: And you sound concerned as you mention her.

Jane immediately seems more emotionally aroused. At this point, Amina could have asked Jane to put the concern over her sister somewhere safe and returned to her previous question to see if other concerns arise.

J: Well, I told you about the cancer last time, but I just had this really horrible memory. Must have been last November, after they knew it wasn't IBS, and they found something was blocking an ovary and that they needed to operate to remove it. I hadn't actually seen her for months, but I went to visit her in hospital after the operation and I was just shocked, she looked so ill. Just withdrawn and pale. It didn't look like her.

As Jane starts to talk with urgency about her sister, Amina abandons clearing a space and follows her client empathically.

A: You remember when you came in to see her at the hospital, it was a real shock to see her so pale and withdrawn, almost like it wasn't your sister.

J: [Wiping tears.] And then she told me they'd found cancer, and it was serious. I had to keep pulling myself together and act normal for her, even though I was feeling sick. I didn't want to think that she might die, but I didn't want her to see that.

A: That must have been so hard. Your reaction was so strong you were feeling physically sick, you were having thoughts that she might die, but you were trying to act normal and not let her see what was going on for you. And I can see the tears now as you recall that moment.

J: [*Cries for 30 seconds*] I had to be strong for her, but I was churning up inside. The worst was actually calling Mum afterwards to tell her the news. I had to hold it together, be strong on the phone, but afterwards I just collapsed.

A: That sounds so painful. You're just coming to terms with the news yourself, then having to tell Mum, and also needing to be strong for her, like you had to be strong also for your sister.

J: I've always been the strong one, I'm always reliable whatever happens, I'm solid. That's always been the case in our family.

This sounds to Amina a little like a meaning protest. It sounds like Jane is asserting a cherished belief about her being strong and solid whatever happens, while on the verge of acknowledging that this isn't always the case.

A: Your mum and sister can always rely on you. You're solid. That sounds really important to you.

Amina doesn't challenge Jane's belief, as this would be threatening to her self-structure. Instead, she maintains a respectful empathic presence in which Jane can feel safe to explore the belief under her own agency.

J: It sounds strange now because obviously I wasn't that strong. I was so upset, I collapsed and cried and didn't sleep that night after calling Mum, but nobody knows that. And look at me now, I haven't even told them I'm having counselling and might be depressed.

A: It's like you're acknowledging now that you're not always strong, you can feel low and be upset and have your own feelings, but somehow you can't let them see that.

J: [*Sighs*] I'm not always strong. I don't know why I can't tell them, I've just always been that person. I can't imagine telling them I'm not coping. I don't want them to have to worry about me.

A: You don't want them to know that you're not coping, so they don't have to worry about you.

J: No, I don't. And I'm not coping. Actually, I haven't told you this, but my sister and I have kind of fallen out. When I was trying to get her to have chemo, trying to protect her, I was just trying to help her. But around Christmas she just, well, lashed out, I guess. She was saying she wanted to live her life, she wanted to take each day and do things, and not feel like she was cooped up in a bubble. She was actually angry with me. It was so hard to hear.

In the rest of the session, and the next, Jane was able to explore her previously firm sense of being the strong, reliable sister and daughter. Gradually she was able to re-evaluate this and confront her reluctance to be open about her experience with her family and friends. Amina's close and genuine empathic responses helped Jane find a new way of understanding herself and how she had impacted those around her. This rebuilding of a shattered belief is known in PCE-CfD as *meaning creation* – a gentle and respectful collaborative process in which the client is fully engaged in finding and revising the new meaning.

Gurpreet and Matt

In our second case example we meet Gurpreet, a 27-year-old British Sikh woman who currently lives in the West Midlands with her husband, Ranveer. Her parents and brother live nearby, just two streets away, and Gurpreet describes the family as close-knit. After studying chemistry at university, Gurpreet worked as a lab technician, but was recently made redundant after her company went through a restructuring process. When her family and friends expressed concern over her low mood, Gurpreet decided to self-refer to her local NHS Talking Therapies service. Initially she was offered six sessions of PCE-CfD, but towards the end of these her PHQ-9 score had just started to improve a little. Following discussion, her therapist, Matt, was able to secure an additional six sessions. Matt graduated with a diploma in counselling on a person-centred course three years ago and worked in the voluntary sector before joining the NHS Talking Therapies service, where he works three days a week. He recently completed additional training in PCE-CfD. The extract below is from the middle of their eighth session, starting about eight minutes in. The example illustrates how empathic responses in PCE-CfD can help clients experience their emotions more fully, through their evocative and process-facilitative nature. Again, the commentary is in italics.

Gurpreet: So, it's like at that time, when I was that young, I think my older brother just knew what I needed and what was the right thing to do, and he would just kind of speak for me and I was happy for him to do that. And it's strange to think that's kind of what continued to happen at uni, just with other people, as I said before. And it's kind of what's also happening now. In a way, I'm still doing that now with Ranveer. It's like throughout my whole life I've just been waiting for other people to decide things for me, it's strange, I guess, I'm just becoming more aware of it.

Gurpreet is summarising her emerging appreciation of how she has avoided making decisions for herself in various contexts throughout her life to date.

Matt: You're starting to see this pattern more clearly. You can see it back in your childhood and all through to now, where you hold back from making choices or speaking up, and wait for others to take the lead, and it feels so strange now, in some way, just noticing this and thinking about it?

By picking up on the 'strangeness' felt by Gurpreet in expressing this broader understanding, Matt helps her to be more aware of her process and facilitate greater specificity in her appreciation and expression of her experience in the moment.

G: Yeah, like… uh, I've always been like this, and can see it now, it's so… obvious in a way, but somehow, I'm only just realising. It's like I'm looking at myself and noticing these things. I never… like to upset people or go against their plans.

M: So it's easier to just let them decide, because then you don't risk upsetting them, which might feel uncomfortable, or, I don't know if this is right, a little scary maybe?

Matt picks up on the way Gurpreet says she never likes to upset people, her tone of voice and general expression, to get a sense of her underlying feelings beneath her narrative at this point, attempting to approach her core meanings in this empathic response.

G: Yes, exactly. I am really afraid that, if I choose, then maybe I'll get it wrong. And I think then it'll be my fault because I got it wrong. If the other person decides, then whatever, it doesn't matter. I think that's why that happens a lot in my relationship. I don't take control of what we're actually doing day-to-day, sort of thing. Even just things like what time we get up and what time to go to bed. I don't say, 'Oh I'm getting tired, shall we go to bed,' I'll always wait for Ranveer to say.

M: You might be sitting there actually feeling tired, maybe you want to go to sleep and consider suggesting this, but you don't dare to actually say it in case you get it wrong somehow, like if Ranveer wants to stay up later? I can really sense that fear, it feels so powerful, it's so much safer just to let him decide.

Matt is paying close attention to the emotional aspects inherent both explicitly and implicitly in Gurpreet's communication. This emotion focus allows him to make an empathic conjecture about the strength and role of fear for the client here.

G: Yes, I remember when I have made mistakes before, like, when navigating in the car and I've made us take a wrong turn and it's added lots of time to the journey, and I just feel so bad. I withdraw and kind of freeze and feel really small. So then, instead of saying 'Right, we've gone the wrong way, let's fix it by going this way, let's get back on track,' I just get tongue tied and I don't know why, and Ranveer has to pull over and look at the map himself. Then he gets frustrated and, well, annoyed with me.

M: He gets annoyed after you've made a wrong turn. You feel so bad and it sounds like you go into this place, this state where you're frozen and feeling small and can't speak up clearly and say what you want to say. And at the same time Ranveer is frustrated with you. It's petrifying?

Matt recognises the description of possible trauma-related dissociation but places this awareness to one side as he wants to stay empathically attuned with the client's unique and rich experience, avoiding any labelling that may take something away from this. He also senses a possible significance in how Gurpreet mentions her husband's frustration and annoyance.

G: Exactly, that's the fear. [*Silence for 16 seconds*] I get like that in different situations. Actually, I got a bit like it just yesterday thinking about the job and the interview. It's been over a week now and I still haven't heard from them. If I don't get it, I don't know what I'll do. I keep looking for other jobs but there's so little around here right now. Oh… I feel like such a failure sometimes.

M: It's so difficult, it's like you're running out of options, the opportunities aren't there, you're worried you may not have got this one, it just feels like you've failed. And, while thinking about this yesterday, you found yourself with that familiar fear?

The client has shifted focus to the job interview that was discussed in previous sessions. Matt tracks this, trying to stay in her frame of reference and picking up on the sense of distress and failure.

G: It was after I tried talking to Ranveer about it in the kitchen. [*Tearing up*] I think he, he would be happy, you know, if I was a sort of housewife. That's what he told me, that I didn't really have to have a job, I could look after the cleaning, laundry, cooking sort of thing. And it was after that that, yes, I felt… that feeling.

M: You were there in the kitchen, trying to tell him about your concerns, when he started saying you didn't have to worry about it because you could be a housewife, and it felt like he was almost, I don't know, welcoming or almost encouraging you to consider this? Like he wants that for you? And then…

This evocative empathic response allows Gurpreet to stay connected with the details of her recollection and reflect on her related feelings, noticing what comes up. It is facilitative of her process.

G: That's the thing. The truth is, I really, really, really don't want that for me. [*Starts crying, pause 12 seconds*] I – I want to keep working… at my job… it's really important. I'd even consider moving to London or somewhere where there are more options. But here's the thing, I can't imagine ever being able to say that to him.

M: 'I want to keep working…' There's a real sense of anger as you say that.

Matt clearly senses anger and brings this into his response, thereby helping Gurpreet maintain her emotion regulation at a level where she can continue to process her feelings.

G: I mean why can't I…? Yes, I am angry, with him and also with… myself, for being so weak. Why can't I stand up for myself?

M: You're able here and now to say how you truly feel, but when you're with him, it's like your confidence just falls away, and right now you feel so angry with yourself for not being stronger.

G: You know, sometimes I look at myself in the mirror and it's almost like 'Who is that?' Almost like I feel disgusted with myself.

The above extract shows Matt following Gurpreet with a consistent empathic presence. A lot of elements are coming into play, with various new or revised understandings emerging for Gurpreet as she faces her painful feelings, thoughts and memories. The point here is that sometimes a consistent and deep empathic attunement can be highly facilitative of a client's process, and for some clients this can be as helpful as other forms of process-facilitation responses. At various points in this example, Matt could have chosen to suggest a different approach, such as systematic evocative unfolding or dialogue with a significant other or between aspects of herself. Sensing that this might disrupt Gurpreet's flow, he instead maintains a solid and attentive empathic connection as she unfolds her experiencing.

Training

Following the development of a CfD curriculum (Hill, 2011b), training in PCE-CfD has been offered as continuing professional development to qualified counsellors with a background in humanistic counselling and the person-centred approach. The course is currently offered at four sites across England, and includes a five-day programme, following which trainees engage in course-specific PCE-CfD supervision and must log 80 client hours using the approach. Recorded sessions are submitted for assessment, four of which must reach the threshold for adherence to the model in order to gain the qualification. Training sites often offer additional 'refresher' days, or similar, throughout the year, which are open to current trainees. Supervision of PCE-CfD practice requires a highly specialised understanding and appreciation of the approach, and a dedicated training is offered in PCE-CfD supervision. Supervisors take a partly pedagogical approach, reviewing recordings with trainees and helping them select ones to submit for assessment.

Recordings submitted during this training are assessed using a standardised tool: the Person-Centred and Experiential Psychotherapy Scale (PCEPS-10) (Freire et al., 2014; Westwell, 2018). Originally developed for the purpose of assessing the fidelity of PCE therapy interventions in randomised controlled trials (RCTs), the version used in this training is scored over 10 items: client frame of reference/track, psychological holding, experiential specificity, accepting presence, content directiveness, emotion focus, dominant or overpowering presence, clarity of language, core meaning and emotion regulation sensitivity. Each item is scored from 1–6, and an overall score of 40 or more indicates that the assessed recording has reached adherence to the PCE-CfD model.

Most therapists taking the training are already employed in NHS Talking Therapies services – environments where CBT approaches and medical-model thinking are dominant. In the words of two experienced PCE-CfD trainers (Proctor & Hayes, 2017): 'Regardless of initial qualification, most therapists attending the training have been influenced heavily by a solution-focused, outcome driven, toolbox-based approach to therapy' (p.4). A consequence of this is that training must allow trainees to reorient themselves back towards a person-centred stance and affiliation with the attitudes associated with the approach.

Drewitt and colleagues (2018) surveyed and interviewed PCE-CfD trainees and found that participants were positive about the model and five-day training, but sometimes perceived a lack of understanding and support from their employing service. Nye and colleagues (2019) explored the experiences of counsellors who trained in PCE-CfD within their IAPT service, and identified factors affecting their completion of the training, such as flexibility and readiness to change. Views of PCE-CfD tutors have been reported by Haake and colleagues (2021), indicating some apparent differences in approach between training centres, as well as highlighting the tensions between the individualism of the person-centred approach and the standardisation expected by IAPT.

As reported earlier in this chapter, a new development is the piloting of a three-year professional training in PCE-CfD funded by the NHS. Students work for between two and three days per week alongside their course in an NHS Talking Therapies service and are paid a full-time salary throughout. This matches the existing NHS-funded training offered to CBT practitioners who wish to train to work in NHS Talking Therapies and is intended to increase access to counselling in NHS primary care. The scheme, currently being piloted at Metanoia Institute, leads (on successful completion) to the award of a postgraduate diploma in high-intensity psychotherapeutic counselling.

Research

There has been a growing body of research of relevance to PCE-CfD. For more than a decade now, the NHS has published detailed annual reports of IAPT/NHS Talking Therapies datasets, including information about the different types of therapy offered for specific conditions. These data have been analysed in a number of studies comparing CBT and counselling as practised in IAPT/NHS Talking Therapy services in relation to the treatment of depression. Two studies used multilevel modelling to assess the variability of effectiveness in terms of outcomes for both modalities (Pybis et al., 2017; Saxon et al., 2017). The findings indicate that, in practical terms, counselling is as effective as CBT for people routinely accessing NHS psychological therapies for the treatment of both moderate and severe depression. Barkham and colleagues (2017) reviewed and discussed the evidence base relevant to the NICE guidelines for depression, including meta-analyses and randomised controlled trials (RCTs), and argued for the inclusion of a broader range of sources of evidence, such as the practice-based studies using the IAPT datasets. Indeed, the value of RCTs for psychological therapies is affected by the impossibility of single or double-blinding therapeutic interventions in trials, and both therapist and client expectations cannot be separated from other factors contributing to the outcomes (Evans & Carlyle, 2021). A qualitative research study has examined clients' perspectives of the effectiveness of PCE-CfD (Goldman et al., 2016). Participants found the therapy helpful, reporting that they felt understood and able to work through issues within the counselling relationship, although some disliked the limit on the numbers of sessions.

An important quantitative study is the PRaCTICED trial: a pragmatic, randomised non-inferiority trial that examined whether PCE-CfD is cost-effective and comparable with CBT in the treatment of moderate and severe depression within an IAPT service in Sheffield (Barkham et al., 2021). This was a relatively large study, randomly assigning 510 participants to receive either CBT or PCE-CfD (described as Person-Centred Experiential Therapy (PCET)) and had a balanced researcher allegiance. The PCEPS-10 was used to ensure the PCE-CfD therapists in the trial were adhering to the model, and PHQ-9 scores were used to determine the outcomes. The results supported the hypothesis that PCE-CfD was not inferior to CBT in terms of changes in PHQ-9 scores at six months post-randomisation. However, at 12 months, the 95% confidence interval did exceed the non-inferiority margin, indicating that in this trial PCE-CfD was slightly less effective than CBT on this measure at this time point. It is worth noting that the analyses were made at six and 12 months following the randomisation of the participants, rather than following the completion of the course of therapy. Following randomisation, participants did not begin therapy immediately; they waited varying lengths of time for their first session and then had between four and 20 therapy sessions spread over varying timescales, meaning that the data analysis time points of six and 12 months post-randomisation were not consistent between clients in relation to the start or end of their therapy. It is not known whether a different choice for 'time zero' would have led to different results.

Conclusions

In this chapter, we have described the theory and current practice of PCE-CfD, presenting it as being at odds with the medicalised environment in which it is most commonly practised. The continued development of this therapy and training of practitioners has secured, at least for the time being, a place for the PCE approach within the publicly-funded healthcare system in England. The combination is perhaps not a comfortable fit, and some will question if it is possible to maintain the integrity of the person-centred paradigm within the NHS. Others may value the availability of a form of person-centred therapy free at the point of access, and the training and employment opportunities for counsellors that come with this. The research studies providing evidence to support the approach are gradually growing in number, although still far behind the wealth of trial data supporting some other therapy modalities – most notably, CBT. If PCE-CfD is to survive and have a healthy future, further research will be needed. A broader cultural transformation in our understanding of the nature of psychological distress may be possible, if PCE therapists working with the system can hold onto the approach and effect change from within.

Resources

- The BACP *Manual for the Selection, Training and Supervision of Counsellors in the IAPT Programme* is available at www.bacp.co.uk/media/5751/iapt-pce-cfd-national-curriculum.pdf
- Murphy, D. (2019). *Person-centred experiential counselling for depression* (2nd ed.). Sage. The revised and updated edition of the first book on the topic (Sanders & Hill, 2014).
- The Person-Centred and Experiential Psychotherapy Scale (PCEPS-10) (Freire et al., 2014) can be downloaded from the BACP website at: www.bacp.co.uk/media/5752/pceps-therapy-adherence-scale.pdf
- The UCL *Counselling for Depression Competence Framework* can found downloaded from the UCL website at: www.ucl.ac.uk/pals/research/clinical-educational-and-health-psychology/research-groups/core/competence-frameworks-7

References

American Psychiatric Association. (APA). (2013). *Diagnostic and statistical manual of mental disorders* (5th ed.) (DSM-5). APA.

Baker, N. (2012). Experiential person-centred therapy. In P. Sanders (Ed.), *The tribes of the person-centred nation: An introduction to the schools of therapy related to the person-centred approach* (2nd ed.) (pp.71–102). PCCS Books

Barkham, M., Moller, N.P. & Pybis, J. (2017). How should we evaluate research on counselling and the treatment of depression? A case study on how the National Institute for Health and Care Excellence's draft 2018 guideline for depression considered what counts as best evidence. *Counselling Psychotherapy Research, 17*(4), 253–268.

Barkham, M., Saxon, D., Hardy, G.E., Bradburn, M., Galloway, D., Wickramasekera, N., Keetharuth, A.D., Bower, P., King, M., Elliott, R., Gabriel, L., Kellett, S., Shaw, S., Wilkinson, T., Connell, J., Harrison, P., Ardern, K., Bishop-Edwards, L., Ashley, K., Ohlsen, S, Pilling, S., Waller, G & Brazier, J.E. (2021). Person-centred experiential therapy versus cognitive behavioural therapy delivered in the English Improving Access to Psychological Therapies service for the treatment of moderate or severe depression (PRaCTICED): a pragmatic randomised, non-inferiority trial. *Lancet Psychiatry, 8*(6), 487-499.

Centre for Economic Performance Mental Health Policy Group (CEPMHPG). (2006). *The depression report: A new deal for depression and anxiety disorders*. London School of Economics and Political Science.

Drewitt, L., Pybis, J., Murphy, D. & Barkham, M. (2018). Practitioners' experiences of learning and implementing Counselling for Depression (CfD) in routine practice settings. *Counselling & Psychotherapy Research, 18*, 3–13.

Elliott, R. & Greenberg, L. (2021). Emotion-focused counselling in action. Sage.

Elliott, R., Watson, J.C., Goldman, R.N. & Greenberg, L.S. (2004). *Learning emotion-focused therapy: The process-experiential approach to change*. American Psychological Association.

Evans, C. & Carlyle, J. (2021). *Outcome measures and evaluation in counselling and psychotherapy*. Sage.

Freire, E., Elliott, R. & Westwell, G. (2014). Person-Centred and Experiential Psychotherapy scale (PCEPS): Development and reliability of an adherence/ competence measure for person-centred and experiential psychotherapies. *Counselling & Psychotherapy Research, 14*, 220–226.

Gendlin, E.T. (1962). *Experiencing and the creation of meaning: A philosophical and psychological approach to the subjective*. Free Press of Glencoe.

Gendlin, E.T. (1978). *Focusing*. Bantam.

Goldman, S., Brettle, A. & McAndrew, S. (2016). A client-focused perspective of the effectiveness of Counselling for Depression (CfD). *Counselling & Psychotherapy Research, 16*, 288–297.

Greenberg, L.S. (1984). A task analysis of intrapersonal conflict resolution. In L.N. Rice & L.S. Greenberg (Eds.), *Patterns of change: Intensive analysis of psychotherapy process* (pp. 67–123). Guilford Press.

Greenberg, L.S. & Safran, J. (1989). Emotion in psychotherapy. *American Psychologist, 44*(1), 19–29.

Haake, R., Hardy, G.E. & Barkham, M. (2021). Person-centred experiential therapy: Perceptions of trainers and developers. *Counselling & Psychotherapy Research, 21*, 460– 470.

Health Education England (2023). *NHS Talking Therapies for Anxiety and Depression workforce census national report.* www.hee.nhs.uk/sites/default/files/documents/HEE%20NHS%20Talking%20Therapies%20for%20Anxiety%20and%20Depression%20Workforce%20Census%202022%20-%20National%20Report.pdf

Higgins, E.T. (1987). Self-discrepancy: A theory relating self and affect. *Psychological Review, 94*, 319–340.

Hill, A. (2011a). *The competences required to deliver effective Counselling for Depression (CfD).* University College London. www.ucl.ac.uk/clinical-psychology//CORE/Counselling_for_depression/Counselling%20for%20depression%20clinician's%20guide.pdf

Hill, A. (2011b). *Curriculum for Counselling for Depression: Continuing professional development for qualified therapists delivering high intensity interventions.* National IAPT Programme Team.

Levitt, B.E. (2019). *Questioning psychology.* PCCS Books.

Mearns, D. (1999). Person-centred therapy with configurations of the self. *Counselling, 10*(2), 125–130.

Moncrieff, J., Cooper, R.E., Stockmann, T., Amendola, S., Hengartner, M.P. & Horowitz, M.A. (2022). The serotonin theory of depression: A systematic umbrella review of the evidence. *Molecular Psychiatry, 28*, 3243–3256. https://doi.org/10.1038/s41380-022-01661-0

Morriss, R., Tyrer, F., Zaccardi, F. & Khunti, K. (2021). Safety of antidepressants in a primary care cohort of adults with obesity and depression. *PLoS ONE, 16*(1), e0245722.

Murphy, D. (2017). Person-centred experiential counselling psychology. In: D. Murphy (Ed.), *Counselling psychology: A textbook for study and practice* (pp.72–87). John Wiley & Sons.

Murphy, D. (2019). *Person-centred experiential counselling for depression* (2nd ed.). Sage.

National Collaborating Centre for Mental Health. (2023). *The Improving Access to Psychological Therapies manual, version 6.* NHS England. https://www.england.nhs.uk/publication/the-improving-access-to-psychological-therapies-manual

National Institute for Clinical Excellence. (2004). *Depression: Management of depression in primary and secondary care.* Clinical guideline 23. National Institute for Health and Clinical Excellence.

National Institute for Health and Clinical Excellence. (2009). *Depression: Treatment and management of depression in adults.* Clinical guideline 90. National Institute for Health and Clinical Excellence.

National Institute for Health and Care Excellence. (2022). *Depression in adults: Treatment and management.* NICE guideline NG222. NICE. www.nice.org.uk/guidance/ng222

Nye, A., Connell, J., Haake, R. & Barkham, M. (2019). Person-centred experiential therapy (PCET) training within a UK NHS IAPT service: Experiences of selected counsellors in the PRaCTICED trial. *British Journal of Guidance & Counselling, 47*(5), 619–634.

Pybis J., Saxon, D., Hill, A. & Barkham M. (2017). The comparative effectiveness and efficiency of cognitive behaviour therapy of depression: Evidence from the 2nd UK National Audit of psychological therapies. *BMC Psychiatry, 17*, 215.

Proctor, G. & Hayes, C. (2017). Counselling for Depression: A response to counselling education in the twenty-first century. Ethical conflicts for a counselling approach operating within a medicalised bureaucratic health service. *British Journal of Guidance & Counselling, 45*(4), 417–426.

Rogers, C.R. (1951). *Client-centered therapy: Its current practice, implication and theory.* Houghton Mifflin.

Rogers, C.R. (1957a). A note on the nature of man. *Journal of Consulting Psychology, 4*(3), 199–203.

Rogers, C.R. (1957b). The necessary and sufficient conditions of therapeutic personality change. *Journal of Consulting Psychology, 21*(2), 95–103.

Rogers, C.R. (1959). A theory of therapy, personality, and interpersonal relationships as developed in the client-centered framework. In: S. Koch (Ed.), *Psychology: A study of a science. Vol. 3: Formulations of the person and the social context* (pp.184–256). McGraw-Hill.

Rogers, C.R. (1961). *On becoming a person: A therapist's view of psychotherapy*. Constable.

Rogers, C.R. (1963). The actualizing tendency in relation to 'motives' and to consciousness. In: M. Jones (Ed.), *Nebraska symposium on motivation* (pp.1–24). University of Nebraska Press.

Rogers, C.R. (1976). Interview with Anthony Clare. *All in the Mind*. BBC Radio.

Roth, A., Hill, A. & Pilling, S. (2009). *The competences required to deliver effective humanistic psychological therapies.* University College London. www.ucl.ac.uk/pals/research/clinical-educational-and-health-psychology/research-groups/core/competence-frameworks-4

Sanders, P. (2017). Principled and strategic opposition to the medicalisation of distress and all its apparatus. In S. Joseph (Ed.), *The handbook of person-centred therapy and mental health: Theory, research and practice* (pp.11–38). PCCS Books.

Sanders, P. & Hill, A. (2014). *Counselling for depression: A person-centred and experiential approach to practice.* Sage.

Saxon, D., Firth, N. & Barkham, M. (2017). The relationship between therapist effects and therapy delivery factors: Therapy modality, dosage, and non-completion. *Administration and Policy in Mental Health and Mental Health Services Research, 44*(5), 705–715.

Spitzer, R.L., Kroenke, K., Williams, J.B.W. & Löwe, B. (2006). A brief measure for assessing generalized anxiety disorder: The GAD-7. *Archives of Internal Medicine, 166*(10), 1092–1097.

Tudor, K. & Worrall, M. (2006). *Person-centred therapy: A clinical philosophy*. Routledge.

Watson, N., Bryan, B.C. & Thrash, T.M. (2010). Self-discrepancy: Comparisons of the psychometric properties of three instruments. *Psychological Assessment, 22*(4), 878–892.

Westwell, G. (2018). *Articulating person-centred experiential practice: The development of the PCEPS-10. A competence/adherence measure for PCE therapy*. Paper presented at PCE 2018, Conference of the World Association for the Person-Centered and Experiential Psychotherapies and Counselling, Vienna, July.

Wilkins, P. (2019). Assessment and 'diagnosis' in person-centred therapy. In: Joseph, S. (Ed.) *The handbook of person-centred therapy and mental health: Theory, research and practice* (pp.134–153). PCCS Books.

7. Motivational interviewing

William R. Miller

In the footsteps of Carl Rogers

Motivational interviewing (MI) arose from a series of happenstance events. My clinical psychology training was at the University of Oregon, where the programme was strongly committed to behaviour therapy at a time when even cognitive therapy was controversial. Oregon required a preparatory two-semester seminar on how to talk with clients, and in 1972 none of the behaviourist clinicians chose to teach it, so they reached across the campus to the counselling psychology faculty to find an instructor. They chose Susan Gilmore, a student of Leona Tyler and thus an academic grandchild of Carl Rogers, and she introduced us to a person-centred approach (PCA) to therapeutic relationship. Thus, I was developing skills in accurate empathy before I ever sat down in a therapist's chair, for which I am profoundly grateful. Once I began practising cognitive-behaviour therapy (CBT), I naturally did so in a person-centred way, with a humanistic rather than behaviouristic orientation.

When I joined the clinical faculty at the University of New Mexico in 1976, I was already studying therapies to help people change alcohol use behaviours. Having no external funding for research, I was training our psychology students to be the therapists in a series of clinical trials. I coached them in empathic listening skills as well as the specific behavioural procedures that we were studying. I also began teaching a required first-year seminar for our clinical students on the person-centred approach (PCA) as a foundation for doing psychotherapy – a course I would continue teaching until I retired in 2006.

In one clinical trial, three supervisors independently observed the nine therapists treating people who were struggling to manage their alcohol consumption. We documented the specific behavioural procedures used by the therapists and also rated their listening skills using the accurate empathy rating scale developed by Truax and Carkhuff (1976). When treatment was done and we had collected our follow-up data, we analysed predictors of subsequent alcohol use. There were no differences based on the length and types of behaviour therapy we were comparing, but the quality of therapists' empathic listening accounted for two-thirds of the variance (*r*=.81) in clients' likelihood of continued drinking six months after treatment (Miller et al., 1980), and this predictive relationship remained significant at 12 and 24 months (Miller & Baca, 1983).

With these unexpected findings in hand, I took a first sabbatical leave in 1982 to work at an alcoholism hospital – the Hjellestad Clinic near Bergen, Norway – lecturing on behavioural treatment of alcohol disorders. The medical director asked if I would also be willing to meet periodically with their psychologists and social workers, many of whom were recent graduates, and I gladly agreed. They were treating patients with fairly severe alcohol problems, and they wanted me not only to teach them about my approach but also to demonstrate it. I was teaching both empathic listening and behaviour therapy, and they would role-play (fortunately for me, in English) the patients they were seeing that they found challenging. I was surprised when, unlike my American students, they began interrupting me in mid-interview to ask thoughtful questions:

'You asked the client a question just now, but you could have asked about many different topics. Why did you choose that particular question?'

'You just reflected something that the client said. Of all the things he said, why did you reflect that part?'

'The client seems to be resisting; why didn't you push harder on that subject?'

'How do you decide what you're going to ask or reflect?'

In the process, we discovered some decision rules that I seemed to be using, but of which I had been unaware:

- Ambivalence about change is normal – it's a balancing of conflicting motivations.
- It should be the client rather than the counsellor who voices the arguments for change.
- Don't push back if you feel resistance, but listen to it.
- Believe in clients' wisdom and ability to choose a positive path, given sufficient support.
- Affirmation strengthens client self-esteem and self-efficacy.
- Reflective listening is not passive mirroring but selectively shines light on particular aspects of what clients say.

We were, in essence, mirroring the early steps of Carl Rogers and his colleagues, paying close attention to the practice of counselling in order to develop testable hypotheses about underlying processes that influence client outcomes (Kirschenbaum, 2009).

I was particularly interested in hearing clients' self-motivational statements regarding change, which we later termed 'change talk'. These are indications of the person's own desire, ability, reasons, need and willingness to change. We consciously arranged conversations to invite such change talk from clients. I wrote up what Rogers called an informal 'discussion paper' describing the method and mailed it to several colleagues for comments. One was Ray Hodgson in Cardiff, Wales, who replied, to my surprise, that he would like to publish it as an article in the journal he edited, *Behavioural Psychotherapy*. I sent him a reduced manuscript and he sent it to a young colleague named Steve Rollnick for anonymous review. The article was accepted and appeared in print the following year as the first published description of motivational interviewing (MI) (Miller, 1983). Seven years later, on a second sabbatical leave in Sydney, Australia, I met Steve Rollnick, who also happened to be at the National Drug and Alcohol Research Centre, doing research on smoking cessation. He encouraged me to write more about the method and we decided to co-author the first MI text (Miller & Rollnick, 1991).

Subsequent research found that clients' in-session change talk does predict positive change during and after treatment. This is true in MI and in other therapies, such as CBT (Lombardi et al., 2014; Moyers et al., 2007). It is also the case that clients' expressed arguments for the status quo (which we later termed 'sustain talk') predict that less change will occur (Magill et al., 2018, 2019). Actually, it is the ratio of change talk to sustain talk that best predicts outcome: the more clients themselves argue for rather than against change, the more likely it is that change will occur. It makes sense clinically that clients who sound 'motivated' are more likely to get better, but it's not just a matter of their spontaneous motivation. Therapists strongly influence how much change talk versus sustain talk clients will express. In correlational, longitudinal and experimental studies, therapists can increase or decrease this motivational ratio by what they ask, reflect, affirm and summarise. In other words, it matters what clients say during treatment sessions, and therapists strongly influence it.

A close parallel in PCA research is clients' experiencing (Gendlin, 1961) as measured from what they say during therapy sessions (see Chapter 4, this volume). Clients who express high experiencing tend to show more positive change during and after various kinds of therapy, and their level of experiencing is influenced by therapist responses (Rogers et al., 1967; Wiser & Goldfried, 1998).

Is it proper to use therapeutic skills intentionally to influence what clients will say and experience during treatment sessions? This departs from a classic 'non-directive' perspective on counselling and psychotherapy (see Chapter 2, this volume). However, whether aware of it or not, therapists do influence what clients will say and experience. Rogers himself responded differentially to client content (Truax, 1966). You can never exactly mirror all that a client has said, and it matters what you choose to ask, reflect, affirm and include in summaries. If that is so, and if what clients say and experience during sessions predicts better (or worse) outcomes, then is it ethical not to be aware of and use this knowledge therapeutically?

Kirschenbaum (2009) reports that, in the late 1940s, Rogers:

> began to avoid the term 'nondirective' and to use the 'client-centred' label almost exclusively.... He also realized that nondirective was a 'term of rebellion.... saying what we were against' and did not capture the essence of the approach, which was adopting the client's frame of reference. (p.163)

MI very much seeks to understand a dilemma from the person's frame of reference.

My own perspective on direction has surely been influenced by working primarily in addiction treatment. Psychotherapists recognise that it can be difficult to make much progress on other issues while clients are still dependent on addictive substances or behaviours. When there is a substantial obstacle to someone's wellness and growth, would not a person-centred counsellor help them remove it when it is possible to do so (Miller & Brown, 1997; Miller et al., 2019)? Yet the term 'directive' misrepresents the relational foundation of PCAs, including MI. How can important therapeutic goals be reconciled with a PCA?

It is helpful, I think, to distinguish between being directive and having a conscious direction in counselling and psychotherapy. In the latter case, most therapists hope for clients to change or move in some beneficial way during counselling. A strong working alliance is widely recognised as important in psychotherapy, and its quality consistently predicts client outcomes (Graßmann et al., 2020; Horvath & Symonds, 1991). A key element of a working alliance is having shared goals toward which to move; indeed, how could treatment efficacy be determined without understanding what therapy is meant to effect? I benefitted from working in addiction treatment, where at least some treatment goals seem clear and can be a matter of life and death. You probably haven't done much for clients with substance use disorders if there has been no change in substance use. Having clear goals and a conscious plan for moving towards them is one characteristic of more effective psychotherapists (Miller & Moyers, 2021). In addiction treatment, that typically includes reduction in substance use and related harm. Thus, we began describing MI as person-centred and directional rather than directive (cf. Cooper, 2019).

MI has been criticised as being too atheoretical, although it has been assimilated and combined with various theoretical perspectives (e.g. Christopher & Dougher, 2009; Engle & Arkowitz, 2006; Markland et al., 2005). Like PCA itself, MI did not begin with a theory but by paying close attention to practice and forming testable hypotheses (Kirschenbaum, 2009). Also like PCA, MI is being applied in a wide variety of different languages and cultures and in many fields beyond psychotherapy, including criminal justice, education, health care, leadership, pastoral care and social work. MI includes both interpersonal and technical elements (Miller & Rose, 2009), and the relational component overlaps substantially with core PCA skills that characterise more effective helpers, such as accurate empathy, positive regard and acceptance (Miller & Moyers, 2021).

The practice of motivational interviewing

MI has evolved considerably in the 40 years since it was first described. The first edition of our text (Miller & Rollnick, 1991) centred on addictive behaviours. By the second edition in 2002, MI was already being used in health care and other areas, and so we focused more broadly on preparing people for change. The third edition, in 2013, was no longer just about preparing people for change and introduced the four component processes of MI described below. We placed greater emphasis on the underlying attitude or spirit with which MI is practised, deconstructed the concept of resistance, and introduced new psycholinguistic research on change talk. Then, in 2023, we again completely rewrote the fourth edition (Miller & Rollnick, 2023), describing MI as a way to help people change and grow and incorporating a still larger range of research and areas of application.

MI is a particular way of having constructive conversations about change. Not all counselling and psychotherapy is about change, except in the broadest sense. Sometimes clients are struggling with making a choice, finding meaning in their lives or coping with the chaos of a crisis (Gilmore, 1973). MI has always been primarily about helping people make positive changes in their lives.

The spirit of motivational interviewing

When we began teaching MI in 1991, we soon noticed a problem. Students were using techniques we had described, but as we watched them practise, it felt wrong. It was as if they had learnt the words but not the music. It wasn't their fault; obviously we had left out something important in our teaching, which was the underlying mindset or 'heartset' with which MI is practised. We came to call this 'the spirit of MI,' paralleling what Rogers described as therapeutic attitudes underlying PCA and later as 'a way of being' (Rogers, 1980; Rollnick & Miller, 1995). In our current understanding, we describe this guiding spirit as having four inter-related components:

1. Partnership

Like PCA more generally, MI is a collaborative approach. It is like dancing, not wrestling. The counsellor is not an expert on their clients' lives; they draw on their clients' own expertise about themselves. When the topic of conversation is someone's life, you need their expertise. MI is not about fixing people but helping them to change and grow using their own wisdom and resources. Rather than a therapist implying 'I have what you need, and I'm going to give it to you' (such as insight, rational thought or behavioural skills), the MI practitioner conveys, 'You have what you need, and together we will find it.' Clients bring personal strengths and capabilities to a therapeutic relationship, and you are a companion on the journey.

2. Acceptance

MI starts with and accepts people as they are. Non-judgemental acceptance is widely recognised and empirically demonstrated as a healing factor in helping relationships (Farber et al., 2019). Clients are prized and do not need to earn our respect. In MI we encounter the same paradox that Rogers observed: that when people experience being accepted as they are, it becomes possible for them to change. Acceptance first requires being actively interested in and understanding a person's own experience and frame of reference, without judging.

3. Compassion

We mean here not sympathy but empathy, a benevolent intention to do no harm and to promote the other's wellbeing and happiness. Any method of interpersonal influence can potentially be used in a self-serving manner. MI is not a way of getting people to do what you want them to do. The prime directive is the client's health and best interest.

4. Empowerment

Empowering doesn't mean bestowing on people some power that they didn't have before, but rather helping them to recognise and use what they do have – their own wisdom and strengths. A starting perspective is that clients already have much of the motivation and capability that they need, and your task is to evoke it – to call it forth. MI also honours people's autonomy – their ability and right to choose their own way. Autonomy is not merely recognised but actively encouraged and supported. To honour clients' autonomy is to let go of a power that we never had in the first place.

Four tasks in motivational interviewing

Although we began with a set of five principles (Miller & Rollnick, 1991), since our third edition we have instead described four component tasks, or processes, in MI. These are like stair steps toward change, each building on the foundation of the preceding tasks. They may sound linear: first you engage, then you focus, next you evoke, and finally you plan. In fact, they are recursive: MI involves flexibly moving back and forth on the staircase, observing closely and responding in the moment to the client's experience. Each of the four tasks addresses an underlying question in the therapeutic relationship.

1. Engaging

The engaging task is second nature for PCA practitioners. In this first task of MI, the metaphoric question is, 'Can we take a walk together? Can we go on a journey together?' Engaging is about establishing a relationship of mutual trust and respect, and the basic interpersonal skills are familiar in PCA: asking open questions, affirming clients' strengths and positive efforts, reflecting with accurate empathy, and summarising. From the first contact, MI is person-centred, seeking to understand clients' experience from their own perspective.

2. Focusing

The focusing task involves arriving at shared goals, an agreed set of intentions toward which counselling will move (note that this differs from Gendlin's use of 'focusing' in Chapter 4, this volume). As stated earlier, this is a central element of a working therapeutic alliance that, when measured, predicts client satisfaction, retention and outcome. The underlying question in focusing is, 'Where are we going?' This is the directional aspect of MI. It explores the topics to be discussed and clarifies what the client and therapist intend to accomplish together. Sometimes these mutual goals are informed by the context – in a smoking cessation or pain management clinic, for example. In general practice, focusing is often a gradual process that begins with presenting concerns and clarifies goals and direction for counselling. This often becomes an ongoing process as mutual aims evolve over time.

3. Evoking

The evoking process has been most distinctive and well-developed in MI. As New Year resolutions illustrate, the setting of goals is often insufficient in itself. What are the person's own motivations for this change or growth? Here the counsellor invites clients to voice their own motivations for change, keeping in mind some common forms of change talk:

- *Desire.* What does the person want to happen? Some frequent words used to express desire are 'I want', 'wish', 'would like', or 'hope'.
- *Ability.* This kind of change talk bespeaks the client's perceived ability to accomplish the change, sometimes called self-efficacy. Common words here are 'I can', 'could', or 'am able to'.
- *Reason.* In responding to a question like 'Why would you choose to do this?', people might voice particular reasons for change, which are often expressed in an if–then format. You could ask, 'What are the three best reasons for you to do this?'
- *Need.* Another natural kind of change talk is imperative language that implies importance or urgency without necessarily saying why. Some common forms are 'I have to', 'have got to' and 'must'.

These first four types we call preparatory change talk. It's how people consider or get ready when talking to themselves or others. The other three we call mobilising change talk, and they signal getting closer to actually taking action:

- *Commitment.* This type of change talk is how people make agreements or promises verbally. Just because people say that they want to, could, have good reasons for, or must do something does not mean that they will. Some typical language of commitment includes 'I will', 'am going', 'promise'.
- *Activation.* These are almost commitment, but not quite – 'I'm willing to', 'will consider', 'plan to', 'intend to'. They imply inclination but not exactly commitment to do it. 'I'll try' indicates some desire or willingness plus doubt about ability.
- *Taking steps.* Sometimes clients tell you about things they have already done that are steps on the way to change. 'I poured away all the alcohol in the house', 'filled that prescription you gave me', 'bought a pair of running shoes'. These are successive approximations to the intended change.

A basic skill in MI, then, is asking open questions to which the natural answer is change talk:

- What do you want or hope to do? (Desire)
- How might you go about it in order to succeed, knowing what you do about yourself? (Ability)
- What are some good reasons for you to do it? (Reasons)
- How important would you say it is for you to do this? (Need)
- What are you willing to do? (Activation)
- What have you already done to move in this direction? (Taking steps)

- What do you think you will do? (Commitment)

MI is not about asking these or other clever questions. These are just examples of invitations to be followed with good empathic listening, affirmation and summaries of change talk.

In evoking, it matters what you ask. In general, at least after a good start on engaging, an MI practitioner usually avoids asking questions such as those listed below during the evoking process:

- Why haven't you already done this?
- What's wrong with doing it?
- What do you like so much about the way things are now?

The expected answer to such questions would be sustain talk. Don't go fishing for sustain talk, but when it occurs spontaneously, listen to it.

It also matters what you choose to reflect. Change talk and sustain talk often come intermixed, even in the same sentence or paragraph. People are normally ambivalent about change. Suppose a client said to you: 'I don't need anger management! People just need to stop pissing me off. I know I fly off the handle sometimes, but it's just because they aren't listening.'

What might you say next as a reflection?

- 'You don't really need anger management.'
- 'The problem is other people.'
- 'Sometimes you have over-reacted a bit.'
- 'It's really important for people to listen to you.'

All of these are perfectly good reflections of what the client said. The first two will likely evoke more sustain talk against anger management as a goal, although sometimes reflecting sustain talk does cause the person to voice change talk as the other side of their ambivalence. The fourth will lead to talk about other people's behaviour. The third picks up on the little bit of change talk that was implicit (problem recognition) and invites some elaboration on it.

Basically, you're listening for change talk, and you don't have to just sit there and wait for it to happen. The evoking process invites it with specific questions, and it also matters what you say next when you hear change talk. To hear more change talk, you might reflect it, affirm it, or ask an open question to invite elaboration. In MI you're collecting and remembering change talk. You can give it back in small or larger summaries of all the change talk you've heard so far, as a kind of bouquet of flowers or a box of chocolates. Instead of telling people what you think they should do and why, you are collecting their own motivations for change – their desire, ability, reasons, need, willingness, steps and commitment language, without adding your own material. Clients hear their own change talk, then they hear it again as you reflect and summarise it. There is quite an art to this, but those are the basics.

I am aware, of course, that in some PCA approaches you might always intend to reflect whatever the client offers as change and sustain talk. The evoking process in MI involves differential reflection, and I believe we have solid scientific evidence that it matters.

4. Planning

When there seems to be sufficient motivation, the conversation may migrate naturally from the why to the how of change. This is the planning task. A temptation now is for you to tell clients how to do it, and they might welcome some information about it, but a normal response when told what to do is to not do it, or perhaps do the opposite, even when you agree with the advice (de Almeida Neto, 2017). It's called psychological reactance and is a perfectly normal human response (Brehm & Brehm, 1981). The planning process, then, is one of negotiation, not prescription. What are the client's own ideas? Of various options, which one(s) would be most acceptable or sensible to this person? MI can include offering information and suggestions, but it's done in a particular PCA-consistent way: with permission, honouring autonomy and considering various options (Miller & Rollnick, 2023).

Resistance

Although reluctance to comply with advice is normal, it is sometimes interpreted as resistance from the counsellor's perspective. Within MI, such labelling – even privately in your own mind – is seen as unhelpfully adversarial, suggesting a contest of wills. 'Here I am doing my best to help you, and you're resisting me.' Behaviour regarded as resistant is necessarily interpersonal – an interaction of two or more people. This means that you can increase or decrease clients' motivation or resistance by how you respond (Glynn & Moyers, 2010; Patterson & Forgatch, 1985). Thinking of it as resistance just adds needless baggage and sounds like blaming the client for not changing.

In the third edition of the MI text, we deconstructed the concept of resistance that we had previously been using. Most of our prior examples of resistance were simply client sustain talk, which is a normal part of ambivalence ('I don't need to change;' 'Everything is okay as it is'). After subtracting sustain talk from what counsellors usually mean by resistance, we found a second significant component, which we called discord. This signals dissonance in the therapeutic relationship. Discord often contains the word 'you' ('You aren't listening to me;' 'How could you possibly understand?'). Understood in this way, there is something that you can do (and are already doing) to influence sustain talk and discord. It is important to notice and not respond in a way that exacerbates them, because if they are not addressed these in-session client responses predict no change from the status quo. As mentioned earlier, the prevalence of client sustain talk is a stronger predictor of outcome than is change talk itself. Sustain talk and discord are highly responsive to counsellors' behaviour and do predict how likely it is that change will occur.

Counselling with neutrality

When counselling with neutrality, the conscious intention is not to influence the client's direction of choice or change – a truly 'nondirective' intention that fits some contexts of practice better than others. Sometimes neutrality in counselling (having or favouring no particular change goal) is confused with equanimity (being a calm presence and accepting what clients bring you). Professional neutrality is less fitting in treating addiction, working on a suicide prevention helpline or being a probation counsellor with violent offenders. You can do all of these things in a person-centred way, with empathy and equanimity, even nonchalance, but if you're not working to reduce harmful substance use, suicide risk or victimising others, then you're probably not doing your job. There are clinical situations where it is appropriate to have clear goals and direction for change, ideally shared by client and counsellor. Remember that having clear focus or direction is an attribute of more effective psychotherapists, a strong therapeutic alliance and greater benefit from treatment (Miller & Moyers, 2021).

In other contexts of practice, a non-directive or neutral stance is entirely appropriate, at least until you and your client agree clear goals for treatment. What we have learned from MI research about how to facilitate change in a particular direction also informs how not to do so. It is possible to inadvertently influence decisions about choice or change without either you or the client realising what is happening, by what you choose to ask, reflect, affirm and include in summaries. Just starting down one path with an open question and then following with empathic listening can inadvertently tip the balance. So, what does MI research reveal about how to keep your balance and maintain neutrality?

One way to think about ambivalence is as a balance between the perceived pros and cons of each particular choice (Miller, 2022). The relative weight of pros and cons indicates proximity to decision and change (Prochaska et al., 1994). Exploring this 'decisional balance' (Janis & Mann, 1977) is a way to help people to make difficult decisions without influencing the balance yourself, so that they can feel at peace with the choice they have made, given what they knew at the time. In its simplest form, think of a 2x2 table with two possible choices (e.g. to have children or not) and the advantages and disadvantages of each choice. You would equally ask about, affirm and reflect the pros and cons of each possible choice and offer a balanced summary. You can also offer double-sided reflections that contain both sustain talk and change talk, with an 'and' in the middle. In contrast to a decisional balance approach, MI differentially evokes the pros of change and the cons of the status quo. A decisional balance procedure has sometimes been used in interventions that are intended to encourage change in a particular direction (such as smoking cessation) but doing so seems to decrease commitment to the intended change. This is unsurprising, given that you are clarifying the person's ambivalence (Miller & Rose, 2015).

A first contribution of MI research, then, is to be conscious about whether your task is to be nondirectional or directional, because you would do different things depending on your intention. Furthermore, what we have learned indicates that, to maintain neutrality, it would be appropriate to consciously, intentionally keep your balance by equally evoking, reflecting, affirming and summarising motivations on each side of the decision. A clinical complexity here, I find, is that, while exploring a decisional balance, clients often reach a point where they clearly seem to be leaning in one direction. At this point, discuss whether that is a direction in which the client is deciding to go. If so, then you might switch from non-directivity to the differential evoking approach of MI. Indeed, continuing to revisit reasons for a conflicting choice can be torturous.

Direction in MI

Most often MI helps clients to move in a particular direction because that's what they have asked you to do. In some settings, like addiction treatment or probation, treatment may begin with a provisional change goal about which the client is at best ambivalent (e.g. to reduce substance use or antisocial behaviour). As part of medical rehabilitation, a physical therapist often asks patients to do what is painful in order to recover function, and again ambivalence is a common obstacle: 'I both want to do it and don't want to do it.' Direct persuasion is often insufficient or even countertherapeutic in responding to ambivalence. That is the world in which MI began: helping clients to find their own motivation for a change about which they are conflicted. As it turns out, that is a very common scenario in many helping professions.

An ethical issue sometimes expressed about MI is whether it can be used to make clients do what you (or your agency) want them to do that is contrary to their own will or best interests. This is analogous to fears sometimes raised about post-hypnotic suggestion or subliminal advertising. Rollnick and I have long cautioned against inappropriate applications of MI: for example, to persuade people to sign a consent form, buy a product, or donate an organ (Miller, 1994; Miller & Rollnick, 2002). Nevertheless, is it possible? I know of no scientific evidence that MI can be used to manipulate people in this way. A case in point is a recent report in which the Danish police required monthly 'mandatory motivational interviews' to encourage refugees to leave the country after their application for asylum had been denied (Kohl, 2022). According to police reports, only a few refugees ever signed the form agreeing to voluntary departure, and even those who did rarely left.

In summary, be conscious of your intention to be neutral and non-directional versus your intention to move in a particular direction, and be aware of the reasons for your intention. Again, depending on which you choose, different therapeutic methods are appropriate.

Case study: The conflicted drinker

He came to see me at the insistence of his wife, who had given him an ultimatum: 'Either you do something about your drinking problem, or I'm going to take the children and leave you.' He told me that he did not have an alcohol problem and had come only because he didn't want to lose his family. When I spoke with his wife, she reported no violence, drunk driving, financial difficulties or social embarrassments. 'He's a good father,' she told me, 'but I'm not about to go through what my mother did with my dad. He was an alcoholic.' Mostly they argued about how much he drank and how often.

'I'm no alcoholic,' he told me, 'but you can tell me what you think.'

'I don't care much about labels,' I replied. 'What I care about is you. I don't know enough about your situation yet to have an opinion, but I'm certainly willing to help you think it through.' Two sessions in the first week made it clear that keeping his family together was a top priority for him: 'They are more important to me than anything else, but what should I tell her about drinking?'

What I suggested was what we call a 'drinker's check-up' – an assessment to get more information. The check-up involved about two hours of interview and cognitive and lab tests with a technician, using measures particularly focused on the early effects of alcohol on mental and physical health (Miller et al., 1992). Then I sat down with him to review the results in an MI manner.

A characteristic difference from a more confrontational approach is how you respond when someone baulks at or disagrees with a piece of information. A good example is the first result that I described to him, based on a calendar reconstruction of his usual drinking pattern. All reported alcohol use is converted into standard drink units equal to 15ml of pure alcohol, whether it's in beer, wine or distilled spirits. His reported drinking added up to 96 of these standard drinks in a typical week, or about 13 drinks a day. 'Compared with American men's drinking, that puts you at the 99th percentile,' I explained, 'which means that, out of 100 men on average, you drink more than 98 of them, and there is one guy who drinks as much as you or more.'

He baulked. 'That's crazy,' he said. 'Every guy I know drinks like I do, mostly. That can't be right.' We went back over the calendar of his usual drinking, and he agreed that it looked about right in terms of the numbers.

'It's hard for you to see how it's possible that you could be drinking more than 98% of men. That just doesn't make any sense to you,' I said.

'No, it doesn't,' he replied. 'I mean, I guess if you're counting everybody – old guys and teenagers and church-goers – I'd hold my own against them.'

'But compared with the guys you know, you don't see much difference.'

'No. I probably drink more than some of them. I can hold my liquor better than most.'

And that opened up the next topic – his apparent tolerance for alcohol, which was very high. 'You can drink a lot more than most men and not really feel it,' I guessed. He proudly allowed as to how that was so. 'Okay, I can see how that might be a concern then,' I said.

He raised his eyebrows. 'A concern? What do you mean?' So I explained how a high tolerance for alcohol is actually like not having a smoke alarm to warn you when you're drinking enough to harm yourself. 'People with a high tolerance like you are more likely to do damage without realising it.' He hadn't ever thought of it that way.

The cognitive tests showed similarities to heavy drinkers on subtle neuropsychological tasks that one might not notice in everyday life. Liver function tests were mostly within the lab normal range but pushing the top of that range or, in one case, just over. I told him: 'It looks like so far you've been lucky, but there are some warning signs.'

A result that got his attention was our estimate of what his blood alcohol concentration would be during and after a typical night of drinking at home. It peaked at about three times the legal intoxication level in New Mexico and declined slowly, so that the next morning, when he was driving a company van and sometimes taking his kids to school, he was well over the legal limit. 'But I feel just fine in the morning! So, if I ever got pulled over . . .'

'You do have a high tolerance,' I said.

'But it would still show up on a breath test?'

'Yes. That worries you.'

'I could lose my job.'

I offered him what is a classic empathic bouquet of his own change talk. When doing a summary like this I talk more than is usual for me.

'So you told me the only reason or the main reason you're here is that your family is important to you and you don't want to lose them. You love them, and really don't want to be apart from them. You've noticed that the amount you drink has crept up over the years, but that hasn't really worried you. There were some results from the check-up that you don't like; for example, that you drink more than most men and have a really high tolerance for alcohol. The cognitive test results bothered you some, showing a few early effects of heavy drinking, and the liver tests were a kind of warning light. You didn't realise that you were drinking enough to still be legally intoxicated in the morning when you drive to work or take your kids to school. But really your main concern is that you want your family to stay together. So what are you thinking at this point?'

That last bit is what we call a key question, following from all the change talk and acknowledging the client's freedom of choice. Sometimes I ask, 'So what do you think you'll do?' He talked about quitting drinking, at least on a trial basis.

I reflected it. 'You're thinking, then, that you'll quit drinking, at least for a while, and see how you feel. So, is that what you want to do?' I was looking for commitment language.

'No,' he said.

Various expletives flashed through my mind. I had just given him a classic MI summary of his own change talk. I developed this method, after all, and still he says no? I think I tipped my head slightly to one side and questioned, 'No?'

'No,' he said. 'It's not what I want to do. It's what I'm going to do.' I had asked the wrong question.

He did quit abruptly at the end of the second week of treatment. I cautioned him about possible withdrawal syndrome, but he told me about going for a couple of days recently without alcohol with no problem, and indeed he experienced no significant symptoms. Because he was part of a clinical trial, our research assistants saw him regularly over 12 months following completion of treatment. By perfection standards, he was counted as 'relapsed' because he had occasional days with some drinking, but throughout the year of follow-up his alcohol use decreased by 96% compared with his pre-treatment levels. By *DSM* criteria, he was in continuous remission from month 2 onward.

Case study: The committed smoker

This second case was a recorded demonstration by Dr Theresa Moyers, and to my mind a brilliant example of MI skillfulness. The man she interviewed had initially been engaged as an actor to portray a hypothetical client, but we were running behind schedule and, while waiting, he was taking frequent smoke breaks outside. She wondered if he might be willing to abandon the role he had prepared and instead just talk about his own smoking. He agreed, and here is part of the transcript (from Miller et al., 2013, with permission). This is a conversation that could easily occur during a medical visit. 'I' designates the interviewer and 'C' the client.

I: You've agreed to come in today and talk to me a little about your smoking. Can you tell me a little bit about that?

C: Well, I was thinking about this before we were talking about it, that if I were able to sit down right now and have a cigarette, I would, because I like to smoke. [Sustain talk]

I: So, being in front of the camera makes you feel like you want to have a cigarette. [Reflection]

C: Actually, my whole life is based around a cigarette. When I get in my car, I smoke a cigarette. Of course, in radio or in other fields, you can't usually smoke on your job, so you have to take those breaks, but in the older days I used to be able to smoke anywhere, so it makes it a little bit tougher. But yeah, if I could have a cigarette right now, I would. [Sustain talk]

I: It's that much a part of your life, that you feel like you would have one even right now. [Reflection of sustain talk]

C: Absolutely. And I think you find yourself going out at 10 o'clock, 11 o'clock at night to go to the store to grab a pack of cigarettes when you smoke because it's what you need, physically need it, but you also like it because you enjoy it. [There is some change talk buried in the ambivalence]

I: Right. There's a part of you that really enjoys smoking. [A brilliant little reflection! It does echo his enjoyment by reflecting sustain talk, while 'a part of you' invites the other side of ambivalence without directly asking for it.]

[From here on, the client's change talk is shown in *italic font*]

C: Right. *And then there's a part that says, 'You really don't want to, or you shouldn't.'* And it has nothing to do with people saying you can't. It's the fact that, after a period of time, you start – the flavour or the taste, *the problems become an issue.*

I: Mm-hmm. On the one hand you really like it, and it's good for you – helps you, and on the other hand you're noticing some things you don't like about it, like you have to go out at night and get it; you have to look for a break, and then there's also something about the flavour and the taste, you said. [Double-sided reflection]

C: *Yeah. You just get to a point where it's not enjoyable anymore. You're just doing it strictly out of habit, probably because of the nicotine that you want, but it's really not because you want it. It's because it gets to a point where you have to have it.* And I've never tried to quit. I mean, I've been smoking for a long time and I never once said, 'You know what, I'm going to quit smoking.'

I: And why is that, do you think? [Asking about sustain talk]

C: I think it becomes so much a part of your life, it becomes what you do, it's everything that you are… if you go fishing, you go hunting, you go to sporting events, everything you do – that cigarette becomes part of who you are, even to a point where you can't imagine yourself looking in a mirror without holding a cigarette. It is part of you, part of who your character is, even. [Sustain talk, and a beautiful subjective description of the experience of nicotine dependence]

I: So, cigarettes are now a part of your character. [Reflection]

C: Absolutely. It becomes part of your character. I've had people tell me they can't even imagine me without a cigarette, can't imagine what I'd look like without a cigarette.

I: And you can't even imagine yourself without a cigarette. [Reflection]

C: No, so you just… it becomes who you are. *But at the same time, you know, some things are happening. One is you know that the taste isn't there anymore. The cost is getting really, really high, so now you're finding yourself going to these lesser brands, or making this run to the rez*[1] *so you can bypass… I mean, you have to do so much to smoke a cigarette and to maintain that desire that it gets really ridiculous, quite frankly.* [Within three minutes, his change talk is outweighing his sustain talk]

I: Smoking used to be care-free for you, but now it's actually causing you a lot of trouble. [Reflecting change talk]

C: *It's a challenge now. It's not just 'Go get a pack of cigarettes'. It's now, 'How much do they cost? Which ones are the cheaper ones? Did you pick up a carton at the reservation 'cause it's so much cheaper with no taxes? Did you burn that hole in your clothes? Oh my God, that shirt – I burned a hole.' I mean, you start running into more and more issues. Then you start wondering, 'What's the return of this? What is the value?'*

I: Yeah, I was just going to ask you about that, because you mentioned earlier, sort of, you're smoking more and enjoying it less, and not only that, but then here come all of these sort of burdens or costs. [The interviewer reverses an old cigarette commercial about smoking less and enjoying it more]

C: I would be a terrible smoke commercial. A terrible commercial. [He catches the allusion]

I: It's almost like, if you were trying to convince yourself to smoke, you'd have a hard time doing it.

C: *It would be like the old saying, 'Smoke less and enjoy more,' but it's just the opposite: smoke more and enjoy less, so it would be a terrible advertising campaign. You just get to the point*

---

1. 'The rez' refers to an Indian reservation where there are no federal taxes levied on tobacco sales.

where you finally decide for yourself, you know, somewhere along the line, you know, in the back of your mind, somewhere in the back of your mind, you're saying, 'You know, there's gonna come a time when I'm gonna put these down.' [Preparatory change talk]

I: You're thinking about it. [Reflecting change talk]

C: *Absolutely, because of the involvement, the… how much is involved to smoke. It's too much, besides the fact that it's even considered socially unfair, or whether you want to consider it fair or unfair… unacceptable in so many arenas. People go out of their way to make an example by saying, 'Oh my God, he's smoking. How… could you move that away over here?' People become very rude with it. Yet at the same time, it's sort of a two-edged sword.*

I: Well, it sounds like every time you try to think about one side of it, you have to end up thinking about the other side of it. [Direct reflection of ambivalence itself]

C: Yes. It's just a constant; it's a conversation in your mind. Exactly. *It's not as free as the early days* when you went down and got a pack for 25 cents. For God's sakes, you could go into a building and they would have a cigarette machine. You put a quarter in and it didn't matter how old you were, and pull the lever and pull out your cigarettes, and you smoked and no one thought much of it. I can remember smoking in the theatre, smoking on an airplane, smoking in your job, smoking all the time, whenever you wanted to. It was just considered a norm.

I: Right. You didn't used to think about it very much, and now you're thinking about it all the time. [Reflection]

C: *Now it becomes an issue because it's not enjoyable in many, many areas of the smoking experience. It's not just the smoke, the flavour, it's the social norm; it's what it costs you to buy them; what's all involved. And then, of course, the issue of health, which is the older you get, you begin to realise that it's starting to affect you. And every time you go to the doctor, he says, 'Oh, by the way, have you thought about quitting smoking? You know, you ought to be considering that.' So you're constantly having this little – and friends and relatives and people that don't smoke say, 'You know, I quit 10 years ago. You might want to consider it. It changed my life. Food tastes better.' All that good stuff. You're hearing all these positives when you're dealing with all these negatives.*

I: Let me see if I can see what you've just said. One is, you're worried about your health. [She begins a collecting summary of change talk]

C: *Oh, sure.*

I: Every time you go to the doctor, the doctor says something.

C: *Sure.*

I: Second of all, you're thinking about the social stigma, that people are always just sort of looking down on you 'cause you're a smoker, and saying something like, 'Have you thought about smoking? You should stop smoking.'

C: *Yeah, you have a lot of things coming negative, more than positive.* When you first started – when I first started years and years ago, smoking was considered a positive thing, not a negative. You know, 'I'd rather fight than switch' with Tareyton [cigarette brand]; 'Enter into the cool country' with Salem [cigarette brand]; I mean, everything was built around the advertising campaign to make you feel as though it was okay. And then, of course, your friends did it, and it was part of that passage from being a child to an adult when a guy would have his cigarette, and if you're really good you rolled your own. Then you were just really macho. And then you had the Marlboro guy, and all the guys wanted to look like that really pure type person. So, yeah, from that standpoint, you saw the positives. [A burst of sustain talk, all in past tense.] *Today you see the negatives, and you hear the negatives.*

I: You're seeing the negatives. [She reflects the change talk]

C: *Absolutely.*

I: And you've thought about quitting.

C: *Yes. It's entered my mind many times in the last year or so.*

[He then talked for a while about difficulties of quitting and fear of withdrawal]

C: So that's what you're dealing with. You have to… There's a physical part of that, and then there's a mental part, *so both of those have got to mesh at the same time before you finally say, 'Okay, I don't care if I have to go through 10 days. I've got to quit.' And I think that when finally those two… for me anyway, when those two roads collide, or when those two roads intersect with each other, I think that's when you're finally able to make that choice.* [We call this envisioning the change]

I: And how is that going to happen for you?

C: I think constantly reinforcing in your mind that you want to quit. I think, you know, constantly saying to yourself, '*Gee, this is getting to be a pain.*' Or maybe it could be just that one time when you are sneaking out of the house on a cold winter night at 11:30 with ice on the road, and you're driving to go get a pack of cigarettes, you finally go, 'Wait a minute. *This is insane! This is really insane.*' [More envisioning]

I: Well, I get the feeling that it's coming for you.

C: *It is.*

I: It's on the way.

C: *Right, it is on the way, because it's time. You just know somehow.* [Mobilising change talk]

I: It's time right now. [Reflection, trying out a short timeframe]

C: *It's time.*

I: And you know.

C: *And you know it's time, and the body is saying it's time, and the mind is saying it. That's why I say I think the two roads have to intersect, and when they do, you'll do it.* [He talks about himself in second person 'you' language, but clearly he is talking about himself]

I: And when you look ahead, right – if you look ahead, say, a year, do you see those two roads coming together? [Trying a longer timeframe]

C: *I think I see it sooner than a year. I think I see it sooner.*

I: Even sooner.

C: *Yes. I think there comes a time when you just have to just finally say… I just gave you the reasons why it's so bad to smoke. If you're constantly reinforcing that in your mind, and you're remembering it every time, then eventually you'll say, 'You know what? I think I've convinced myself.'*

I: And is that how it will happen for you – that you will wake up one day and you'll say, 'That's it. I'm ready. I'm done'?

C: *I think that's the way it will happen. And like I said, it should have happened when it's January and there's snow on the ground and you're driving at 11 o'clock to get a pack of cigarettes. That should have been the time, but it's the insanity of it because of that addiction, and it is an addiction, and it is the insanity that you don't want to go through that withdrawal and at the same time you can't imagine yourself without it. But somewhere along the line, you have to make that decision.*

This concentration of change talk would rarely occur by chance. Dr Moyers was primarily using the skill of reflective listening, but there is a clear direction to it and to the questions she asks. This short example illustrates both how PCA skills are used strategically to support change, and also the change talk that practitioners listen for and respond to in client speech.

Research evidence

MI has remained close to Carl Rogers' emphasis on clinical psychology as an empirical science (Miller & Moyers, 2017). One of the few things on which he and the behaviourist B.F. Skinner agreed was 'Believe your data.' Assertions about psychotherapy are testable hypotheses and subject to replication. In the space available here, I will briefly summarise three inter-related lines of research – outcome, process and training studies– paralleling similar extensive lines of PCA work.

Outcome research

There are now more than 2,000 controlled clinical trials involving MI – an outcome literature so large that more than 200 systematic reviews and meta-analyses of MI have been published. When the clinical efficacy of person-centred therapies is questioned, here is an ample source of relevant evidence. The outcome literature for MI is larger than that for all other PCA tribes combined.

Given the size and findings of this literature, a first reasonable conclusion is that MI is an evidence-based treatment with small-to-medium effects on average. Clinical trials generally support the efficacy of MI (usually 1–2 sessions) relative to no additional intervention, placebo or brief advice. When compared head-to-head in randomised trials with other bona fide psychotherapies that are often of greater intensity, outcome differences tend to be small if any (e.g. Hettema et al., 2005; Project MATCH Research Group, 1998a; UKATT Research Team, 2005). This renders MI a reasonable ethical 'minimal treatment' comparison group in pharmacotherapy and psychotherapy trials.

Meta-analyses suggest that MI is more effective when offered in more than a single session (Rubak et al., 2005). There is also good evidence that MI can improve client outcomes when added to other treatment, often as a pre-therapy intervention. A complexity in more recent trials is that MI is now often being combined or intertwined with other evidence-based treatments as a clinical style for practice.

A second clear conclusion is that the effectiveness of MI is highly variable across trials, sites and providers (Lundahl et al., 2010; Rubak et al., 2005). About a quarter of controlled trials have found no effect of MI, and in multi-site trials it has worked at some sites and not others, which also happens with pharmacotherapies and other psychotherapies (Ball et al., 2007). Even when therapists are trained together and their practice is closely monitored, large differences occur in client outcomes by provider (Project MATCH Research Group, 1998b) – also a common finding in psychotherapy research more generally (Miller & Moyers, 2021). These differences have to do in part with the quality of the MI being delivered (Miller & Rollnick, 2014). Trial reports have often provided minimal information about the training, initial skill level and fidelity of therapists in practising MI. As discussed below, there is a large literature on measuring the quality of MI based on human coding of observed practice.

The evidence base for MI also varies according to the clinical concern being addressed. The largest single-diagnosis literature is with substance use disorders, where MI began. There is ample confirmation of the efficacy of MI in reducing alcohol, tobacco and marijuana use and problems, and very modest evidence for MI alone with illicit drugs like stimulants and opioids, where MI is usually combined with other medical and psychological interventions (DiClemente et al., 2017). In health care, significant benefit from MI has been found across a broad range of medical concerns, particularly in managing chronic illnesses such as diabetes (Rollnick et al., 2023). MI has also been effectively applied to increase health behaviours such as medication adherence, physical activity, dietary change and weight loss (Lundahl et al., 2013). In behavioural health, meta-analyses have supported a role for MI in managing anxiety, depression and severe mental disorders (Marker & Norton, 2018; Romain et al., 2020).

Process research

As in the development of PCA (Truax & Carkhuff, 1976), extensive research has focused on therapeutic processes occurring in MI. A first step, of course, is to develop reliable measures of relevant processes occurring in MI, just as occurred for PCA with scales for accurate empathy, positive regard and genuineness (Kirschenbaum, 2009; Truax & Carkhuff, 1976). A variety of measures have been developed to measure MI fidelity and therapeutic processes

(Hurlocker et al., 2020; Moyers et al., 2016). Both client and therapist measures hypothesised in MI to impact treatment outcome do so (Magill et al., 2018; Moyers et al., 2009).

Therapists whose clients show more change are those with fewer MI-inconsistent responses, more MI-consistent responses and a more empathic style, and those whose clients offer more change talk and less sustain talk or discord. The latter could be interpreted as confirming the stereotype that motivated clients get better whereas unmotivated clients do not, but there is also strong correlational, longitudinal and experimental evidence that therapists influence clients' ratio of change talk to sustain talk (Drage et al., 2019; Glynn & Moyers, 2010). It is difficult to separate the relational from the technical components of MI (DiBlasi et al., 2022). Three controlled trials have compared MI with a PCA non-directive condition that mirrors the spirit of MI without trying to evoke change talk. Two of these studies found that MI yielded significantly more change (Sellman et al., 2001) or faster change (Morgenstern et al., 2012), whereas the third found no difference on short-term outcomes (Morgenstern et al., 2017).

Training research

Our first evaluation of MI training yielded two results that were disquieting but should not have been surprising (Miller & Mount, 2001). First, although a two-day clinical workshop on MI received rave reviews on participant questionnaires (quality of training, confidence in practice, how much they were using their new skills), a comparison of pre-training and post-training interviews showed very little actual change in MI practice behaviour – certainly not enough to make a difference to clients. Second, counsellors' self-reported competence in delivering MI was unrelated to observed skill level in practice – findings that I suspect are not unique to MI in continuing professional education.

In any event, our findings suggested a better research question: What does it take to help clinicians develop competence in delivering MI? We began testing two additional training procedures that are commonly used in learning other complex skills such as sports or musical performance. One is objective personal feedback based on observed practice; the other is expert coaching on specific component skills. In our first trial of these two training adjuncts, both significantly improved acquisition and maintenance of clinical skills in MI, as compared with self-study or a training workshop alone (Miller et al., 2004). This finding has been replicated in many studies of training in MI as well as other evidence-based therapies (Miller et al., 2006). The large research literature on teaching and learning MI has been summarised in multiple meta-analyses and systematic reviews. Here are some reasonable conclusions:

- MI is learnable with training but difficult to master through self-study.
- Providers tend to overestimate their proficiency in MI (and probably other skills).
- Personal feedback and expert coaching based on observed practice can improve proficiency and client response.
- The ability to learn MI seems unrelated to degrees or years of education.
- Prior PCA skills (e.g. accurate empathy) facilitate the learning of MI.

Resources

A good starting point is the website of the Motivational Interviewing Network of Trainers (MINT; www.motivationalinterviewing.org), which provides a range of free and updated information including bibliographies of MI research. MINT trainers are listed by nation or state. Also useful are the personal websites of Bill Miller (https://williamrmiller.net) and Steve Rollnick (www.stephenrollnick.com).

Primary texts

There are already more than 100 books about MI. Some time-tested primary texts that have matured beyond a first edition are:

- Arkowitz, H., Miller, W.R. & Rollnick, S. (Eds.). (2015). *Motivational interviewing in the treatment of psychological problems* (2nd ed.). Guilford Press.
- Hohman, M. (2021). *Motivational interviewing in social work practice* (2nd ed.). Guilford Press.
- Miller, W.R. & Rollnick, S. (2023). *Motivational interviewing: Helping people change and grow* (4th ed.). Guilford Press.
- Rollnick, S., Miller, W.R. & Butler, C. (2023). *Motivational interviewing in health care: Helping patients change* (2nd ed.). Guilford Press.

Specifically designed to help you develop skillfulness in MI are:

- Manuel, J.K., Ernst, D., Vaz, A. & Rousmaniere, T. (2022). *Deliberate practice in motivational interviewing*. American Psychological Association.
- Rosengren, D.B. (2018). *Building motivational interviewing skills: A practitioner workbook* (2nd ed.). Guilford Press.

Guilford Press (www.guilford.com) publishes an ongoing series of books on specific applications of MI in helping professions.

References

Ball, S.A., Martino, S., Nich, C., Frankforter, T.L., van Horn, D., Crits-Christoph, P., Woody, G.E., Obert, J.L., Farentinos, C. & Carroll, K.M. (2007). Site matters: Multisite randomized trial of motivational enhancement therapy in community drug abuse clinics. *Journal of Consulting and Clinical Psychology, 75*, 556–567.

Brehm, S.S. & Brehm, J.W. (1981). *Psychological reactance: A theory of freedom and control.* Academic Press.

Christopher, P.J. & Dougher, M.J. (2009). A behaviour-analytic account of motivational interviewing. *Behaviour Analyst, 32*, 149–161.

Cooper, M. (2019). *Integrating counselling and psychotherapy: Directionality, synergy, and social change.* Sage.

de Almeida Neto, A.C. (2017). Understanding motivational interviewing: An eutionary perspective. *Eutionary Psychological Science, 3*(4), 379–389.

DiBlasi, T., Tafrati, R.C. & Kassinove, H. (2022). Core mechanisms of change in motivational interviewing: An attempt to separate relational from technical element effects. *Psihologijske teme 31*(3), 743–761.

DiClemente, C.C., Corno, C.M., Graydon, M.M., Wiprovnick, A.E. & Knoblach, D.J. (2017). Motivational interviewing, enhancement, and brief interventions over the last decade: A review of reviews of efficacy and effectiveness. *Psychology of Addictive Behaviors, 31*(8), 862–887.

Drage, L., Masterson, C., Tober, G., Farragher, T. & Bewick, B. (2019). The impact of therapists' responses to resistance to change: A sequential analysis of therapist-client interactions in motivational interviewing. *Alcohol & Alcoholism, 54(*2), 173–176.

Engle, D. & Arkowitz, H. (2006). *Ambivalence in psychotherapy: Facilitating readiness to change.* Guilford Press.

Farber, B.A., Suzuki, J.Y. & Lynch, D.A. (2019). Positive regard and affirmation. In J.C. Norcross & M.J. Lambert (Eds.), *Psychotherapy relationships that work. Vol. 1: Evidence-based therapist contributions* (3rd ed.) (pp.288–322). Oxford University Press.

Gendlin, E.T. (1961). Experiencing: A variable in the process of therapeutic change. *American Journal of Psychotherapy, 15(*2), 233–245.

Gilmore, S.K. (1973). *The counsellor-in-training.* Prentice-Hall.

Glynn, L.H. & Moyers, T.B. (2010). Chasing change talk: The clinician's role in evoking client language about change. *Journal of Substance Abuse Treatment, 39*(1), 65–70.

Graßmann, C., Schölmerich, F. & Schermuly, C.C. (2020). The relationship between working alliance and client outcomes in coaching: A meta-analysis. *Human Relations, 73*(1), 35–58.

Hettema, J., Steele, J. & Miller, W.R. (2005). Motivational interviewing. *Annual Review of Clinical Psychology, 1*, 91–111.

Horvath, A.O. & Symonds, B.D. (1991). Relation between working alliance and outcome in psychotherapy: A meta-analysis. *Journal of Counselling Psychology, 38*(2), 139–149.

Hurlocker, M.C., Madson, M.B. & Schumacher, J.A. (2020). Motivational interviewing quality assurance: A systematic review of assessment tools across research contexts. *Clinical Psychology Review, 82*, 101909.

Janis, I.L. & Mann, L. (1977). *Decision making: A psychological analysis of conflict, choice and commitment.* Free Press.

Kirschenbaum, H. (2009). *The life and work of Carl Rogers.* American Counselling Association.

Kohl, K.S. (2022). The stalemate: Motivational interviewing at a carceral junction. *Incarceration: An international journal of imprisonment, detention and coercive confinement, 3*(1), 1–18.

Lombardi, D.R., Button, M.L. & Westra, H.A. (2014). Measuring motivation: Change talk and counter-change talk in cognitive behavioural therapy for generalized anxiety. *Cognitive Behaviour Therapy, 43*(1), 12–21.

Lundahl, B.W., Kunz, C., Brownell, C., Tollefson, D. & Burke, B.L. (2010). A meta-analysis of motivational interviewing: Twenty-five years of empirical studies. *Research on Social Work Practice, 20*(2), 137–160.

Lundahl, B., Moleni, T., Burke, B.L., Butters, R., Tollefson, D., Butler, C. & Rollnick, S. (2013). Motivational interviewing in medical care settings: A systematic review and meta-analysis of randomized controlled trials. *Patient Education and Counseling, 93*(2), 157–168.

Magill, M., Apodaca, T.R., Borsari, B., Gaume, J., Hoadley, A., Gordon, R.E.F., Tonigan, J.S. & Moyers, T. (2018). A meta-analysis of motivational interviewing process: Technical, relational, and conditional process models of change. *Journal of Consulting and Clinical Psychology, 86*(2), 140–157.

Magill, M., Bernstein, M.H., Hoadley, A., Borsari, B., Apodaca, T.R., Gaume, J. & Tonigan, J.S. (2019). Do what you say and say what you are going to do: A preliminary meta-analysis of client change and sustain talk subtypes in motivational interviewing. *Psychotherapy Research, 29*(7), 860–869.

Marker, I. & Norton, P.J. (2018). The efficacy of incorporating motivational interviewing to cognitive behavior therapy for anxiety disorders: A review and meta-analysis. *Clinical Psychology Review, 62,* 1–10.

Markland, D., Ryan, R.M., Tobin, V. & Rollnick, S. (2005). Motivational interviewing and self-determination theory. *Journal of Social and Clinical Psychology, 24*, 811–831.

Miller, W.R. (1983). Motivational interviewing with problem drinkers. *Behavioural Psychotherapy, 11,* 147–172.

Miller, W.R. (1994). Motivational interviewing: III. On the ethics of motivational intervention. *Behavioural and Cognitive Psychotherapy, 22*, 111–123.

Miller, W.R. (2022). *On second thought: How ambivalence shapes your life.* Guilford Press.

Miller, W.R. & Baca, L.M. (1983). Two-year follow-up of bibliotherapy and therapist-directed controlled drinking training for problem drinkers. *Behaviour Therapy, 14*, 441–448.

Miller, W.R. & Brown, S.A. (1997). Why psychologists should treat alcohol and drug problems. *American Psychologist, 52*, 1269–1272.

Miller, W.R., Forcehimes, A.A. & Zweben, A. (2019). *Treating addiction: A guide for professionals* (2nd ed.). Guilford Press.

Miller, W.R. & Mount, K.A. (2001). A small study of training in motivational interviewing: Does one workshop change clinician and client behaviour? *Behavioural and Cognitive Psychotherapy, 29*, 457–471.

Miller, W.R. & Moyers, T.B. (2017). Motivational interviewing and the clinical science of Carl Rogers. *Journal of Consulting and Clinical Psychology, 85*(8), 757–766.

Miller, W.R. & Moyers, T.B. (2021). *Effective psychotherapists: Clinical skills that improve client outcomes*. Guilford Press.

Miller, W.R. & Rollnick, S. (1991). *Motivational interviewing: Preparing people to change addictive behaviour*. Guilford Press.

Miller, W.R. & Rollnick, S. (2002). *Motivational interviewing: Preparing people for change*. Guilford Press.

Miller, W.R. & Rollnick, S. (2013). *Motivational interviewing: Helping people change* (3rd ed.). Guildford Press.

Miller, W.R. & Rollnick, S. (2014). The effectiveness and ineffectiveness of complex behavioural interventions: Impact of treatment fidelity. *Contemporary Clinical Trials, 37*(2), 234–241.

Miller, W.R. & Rollnick, S. (2023). *Motivational interviewing: Helping people change and grow* (4th ed.). Guilford Press.

Miller, W.R. & Rose, G.S. (2009). Toward a theory of motivational interviewing. *American Psychologist, 64*(6), 527–537.

Miller, W.R. &. Rose, G.S. (2015). Motivational interviewing and decisional balance: Contrasting responses to client ambivalence. *Behavioural and Cognitive Psychotherapy, 43*(2), 129–141.

Miller, W.R., Moyers, T.B. & Rollnick. S. (2013). *Motivational interviewing: Helping people change*. The Change Companies.

Miller, W.R., Sorensen, J.L., Selzer, J.A. & Brigham, G.S. (2006). Disseminating evidence-based practices in substance abuse treatment: A review with suggestions. *Journal of Substance Abuse Treatment, 31*(1), 25–39.

Miller, W.R., Taylor, C.A. & West, J. (1980). Focused versus broad-spectrum behaviour therapy for problem drinkers. *Journal of Consulting and Clinical Psychology, 48*(5), 590–601.

Miller, W.R., Yahne, C.E., Moyers, T.B., Martinez, J. & Pirritano, M. (2004). A randomized trial of methods to help clinicians learn motivational interviewing. *Journal of Consulting and Clinical Psychology, 72*(6), 1050–1062.

Miller, W.R., Zweben, A., DiClemente, C. & Rychtarik, R. (1992). *Motivational enhancement therapy manual: A clinical research guide for therapist treating individuals with alcohol abuse and dependence, Vol. 2*. National Institute on Alcohol Abuse and Alcoholism.

Morgenstern, J., Kuerbis, A., Amrhein, P., Hail, L., Lynch, K. & McKay, J.R. (2012). Motivational interviewing: A pilot test of active ingredients and mechanisms of change. *Psychology of Addictive Behaviours, 26*(4), 859–869.

Morgenstern, J., Kuerbis, A., Houser, J., Levak, S., Amrhein, P., Shao, S. & McKay, J.R. (2017). Dismantling motivational interviewing: Effects on initiation of behaviour change among problem drinkers seeking treatment. *Psychology of Addictive Behaviours, 31*(7), 751–762.

Moyers, T.B., Martin, T., Christopher, P.J., Houck, J.M., Tonigan, J.S. & Amrhein, P.C. (2007). Client language as a mediator of motivational interviewing efficacy: Where is the evidence? *Alcoholism: Clinical and Experimental Research, 31*(10 Suppl.), 40s–47s.

Moyers, T.B., Martin, T., Houck, J.M., Christopher, P.J. & Tonigan, J.S. (2009). From in-session behaviors to drinking outcomes: A causal chain for motivational interviewing. *Journal of Consulting and Clinical Psychology, 77*(6), 1113–1124.

Moyers, T.B., Rowell, L.N., Manuel, J.K., Ernst, D. & Houck, J.M. (2016). The Motivational Interviewing Treatment Integrity code (MITI 4): Rationale, preliminary reliability and validity. *Journal of Substance Abuse Treatment, 65*, 36–42.

Patterson, G.R. & Forgatch, M.S. (1985). Therapist behaviour as a determinant for client noncompliance: A paradox for the behaviour modifier. *Journal of Consulting and Clinical Psychology, 53*(6), 846–851.

Prochaska, J.O., Velicer, W.F., Rossi, J.S., Goldstein, M.G., Marcus, B.H., Rakowski, W., Fiore, C., Harlow, L.L., Redding, C.A., Rosenbloom, D. & Rossi, S.R. (1994). Stages of change and decisional balance for 12 problem behaviors. *Health Psychology, 13*(1), 39–46.

Project MATCH Research Group. (1998a). Matching alcoholism treatments to client heterogeneity: Treatment main effects and matching effects on drinking during treatment. *Journal of Studies on Alcohol, 59*, 631–639.

Project MATCH Research Group. (1998b). Therapist effects in three treatments for alcohol problems. *Psychotherapy Research, 8*, 455–474.

Rogers, C.R. (1980). *A way of being*. Houghton Mifflin.

Rogers, C.R., Gendlin, E.T., Kiesler, D.J. & Truax, C.B. (Eds.). (1967). *The therapeutic relationship and its impact: A study of psychotherapy with schizophrenics.* Greenwood Press.

Rollnick, S. & Miller, W.R. (1995). What is motivational interviewing? *Behavioural and Cognitive Psychotherapy, 23*, 325–334.

Rollnick, S., Miller, W.R. & Butler, C.C. (2023). *Motivational interviewing in health care* (2nd ed.). Guilford Press.

Romain, A., Bernard, P., Akrass, Z., St-Amour, S., Lachance, J.-P., Hains-Monfette, G., Atoui, S., Kingsbury, C., Dubois, E., Karelis, A. & Abdel-Baki, A. (2020). Motivational theory-based interventions on health of people with severe mental illness: A systematic review and meta-analysis. *Schizophrenia Research, 222*, 31–41.

Rubak, S., Sandbaek, A., Lauritzen, T. & Christensen, B. (2005). Motivational interviewing: A systematic review and meta-analysis. *British Journal of General Practice, 55*(513), 305–312.

Sellman, J.D., Sullivan, P.F., Dore, G.M., Adamson, S.J. & MacEwan, I. (2001). A randomized controlled trial of motivational enhancement therapy (MET) for mild to moderate alcohol dependence. *Journal of Studies on Alcohol, 62*, 389–396.

Truax, C.B. (1966). Reinforcement and non-reinforcement in Rogerian psychotherapy. *Journal of Abnormal Psychology, 71*, 1–9.

Truax, C.B. & Carkhuff, R.R. (1976). *Toward effective counselling and psychotherapy: Training and practice.* Aldine Transaction.

UKATT Research Team. (2005). Effectiveness of treatment for alcohol problems: Findings of the randomized UK alcohol treatment trial (UKATT). *British Medical Journal, 331*(7516), 541–544.

Wiser, S.G. & Goldfried, M.R. (1998). Therapist interventions and client emotional experiencing in expert psychodynamic-interpersonal and cognitive-behavioural therapies. *Journal of Consulting and Clinical Psychology, 66*(4), 634–640.

8. Existentially informed person-centred therapy

Siebrecht Vanhooren and Mick Cooper

Aisha, a client of Siebrecht, was a 23-year-old Belgian student who suffered from depression and bulimia (Vanhooren, 2023). Aisha could hardly get out of bed. She could not motivate herself to study and would frequently binge eat. She worried about her future and wanted to achieve something important in her life in order not to be forgotten. This was in stark contrast with the fact that she could not motivate herself to get things done. Likewise, she hoped to be happily married at some point, but had a hard time maintaining intimate partner relationships. Life seemed meaningless to her, and the fact that we all have to die one day made her feel that human efforts were pointless.

Aisha felt stuck, did not know how to change her situation, but wanted it to change. Although initially she found it 'silly' to explore her experiences in therapy – having and expressing feelings was a sign, for her, of weakness – something in the therapeutic encounter made her feel at ease and curious. She wanted to give it a chance.

In this chapter, we will use the case of Aisha to explore and illustrate an existentially informed approach to person-centred therapy. In recent decades, several writers and practitioners associated with the person-centred community have described a practice that draws on existential thinking (e.g. Stumm, 2005; Vaidya, 2013). Mick (the second author here) has outlined existential contributions and challenges to person-centred therapy (Cooper, 2003a), and wrote the first two versions of this chapter in the previous editions of this book (Cooper, 2004, 2012). Others, such as Madison (2010), Leijssen (2007) and Siebrecht, the first author (Vanhooren, 2018), have developed an existentially informed, focusing-oriented practice called experiential-existential psychotherapy (see Chapter 4, this volume). This practice not only draws on Rogers and existentialism, but also on the work of Eugene Gendlin, and of Otto Rank (1936), who can be identified as the grandfather of all humanistic and experiential therapies (Kramer, 2019). The present chapter builds on Mick's chapters in the previous editions, but here, rather than comparing and contrasting the different tribes of existential therapy against the classical person-centred approach (as the chapters in the previous editions did), we focus more specifically on the theory and practice of an existentially informed person-centred approach.

The aim of this chapter, then, is to discuss and demonstrate the nature of a person-centred therapy that has existential themes, dynamics and processes implicitly and explicitly running through it. The chapter begins with an introduction to existential philosophy, and then details the givens of human existence from an existential standpoint, drawing out implications for practice.

Existential philosophy: An introduction

Existential philosophy is a diverse and heterogeneous set of ideas, identified with 19th and 20th century philosophers such as Kierkegaard, Heidegger and Sartre. The essence of existential thinking is to try to understand and honour *existence*: to know what it means to be a person and to exist in the world. Existential philosophers believe in the uniqueness of each human being (Cooper, 2017), but argue that each of us has to deal with the same questions of life. Tillich (1952), for instance, states that people are primarily concerned not to disappear into *non-being*. He argues that human beings can experience angst and despair when they are confronted with different forms of loss. For example, someone might experience anxiety when they are confronted with death, existential isolation and a loss of meaning. Yalom (1980) calls these experiences of loss, along with the challenges of freedom and responsibility, *existential givens*. Other scholars have emphasised different existential givens, such as embodiment, (in-)authenticity, time, and life as a process (e.g. Cooper, 2015; Hoffman, 2009; Vanhooren, 2023). For the purpose of this chapter, we will explore the following:

- existence as a unique experience
- existence as being-in-the-world
- existence as meaning-oriented
- existence as freely choosing
- existence as finite and limited.

It is important to realise that these givens are actually only concepts that may help us to explore the existential layer of our clients and ourselves. The existential realm itself is a living and continuous process that stretches beyond the world of theoretical concepts (Gendlin, 1973). Regardless of how many existential givens there are that might describe the essence of what it means to be human, there is a consensus that deepening the awareness of our existence can make life more meaningful.

Such existential awareness often comes with what Jaspers (1951/2003) called *limit situations*. Traumatic experiences are examples of these limit situations and are often accompanied by a heightened existential awareness and more concrete mortality salience

– that is, the awareness of being mortal and that our existence is finite (Arredondo & Caparrós, 2019). They can serve as a 'wake-up call' to reconsider what really matters to us and, as a consequence, make us re-evaluate our life choices and so lead to 'post-traumatic growth' (Tedeschi & Calhoun, 2004). Equally, positive or 'peak' experiences (such as the birth of a child or experiencing awe while star-gazing) can also raise existential awareness and prompt a new search for meaning (Vanhooren, 2023).

Although both positive and negative limit situations can lead to a deepening of our existence, there are also people who struggle with existence itself. Existential suffering can arise in people's everyday life experiences (the 'ontic' level (Holzhey-Kunz, 2014)); but there is also a more profound suffering in relation to the existential givens (the 'ontological' level (Holzhey-Kunz, 2014)). Research shows that there is a robust association between psychological distress and existential suffering (e.g. Vanhooren et al., 2022). For example, anxiety disorders are associated with death anxiety, and psychopathology is associated with feelings of meaninglessness, existential loneliness and a sense of helplessness or 'external locus of control' (Vanhooren, 2023). Concretely, Aisha not only suffered from depression and bulimia (the ontic level), but also from a sense of meaninglessness, existential loneliness and anxiety about making life choices (the ontological level). The approach of an existentially informed person-centred practitioner will differ from that of a classical person-centred therapist in that they will explore not only the client's ontic daily living but also how the client experiences those existential givens that transcend their individual story.

Existence as a unique experience

Paradoxically, perhaps, one of the foremost universal characteristics that existential philosophy has emphasised is the fact that each human being – within the givens of existence – is fundamentally and ineradicably unique. From Kierkegaard onwards, existential philosophers have emphasised the diversity and difference of each human being: that we are all individual, distinctive and irreplaceable. This contrasts somewhat with a scientific worldview, which tends to reduce human beings to a set of common elements, such as Watson's 'stimulus' and 'reaction' construct (1925), or Freud's concepts of the 'id', 'ego' and 'superego' (1923). This emphasis on the uniqueness of each human being is very similar to a classical person-centred approach, which tends to avoid generalised theories of human behaviour, preferring instead to focus on the individuality of the client (see Chapter 2, this volume).

Rank (1936), who strongly influenced Rogers (1942) and the entire field of humanistic psychology (Kramer, 2019), suggested that we need to create a new theory and therapy for every client situation. For Rank, every person is a mixture of what he called 'the individual and the universal': he saw it as essential to start from the client's experiences, and to try to understand these experiences from the client's point of view.

The awareness of the other person's uniqueness can help therapists not to assume that they will be able to 'understand' the client. It can help the therapist to embrace a phenomenological stance to what are often assumed to be 'common understandings', such as what we are supposed to do in therapy. It evokes a sense of curiousness about the other. As we are unique beings, May (1983) speaks of the 'therapeutic encounter' – a meeting of two different beings – instead of the 'therapeutic relationship' or 'alliance'. Although Aisha and I were two human beings who shared the same human condition, we were two very different and unique expressions of our human-beingness. It made me curious to know who she was or who she would become.

Uniqueness as an existential concern also had a part in Aisha's story. She struggled to find her place in the world. Although she really wanted to be part of her group of friends, she wanted to be seen, valued and accepted as a distinct individual, with her own talents. Although she knew it was somehow unrealistic, she hoped to be experienced by others as the prettiest, smartest, funniest person around. A shift in her friends' attention to another person could elicit feelings of a groundless loneliness. Yalom (1980) terms this experience existential loneliness: the darker side of our uniqueness. Aisha also sensed worthlessness and jealousy at those moments. She felt embarrassed and vulnerable acknowledging these feelings.

Existence as being-in-the-world

From an existential perspective, as with the relational approach to person-centred therapy (see Chapter 3, this volume), a person is unique but not separate from their environment. In contrast to a classical person-centred perspective, the environment is not just something that either nourishes or fails to nourish the individual's 'internally determined' path. Here, Heidegger (1962) uses the term *dasein* – 'being-there' or 'being-here', usually translated as 'being-in-the-world' – to describe human existence. With *dasein*, Heidegger underlines the fundamental connection between 'self' and world. For Heidegger (1962) and some of the later existential philosophers (such as Merleau-Ponty, 1962), existence is not something that is 'inside' of us; it is the self-environment that we experience. For this reason, many existential thinkers and practitioners (for instance, Boss, 1963) are wary of using terms like 'inner experiences' or 'inner feelings'. Rather, they prefer terms such as 'lived experiences' (Spinelli, 2006), which do not necessarily imply that the experiences are inside of the individual.

Inspired by Heidegger, Gendlin (1973) states that what we experience is not 'inside' but our ongoing embodied experience of the interaction that we have with our environment. In other words, we are interaction, or we are our situation. Therefore, what the client experiences in therapy is not just themselves or even the 'felt sense' of their problem. What they experience, is themselves in interaction with the therapist. The therapist is part of their situation in the present. That is why 'the problem' might already feel different once they enter the therapy room. For the same reason, the therapist can be aware of the felt sense or the unspoken words of the client, precisely because what the therapist senses is not just themselves but their situation, which includes the client's presence.

For Heidegger (1962), being is not only in-the-world but also 'with-others'. Human beings are conceived of as ultimately inseparable from others: even if we were abandoned on a desert island, we would still be thinking about others, and using the socially-constructed medium of language to think with (see Chapter 3, this volume). Another existential philosopher who has put a great emphasis on our intrinsic interrelatedness with others is Buber (1958). What Rogers takes from Buber, however, is not so much the idea that the 'I' is always connected to another, but Buber's distinction between the humanising 'I-Thou' attitude to others as opposed to the de-humanising 'I-It' attitude. For Buber, this I-Thou attitude is characterised by an acceptance of the other, an openness to the whole of who they are, and a willingness to take the risk of fully engaging with them with the totality of one's own being — a way of relating that has clear parallels with Rogers' (1957) conditions of acceptance, empathy, and congruence.

However, Buber puts more emphasis on the need for the 'I' to bring their own 'otherness' into the relationship with the other. After all, argues Buber, if the 'I' simply becomes a reflecting mirror to the other, then there is no difference across which dialogue can take place. This latter standpoint, while differing from the classical person-centred approach, has come to be more prevalent in the person-centred field through the development of relational depth theory (Mearns & Cooper, 2018), which adopts a strongly intersubjective perspective (see Chapter 3, this volume). In his conversation with Buber, Rogers highlights that therapy can help the client to build a new or different 'relationship' with their self (Anderson & Cissna, 1997). When Rogers states that we can meet our self and learn to relate to ourselves in a different way, he echoes Kierkegaard's (1843/2013) idea that the self is a relationship that has a relationship to itself (Anderson & Cissna, 1997).

How did *dasein* become apparent in the case of Aisha? Aisha's feelings of worthlessness and jealousy were clearly relational, as they referred to how she experienced her being-with-others at significant moments. Interestingly, it was through her sense of an 'I-Thou' relational safety within this therapeutic relationship that she felt courageous enough to explore these feelings. In this therapeutic encounter, she could experience herself as different: she was not crawling into her bed; nor was she trying to get rid of her feelings by binge eating. From an existential point of view, it is precisely this different interaction that precedes a shift in 'the problem', because interacting differently with the other or with ourselves can evoke a change in our experience of our unique being-in-the-world.

As a therapist, I opened myself to sense how Aisha's sense of worthlessness and jealousy felt to me. As my being-in-the-world encompassed my being-with-my-client at that precise moment, I could attune to the effect her experiences had on my being. I could sense a kind of helplessness and warmth – my own reactions to her feelings of worthlessness – but also a sense of emptiness, a void, a stillness, something like a vacuum in her. This is what Ikemi (2017) calls 're-experiencing': my experience of her experience. And giving words to my re-experiencing and communicating them to the client would enable what Gendlin calls 'crossing' (Ikemi, 2017). My experience of her being-in-the-world would cross (in its sense of 'influence or merge') with her experience of being-in-the-world, and thus deepen or broaden her experience and process – or not. And indeed, my voicing of the words 'emptiness', 'stillness' and 'void' corresponded with her experience and helped her to become more aware of her own experiencing. She could recognise that it was this sense of emptiness that made her binge eat and made her feel so exhausted that she just wanted to crawl into bed.

By my opening up to her being-in-the-world and giving it space in my experiencing – or existence – Aisha was able also to give more space to notice and allow these feelings. Every session, Aisha stayed a little longer with her experience of being-herself-in-the-world. Eventually, by focusing (Gendlin, 1996), she became aware of a profound sadness. As she was able to experience this sadness more, her depression made space for tears. What the tears meant was not entirely clear yet. However, for Aisha there was a link with the sense that her life felt meaningless.

Existence as meaning-oriented

While existential philosophy and therapy are often associated with an emphasis on the here-and-now, existential philosophers have, in fact, tended to put a greater emphasis on the future (see, for instance, Heidegger, 1962). It has been argued that human beings are inherently orientated towards particular goals, purposes, projects or meanings, and that this orientation has a great effect on how we think, feel and behave in the present, as well as how we make sense of our past. Such a view of human existence as future- and meaning-orientated is entirely compatible with a classical person-centred perspective; indeed, some person-centred authors have specifically highlighted the value of empathising with a client's orientation towards the future (for instance, Bohart, 2001). In contrast to some existential approaches, however, person-centred thinking does not put any great emphasis on the human *need* for meaning, although it would not in any way deny that this may be central for some clients. Between the person-centred and some existential approaches, then, is something of a debate about whether the most fundamental human need is for *meaning* or for *actualisation*. From a person-centred perspective, for instance, one might argue that the need for meaning is one part of the wider need for actualisation. By contrast, from an existential perspective, one might argue that the need for actualisation is actually only a sub-need of the need for meaning.

Within the existential approach itself, however, there is also substantial debate over the question of whether there are any actual, given meanings to life, or whether we have to create our own meanings. That is, is there some meaning or purpose to our lives that we can find or discover (as suggested by Buber, 1958; Marcel, 1949), or do we have to construct these for ourselves, and so they will never have any ultimate, solid or extrinsic value (as suggested by Camus, 1955; Sartre, 1958)? Again, a classical person-centred position would not necessarily take either of the sides in this debate, but the latter position – that life has no extrinsic value – presents some serious challenges to its perspective. Most significantly, it asks, 'So what?' 'So what if we actualise our potential?' 'What does it matter?'

Rogers' (1961) and Gendlin's (1962) thinking about meaning is closely connected to their concept of *openness to experience* and their process view on existence. As Rogers (1961) observes, once clients are able to open up to the whole horizon of felt experiences, they often experience life as more meaningful, and they also shift priorities in life and experience themselves and their relationship with others as more meaningful. Not only are there some remarkable links with Daseinsanalysis – an existential therapy informed by the work of Heidegger – but there are also similarities with Buber's philosophy in which moments of authentic I-Thou meetings make one's life more meaningful. As Rogers remarks in his dialogue with Buber, moments of true existential meetings with one's self can also evoke a profound change (Anderson & Cissna, 1997). Echoing Rank (1936), in Buber's, Rogers' and Gendlin's point of view, it is the way we meet ourselves, the other, and existence as such, that creates meaning and purpose.

The connection between the experience of meaning and the quality of relatedness is not only confirmed by empirical research (e.g. Delle Fave, 2020). Recent studies also show that the therapeutic relationship might be a source of meaning for clients, and that this meaning in its turn reduces psychological distress (Fortems et al., 2022; Rim et al., 2022). Another source of meaning – in therapy and in daily life – is the search for meaning or the reflection on meaning itself (Rim et al., 2022). Therapy can be understood as a continuous search for meaning, as client and therapist are searching together to understand and make sense of the client's (and therapist's) experiences.

In the Belgian experiential-existential approach, a didactical model is used to explore different levels of meaning (Vanhooren, 2019). The model builds on Holzhey-Kunz's (2014) differentiation between our *ontic* experiencing (such as being stuck in a traffic jam and feeling frustrated) and our *ontological* experiencing of our situation (such as experiencing being stuck in a traffic jam as an expression of the limitations of life). On the ontic level, we further distinguish a *micro-dimension* (i.e. the felt sense and meaning of our here-and-now experiences) and a *meso-dimension* (i.e., our consolidated experiences or constructs, such as our self-image, identity, life-narrative, family stories, world assumptions and values). The ontological or *macro-dimension* stands for our existential awareness and how we give or derive meaning to our human condition.

Person-centred therapies engage strongly in meaning-making on the micro- and meso-dimension, but they do so less explicitly when it comes to this macro-dimension. In contrast to this, most existential therapies pay less attention to meaning-making processes on the micro-dimension. Person-centred existentially informed practices try to explore these different areas of meaning and to engage explicitly in a multi-level meaning-making process (Vanhooren, 2019). During the therapy with Aisha, this model helped us explore her sensed meaninglessness and facilitated meaning-making.

At the micro-dimension, Aisha seemed not to have a direct access to her felt experiences. She also had a hard time finding words that would symbolise her experiences. As Gendlin (1962) explains, experiencing the *felt sense* of our situation and having the capacity to *symbolise* this felt sense makes the meaning of our existence explicit. This micro-dimensional experience serves as a 'bottom-up' meaning-making process. Finding words or symbols for what we experience is an act of meaning-making. Problems at this basic level can lead to a chronic state of not being able to make sense of one's experiences (Warner, 2013).

Aisha could indeed not directly experience her felt sense during those first sessions, and nor could she symbolise and thus 'make sense' of her situation. She described her inner experiences as an undifferentiated 'nothingness' or 'emptiness'. Through focusing, re-experiencing and crossing (Gendlin, 1996; Ikemi, 2017), Aisha's awareness of her bodily felt experiences grew. She could discern something more than emptiness. She could sense that there was something really sad inside, and once she allowed herself to experience this sadness, some sessions later, she no longer felt constantly tired. It was a significant bodily felt shift. On this micro-dimension, the emptiness changed into a deep sadness. As her tears started to flow, and as she could listen and give words to her tears, words like 'a meaningless life' and 'a terrible loneliness' came to her. Quite literally, as she was crying during the sessions, something started to flow again. The words 'meaninglessness' and 'loneliness' were more meaningful to her than her – already former – depression where emptiness and exhaustion prevailed.

On the *meso-dimension*, Aisha had certain assumptions that informed her view of what kind of life was worth living. When we explored what kind of life would feel meaningful, her immediate answer was: 'A pleasant life'. But she also thought that being important or doing something extraordinary would make her existence meaningful. As Rogers (1942, 1961) observed, clients often present with rigid self-structures or unrealistic expectations at the beginning of therapy. However, as meso-dimensional experiences are based on recurrent life experiences or significant life events, these assumptions are there for a reason. Meaning-making processes at this level often consist of self-reflection and exploring these assumptions and/or significant (often unresolved) life events.

When we explored what made Aisha feel or think that she had to do something exceptional, she came to realise that there were a lot of family expectations. Excelling above the average was highly valued. As she became aware of the background to her own expectations of herself and life, she started to question them.

As for life having to be pleasant to be meaningful, we explored where this assumption might have come from. Over time, Aisha realised that it had something to do with her early experiences when her parents constantly argued. She did not want to lead such a life, and so it was important to her that her life had to be pleasant. However, she also became aware that, by avoiding unpleasant experiences such as possible conflicts, her life often felt empty and inauthentic. In contrast to a more classical person-centred approach, I suggested to her that there were different ways of deriving meaning. Delle Fave (2020), like many other scholars involved in meaning research, makes a difference between *hedonic* meaning and *eudaimonic* meaning: hedonic meaning is mainly derived from pleasure; eudaimonic meaning is derived from goals that relate to the other or the world. Aisha felt inspired by the idea of eudaimonic meaning. When she met up with her friends, she wondered how she could contribute to making these friendships more durable and meaningful, instead of only seeing them as a source of pleasure. Just as working on the micro-dimension made it possible for new felt meanings to emerge, working explicitly on this meso-dimension helped her to experience a wider range of meaning in her daily life.

On a macro-dimension, Aisha openly questioned the meaning of life. For her, it did not make any sense: we come out of nothing, and we will just disappear again. Aisha openly wondered about life's meaning during the first sessions. But as she did not seem to have any resources to cope with her sense of meaninglessness at that time, I decided not to explore this ontological experience yet. All she would have found at the macro-dimension would have been a general stuckness, often experienced as angst or despair (Kierkegaard, 1843/2013). During those first sessions, I conveyed my openness towards her ontological questions by simply paraphrasing what she said, and when her experience of life started to shift on the micro- and meso-dimension later on, I empathically reflected and 're-experienced' her experiences. When she raised life's meaninglessness, I shared my sense that there was a lot of loneliness when she talked about these matters, as if she was in a kind of vacuum with nobody around her.

Instead of tumbling together into the pitfall of having a philosophical conversation, my *existential empathy* (Vanhooren, 2022) helped her to become more aware of *how* she experienced life at her core. Existential empathy can be understood as the capacity of the therapist to attune to and resonate with the existential layer of the client's experience, and also to symbolise and communicate this back to the client (Vanhooren, 2022). Through existential empathy and ontological re-experiencing, I tried to facilitate her meaning-making process about life. In this instance, existential empathy goes beyond the concrete situation of the client and stretches to a caring and empathic understanding of the human condition. As Rank (1936) and Rogers (1980) have written, for the client, it is precisely the feeling of being understood that makes existential experiences more tolerable, and even in the case of meaninglessness, the experience of sharing the meaninglessness makes it, in a way, more meaningful.

Aisha's ontological question about the meaning of life and my re-experiencing of her to be really alone when she wondered about the meaning of life made her realise that her sadness and her tears (micro-dimension) had something to do with the sense that she did not have the right to exist just as she was. Her experience of the meaning of life was intertwined by not feeling worthy of living. Rogers (1980) aligns with Buber in arguing that the empathic relationship can create an I-Thou experience through which the client can feel confirmed as having the right to be and to become their self. Aisha experienced this acceptance. By exploring how she felt when she raised the question 'Am I worthy of living?', she realised that this was that feeling she was trying to get rid of by binge eating. At those instances she felt like an abandoned little girl who needs comforting. As Buber remarks, feeling confirmed as a person by another person is an important first step but does not conclude this process. A second necessary second step is *self-confirmation* (Buber, in Anderson & Cissna, 1997), or, in the words of existential therapist Längle (2018), 'to live with an inner consent'.

Over the next few weeks, Aisha tried to take care of that little girl and give her some caring attention. With all the shifts she experienced through this multi-layered meaning-making process, she did not feel stuck any longer. Instead, she experienced more freedom, but wondered what to do with it.

Existence as freely choosing

At the heart of almost all existential philosophies and therapeutic practices is a belief that human beings are fundamentally and ineradicably free. Sartre (1958), for instance, argues that even prisoners are ontologically free, in the sense that they can still decide whether to try to escape or stay put. Furthermore, he tends to argue that everything we do and think is a choice – even what we feel (see Sartre, 1962).

This is possibly one of the biggest contrasts between existential and classical person-centred views of human being. Rogers was very concerned to emphasise the human capacity for freedom (see, for instance, Rogers, 1961, 1977; Rogers & Freiberg, 1994), but he tends to present freedom as something that human beings can attain, rather than something that is intrinsic to our very being at every moment in time. Furthermore, within the person-centred field, there is a tendency to see growth as something that has a large, non-conscious, spontaneous element to it. In the chapter on the classical person-centred approach in this present book (Chapter 2), for instance, Merry and Haugh write: 'The process of actualisation is not regarded as a conscious "activity" in which the individual makes choices between alternatives, but as a process in which the total organism is involved at both conscious and non-conscious levels' (p.33).

By contrast, existential philosophers and therapists have tended to put a greater emphasis on conscious deliberation in the process of human development (see, for instance, Sartre, 1958). From an existential perspective, human development is like coming to a series of crossroads, each of which forces us to make decisions about the way we want to go, or be (Cooper, 2003b; 2015). So, for instance, if I and my partner are deciding whether or not to try for another child, the conscious decisions that we make will have a great impact on who we become in the future.

Furthermore, while an existential approach would not necessarily argue that such decisions are always consciously made, it would hold that our movement through life is an agentic, directional one (Cooper, 2019). From an existential perspective, then, there is no actualising force within us that drives us towards self-enhancement and self-maintenance. It is something that we actively have to choose to do. Similarly, in contrast to a classical person-centred perspective, there is no belief that we have an innate tendency to move towards constructive and pro-social behaviours – rather, we must actively and deliberately choose good over evil (see Rogers' correspondence with May in Kirschenbaum & Henderson, 1990; also Laing's comments on Rogers in Mullan, 1995). From an existential perspective, there are no inner drives or tendencies that cause us to be who we are and no 'process' we can trust. Rather, who we are is shaped by the choices that we make.

However, knowing that you can steer your life in a multitude of directions at any moment can feel overwhelming. It can even give us a sense that our existence is groundless (Yalom, 1980). To avoid this overwhelming and anxiety-provoking realisation, from an existential standpoint, people do not always acknowledge that they have choices in a particular situation. Bugental (1999) talks about self-imposed limitations that create a wall against the vast freedom we have. However, we are not always aware of the fact that these limitations are self-imposed. We give ourselves a fixed and rigid identity or personality – like being shy, or an introvert – so that we do not ever really have to think through the complexities and uncertainties of being a being-in-flux.

As with classical person-centred thinking, then, there is a belief in existential philosophy that human beings have the capacity to distort or deny certain self-experiences or understandings of their own existence. There is a significant difference here, however, between the existential and classical person-centred views. From a classical person-centred perspective, it is argued that the tendency to deny or distort certain experiences arises out of our tendency to introject external values (Rogers, 1951), and particularly the values from others as to which of our experiences are worthy of positive regard (Rogers, 1957). Here, then, is a belief that denial and distortion arise from external sources and that, if individuals were left to their own devices, they would have little need to defend themselves against their own experiences. By contrast, from an existential perspective, denial and distortion are seen as arising from *within* the individual, as well as from the individual's encounter with other people. So, for instance, existential philosophers and therapists would argue that people may have a tendency to deny the fact that they are going to die (see, for example, Yalom, 1980), and this is not principally to do with introjecting a belief from others that dying is wrong, or that they will not be positively regarded if they are on their death-bed. Rather, their denial of death comes about because of the sheer terror of the thought that their existence and projects will come to an end.

While in both approaches denial and distortion of experiences are seen as bringing temporary relief, it is argued that they ultimately cause more problems than they alleviate. From an existential perspective, our awareness of the reality of human existence – like denied self-experiences – does not go away. Rather, it piles up, demanding to be heard, overwhelming us with feelings of anxiety and helplessness. And, by not facing up to this reality, it is argued that we cannot make the most of the possibilities we do have. We pretend to ourselves that we will go on living for ever, so we put off doing things now, or we invite someone else to make our choices for us and end up feeling frustrated and victimised. So the existential approach, like the classical person-centred approach, argues that, although acknowledging the truth of our existence can be difficult, it can also bring with it great vitality, passion and an unrivalled intensity of living. Indeed, while existential philosophy does emphasise the more discomforting aspects of life, it is ultimately part of an attempt to help people live life more fully and intensely.

For Aisha, having more access to her experiencing (micro-dimension), being more aware that she did not have to follow her family's opinions on how to live her life (meso-dimension), and feeling somehow differently connected to life as such (macro-dimension), meant that she could ask herself what was important while she was with others. She became aware that she cared for others, and she made an effort to be a better friend. She also noticed that she cared for the planet and decided to go on rallies and marches to make people aware of climate change. Furthermore, she became aware that she had never made the choice to follow her dreams. May (1996) suggests that, when we come close to realising ourselves, instead of making the choice to do so, often we run away. Aisha had never pursued her dream to become a medical doctor because she was afraid she would fail and look stupid in the eyes of her family. Likewise, she also realised that she never made a real commitment to be in an intimate partner relationship because it might turn out to be a failure. Instead, she had been playing safe in order not to be laughed at.

As Aisha felt more connected to herself and more aware of what seemed to be worth living for, she courageously engaged in a long-term relationship. It really felt like making a choice to her. Also, she decided to quit her current studies. As she was close to finishing her degree, quitting looked foolish to others. However, she knew she would never do something with that degree. Instead she made the choice to become a medical doctor. However, there was no guarantee that either of these two decisions would lead to 'success'. From an existential point of view, although we can make choices, we are still limited beings, and other circumstances have a major influence on our path of life.

Existence as finite and limited

Existential philosophers and therapists, then, see human beings as fundamentally free, but it would be a mistake to assume that they think that people can do whatever they want. Far from it. Existential philosophers have been no less concerned with the fundamental limitations that human existences face, such as the fact that we are going to die, the fact that we are born into a world that is not of our making, and the fact that we are surrounded by numerous economic, social, cultural, political and environmental givens over which we have no influence or control.

In contrast, classical person-centred therapy tends to put less emphasis on the limitations of human existence – apart from the surmountable limitation of conditional positive regard. With its more optimistic outlook, it tends to focus on what human beings can achieve, rather than on those things that are beyond our capacities. Indeed, Rogers explicitly states that such issues as death are no subjects to be dwelt upon (Swildens, 2002).

Paradoxically, then, existential thinking places more emphasis on both the freedoms and limitations of human existence than the classical person-centred approach. In metaphorical terms, its view of human existence is less like a sprouting seed and more like a goldfish in a tank (Cooper, 2003b): confined on all sides, but able to move freely within its boundaries. To take these metaphors further, while the sprouting seed, like the goldfish, is affected by its external environment (such as a lack of sunlight), in the right conditions it can grow to its fullest extent. By contrast, the goldfish can never move outside of its tank; it can never exceed its imprisonment and restrictions. Here, then, the external limitations are conceptualised as being more fixed and inescapable, and more indifferent to the organism's plight.

To illustrate this with a more familiar example, take the instance of a person-centred community meeting. Here, in our experience, there often seems to be an assumption that, if all the participants can express what they want, then as many needs as possible can be met. From an existential perspective, on the other hand, there is more of an acknowledgement that the limits of the situation – such as time boundaries – mean that there must inevitably be compromises, frustrations and feelings of disappointment. Indeed, from an existential standpoint, one of the paradoxes of this situation is that the more each person's needs are talked about, the more likely it is that some people – such as those who 'want to get on with things' – may find that their needs are frustrated.

Aisha's choice to study medicine and her investment in her partner relationship came with new frustrations, questions and fears. After being with her partner for a while, she started to wonder whether this was the right person for her. By studying medicine, she was confronted with the fact that she did not get the highest grades of her cohort. Her new choices, which were the result of this therapy, confronted her with her own limitations and the limitations of life. Likewise, she started to feel that this therapy had offered her what it could, but that it was her job to make choices and engage with life as it was. Therapy would not turn her life into a Garden of Eden; therapy and my capacities as a therapist were limited. Viewing therapy and the meeting between client and therapist as a form of existence, Rank (1936) emphasised the importance of meeting the limitations of life in therapy as well. For this reason, Rank would limit the number of sessions. He believed this not only symbolised the fact that therapy, like life, is finite; it also fuelled therapy with a vitality that came from the awareness that it was limited. Rank (1936) also emphasised the reality that the therapist is limited too. By discovering that the therapist is just a human being, the client might be encouraged to leave the therapeutic space and take their own path.

Aisha's life was not perfect. Although therapy did not turn every moment into a meaningful experience, it had made a difference. Not only did she not suffer anymore from depression and binge eating, she was more aware of her existence with all its limitations and opportunities. She had found a new way to be with the existential givens, and now tried to live her life as truly and meaningfully as possible. Finally, Aisha closed the door of the therapy room behind her and stepped into her future.

Concluding thoughts

That the numbers of existentially informed person-centred practitioners are growing might not be a surprise. Although meaning in life – and other existential concerns – have always been at the core of the larger humanistic psychology movement (Vanhooren et al., 2022), global concerns such as climate change, mass migration and pandemics make people increasingly aware of the limitations of life. At the same time, one-third to two-thirds of our clients have questions about life's meaning when they start therapy, implicitly or explicitly (Golovchanova et al., 2021). Existential concerns in our times might ask for a more explicit approach, and that is precisely what person-centred existentially informed therapy offers.

Openness towards the existential is not always evident in the person-centred nation. In one of our recent qualitative studies, even seasoned person-centred therapists were found to be reluctant to engage with such issues as high levels of meaninglessness in their clients (Pellens et al., 2023). By contrast, person-centred therapists who have been additionally trained in the existential approach report that their capacity to be with clients who are in existential distress has expanded (Frediani et al., 2022). Engaging with our own existential layer – through life or through training – may prompt a search for meaning through which we, as therapists, re-evaluate our unacknowledged ways of coping with our own existential challenges. This might enlarge our capacity to be with and to explore the existential concerns of our clients and humankind. As a result, existentially informed person-centred trainees feel more at ease with the existential, and experience having more 'language' for it at the end of their training (Vanhooren, 2018). It extends their existential empathy.

Besides existential empathy and explicitly facilitating ontological meaning-making process through self-exploration and re-experiencing, specific existentially informed person-centred interventions might also help clients to make sense of their existence. Proponents of the experiential-existential approach have been developing and studying new interventions to facilitate existential awareness and meaning-making (e.g. Missiaen & Vanhooren, 2021; Vanhooren, 2023; Verdegem et al., 2022). However, as Gendlin (1990) warned, interventions cannot and should not replace being with the client and their pains or joys. Likewise, specific experiential-existential interventions should only serve to enable us to engage with our own existential layer and that of others, in order to find new meaning and the courage to engage with life again. Or, as Bugental (1978) elegantly puts it, to help the client to be more present in their own existence.

Resources

Key reading

- Buber, M. (1958). *I and thou* (R.G. Smith, Trans.) (2nd ed.). T & T Clark Ltd.
  Classic relational philosophy text.
- Cooper, D.E. (1999). *Existentialism*. Blackwell.
  One of the best introductions to existentialism.
- Cooper, M. (2015). *Existential psychotherapy and counselling: Contributions to a pluralistic practice*. Sage.
  Contemporary overview of existential practices, from a relational standpoint.
- Cooper, M. (2018). *Existential therapies* (2nd ed.). Sage.
  Introduces the different schools of existential therapy.
- Spinelli, E. (2005). *The interpreted world: An introduction to phenomenological psychology* (2nd ed.). Sage.
  Succinct introduction to phenomenology and its meaning for therapeutic practice.
- van Deurzen, E. (2012). *Existential counselling and psychotherapy in practice* (3rd ed.). Sage.
  Basic principles of contemporary existential practice.
- Vos, J. (2018). *Meaning in life*. Palgrave.
  Contemporary introduction to meaning-centred existential practices.

Organisations

- Meaning & Existence: https://ppw.kuleuven.be/meaning-and-existence/eng
  Belgian-based centre for experiential-existential therapy, training and research.
- New School of Psychotherapy and Counselling: https://nspc.org.uk
  Centre of training for existential therapy in the UK.
- Society for Existential Analysis: http://existentialanalysis.org.uk
  UK-based existential therapy association.
- World Confederation for Existential Therapy: www.facebook.com/groups/existentialworldconfederation
  International confederation, hosts a biennial world congress.

References

Anderson, R. & Cissna, K.N. (1997). *The Martin Buber – Carl Rogers dialogue: A new transcript with commentary*. State University of New York Press.

Arredondo, A.Y. & Caparrós, B. (2019). Associations between existential concerns and adverse experiences: A systematic review. *Journal of Humanistic Psychology*. Advance online publication. https://doi.org/10.1177/0022167819846284

Bohart, A.C. (2001). Emphasising the future in empathy responses. In S. Haugh & T. Merry (Eds.), *Rogers' therapeutic conditions: Evolution, theory and practice. Vol. 2: Empathy* (pp.99–111). PCCS Books.

Boss, M. (1963). *Psychoanalysis and daseinsanalysis*. Basic Books, Inc.

Buber, M. (1958). *I and Thou* (R.G. Smith, Trans.) (2nd ed.). T&T Clark Ltd.

Bugental, J.F.T. (1978). *Psychotherapy and process: The fundamentals of an existential-humanistic approach*. Zeig, Tucker & Theisen.

Bugental, J.F.T. (1999). *Psychotherapy isn't what you think*. Zeig, Tucker & Theisen.

Camus, A. (1955). *The myth of Sisyphus* (J. O'Brien, Trans.). Penguin.

Cooper, M. (2003a). Between freedom and despair: Existential challenges and contributions to person-centred and experiential therapy. *Person-Centered & Experiential Psychotherapies, 2*(1), 43–56. https://doi.org/10.1080/14779757.2003.9688292

Cooper, M. (2003b). *Existential therapies*. Sage.

Cooper, M. (2004). Existential approaches to therapy. In P. Sanders (Ed.), *The tribes of the person-centred nation: An introduction to the schools of therapy related to the person-centred approach* (pp.95–124). PCCS Books.

Cooper, M. (2012). Existentially informed person-centred therapy. In P. Sanders (Ed.), *The tribes of the person-centred nation: An introduction to the schools of therapy related to the person-centred approach* (2nd ed.) (pp.131–160). PCCS Books.

Cooper, M. (2015). *Existential psychotherapy and counselling: Contributions to a pluralistic practice*. Sage.

Cooper, M. (2017). *Existential therapies* (2nd ed.). Sage.

Cooper, M. (2019). *Integrating counselling and psychotherapy: Directionality, synergy, and social change*. Sage.

Delle Fave, A. (2020). Meaning in life: Structure, sources and relations with mental and physical health. *Acta Philosophica, 29*(1), 19–32.

Fortems, C., Dezutter, J., Dewitte, L. & Vanhooren, S. (2022). The mediating role of meaning in life between the therapeutic relationship and therapy outcome in person-centred and experiential psychotherapies. *Person-Centered & Experiential Psychotherapies, 21*(1), 73–93. https://doi.org/10.1080/14779757.2021.1938184

Frediani, G., Krieckemans, L., Seijnaeve, A. & Vanhooren, S. (2022). Engaging with the client's existential concerns: The impact on therapists and counselors. *Person-Centred & Experiential Psychotherapies, 22*(3), 283–302. doi: 10.1080/14779757.2022.2133000

Freud, S. (1923). The ego and the id (J. Strachey, Trans.). *The standard edition of the complete psychological works of Sigmund Freud* (Vol. 19, pp.12–59). Hogarth Press.

Gendlin, E.T. (1962). *Experiencing and the creation of meaning: A philosophical and psychological approach to the subjective*. Northwestern University Press.

Gendlin, E.T. (1973). Experiential psychotherapy. In R. Corsini (Ed.), *Current psychotherapies* (pp.317–352). Peacock.

Gendlin, E.T. (1990). The small steps of the therapy process: How they come and how they help them come. In G. Lietaer, J. Rombouts, & R. Van Balen (Eds.), *Client-centred and experiential psychotherapy in the nineties* (pp.205–224). Leuven University Press.

Gendlin, E.T. (1996). *Focusing-oriented psychotherapy: A manual of the experiential method.* Guilford Press.

Golovchanova, N., Dezutter, J. & Vanhooren, S. (2021). Meaning profiles and the perception of the working alliance at the start of outpatient person-centred, experiential, and existential psychotherapies. *Journal of Clinical Psychology, 77*(3), 770–781. https://doi.org/10.1002/jclp.23057

Heidegger, M. (1962). *Being and time* (J. Macquarrie & E. Robinson, Trans.). Blackwell.

Hoffman, L. (2009). Introduction to existential psychology in a cross-cultural context: An East-West dialogue. In L. Hoffman, M. Yang, F.J. Kaklauskas, & A. Chan (Eds.), *Existential psychology East-West* (pp.1–67). University of the Rockies Press.

Holzhey-Kunz, A. (2014). *Daseinsanalysis.* Free Association Books.

Ikemi, A. (2017). The radical impact of experiencing on psychotherapy theory: An examination of two kinds of crossing. *Person-centered & Experiential Psychotherapies, 16*(2), 159–172. https://doi.org/10.1080/14779757.2017.1323668

Jaspers, K. (1951/2003). *Way to wisdom: An introduction to philosophy.* Yale.

Kierkegaard (1843/2013). *Fear and trembling, and the sickness unto death.* Princeton University Press.

Kirschenbaum, H. & Henderson, V. (Eds.). (1990). *The Carl Rogers dialogues.* Constable.

Kramer, R. (2019). *The birth of relationship therapy: Carl Rogers meets Otto Rank.* Psychosozial-Verlag.

Längle, A. (2018). Spirituality in psychotherapy? The relationship between immanence and transcendence in existential analysis. In S. Laengle, & C. Wurm (Eds.), *Living our own life: Existential analysis in action* (pp.35–52). Routledge.

Leijssen, M. (2007). Making space for the inner guide. *American Journal of Psychotherapy, 61*, 255–270.

Madison, G. (2010). Focusing on existence: Five facets of an experiential-existential model. *Person-centered & Experiential Psychotherapies, 9*, 189–204. https://doi.org/10.1080/14779757.2010.9689066

Marcel, G. (1949). *The philosophy of existence* (M. Harai, Trans.). Books for Libraries Press.

May, R. (1983). *The discovery of being.* W.W. Norton & Company.

May, R. (1996). *The meaning of anxiety.* W.W. Norton & Company

Mearns, D., & Cooper, M. (2018). *Working at relational depth in counselling and psychotherapy* (2nd ed.). Sage.

Merleau-Ponty, M. (1962). *The phenomenology of perception* (C. Smith, Trans.). Routledge.

Missiaen, C. & Vanhooren, S. (2021). Facing our existential demons: A focusing-oriented and existential approach. In N. Kypriotakis & J. Moore (Eds.), *Senses of focusing, vol.1* (pp.317–336). Eurasia Publications.

Mullan, B. (1995). *Mad to be normal: Conversations with RD Laing.* Free Association Books.

Pellens, H., Vanhees, V., Dezutter, J., Luyten, P. & Vanhooren, S. (2023). Therapeutic responsiveness in the blank landscape of depression: A qualitative study among psychotherapists. *Psychotherapy Research.* Advance online publication. https://doi.org/10.1080/10503307.2023.2239457

Rank, O. (1936). *Will therapy: An analysis of the therapeutic process in terms of relationships.* Knopf.

Rim, K.L., Hill, C.E. & Kivlighan, D.M.Jr. (2022). Changes in meaning in life, working alliance, and outcome in psychodynamic psychotherapy: What leads to what? *Journal of Counseling Psychology, 69*(6), 835–844. https://doi.org/10.1037/cou0000636

Rogers, C.R. (1942). *Counseling and psychotherapy: Newer concepts in practice.* Houghton Mifflin.

Rogers, C.R. (1951). *Client-centered therapy.* Constable.

Rogers, C.R. (1957). The necessary and sufficient conditions of therapeutic personality change. *Journal of Consulting Psychology, 21,* 59–103.

Rogers, C.R. (1961). *On becoming a person.* Houghton Mifflin Company.

Rogers, C. R. (1977). *Carl Rogers on personal power.* Constable.

Rogers, C.R. (1980). *A way of being.* Houghton Mifflin Company.

Rogers, C.R. & Freiberg, H.J. (1994). *Freedom to learn* (3rd ed.). Macmillan College.

Sartre, J.-P. (1958). *Being and nothingness: An essay on phenomenological ontology* (H. Barnes, Trans.). Routledge.

Sartre, J.-P. (1962). *Sketch for a theory of the emotions* (P. Mairet, Trans.). Methuen.

Spinelli, E. (2006). *Demystifying therapy* (2nd ed.). PCCS Books.

Stumm, G. (2005). The person-centered approach from an existential perspective. *Person-Centered & Experiential Psychotherapies, 4*(2), 106–123. https://doi.org/10.1080/14779757.2005.9688375

Swildens, H. (2002). Where did we come from and where are we going? The development of person-centred therapy. *Person-Centered & Experiential Psychotherapies, 1*(1&2), 118–131.

Tedeschi, R.G. & Calhoun, L.G. (2004). Posttraumatic growth: Conceptual foundations and empirical evidence. *Psychological Inquiry, 15,* 1–8.

Tillich, P. (1952). *The courage to be.* Yale University Press.

Vaidya, D. (2013). Re-visioning Rogers' second condition: Anxiety as the face of ontological incongruence and basis for the principle of non-directivity. *Person-centered & Experiential Psychotherapies, 12,* 209–222. doi: 10.1080/14779757.2013.836128

Vanhooren, S. (2018). Experiential-existential psychotherapy: Deepening existence, engaging with life. In M. Bazzanu (Ed.), *Re-visioning person-centred therapy: The theory and practice of a radical paradigm* (pp.151–163). Routledge.

Vanhooren, S. (2019). Struggling with meaninglessness: A case study from an experiential-existential perspective. *Person-Centered & Experiential Psychotherapies, 18*(1), 1–21. https://doi.org/10.1080/14779757.2019.1572029

Vanhooren, S. (2022). Existential empathy: The challenge of 'being' in therapy and counseling. *Religions*, *13*(8), 752. https://doi.org/10.3390/rel13080752

Vanhooren, S. (2023). *Op de bodem: Existentiële thema's in psychotherapie en begeleiding* [At the bottom: Existential themes in therapy and counselling]. Pelckmans.

Vanhooren, S., Grosemans, A. & Breynaert, J. (2022). Focusing, the felt sense, and meaning in life. *Person-Centered & Experiential Psychotherapies, 21*(3), 250–268. https://doi.org/10.1080/14779757.2022.2028660

Verdegem, S., Dezutter, J., Vandenberghe, J., Debeurme, I. & Vanhooren, S. (2022). Wat kan'k ermee? Existentiële groepstherapie bij mensen met kanker. [What can I with cancer? Existential group therapy with cancer patients]. *Tijdschrift Klinische Psychologie, 52(1), 50–70.*

Warner, M.S. (2013). Difficult client processes. In M. Cooper, M. O'Hara, P.F. Schmid, & A.C. Bohart (Eds.), *The handbook of person-centred psychotherapy & counselling* (2nd ed., pp.343–358). Palgrave.

Watson, J.B. (1925). *Behaviourism*. W.W. Norton & Co.

Yalom, I. (1980). *Existential psychotherapy*. Basic Books.

9. Pluralistic person-centred therapy

Nicola Blunden

> Living in the moment means an absence of rigidity, of tight organization, of the imposition of structure on experience. It means instead a maximum of adaptability, a discovery of structure *in* experience, a flowing, changing organization of self and personality. (Carl Rogers, quoted in Kirschenbaum & Henderson, 1989, p.143)

The person-centred approaches to therapy aspire to a fluidity of being that transcends pre-ordained structures and assumptions. This in-the-moment openness to emergent experience is perhaps the defining and unifying quality of the many different person-centred ways of being that are represented in this book. Since Rogers first drew attention to what he considered to be the optimal personal and interpersonal fluidity of human flourishing, translating it into a range of psychological theories, the person-centred communities have struggled with the paradox of this theoretical inheritance. Theory is, itself, an attempt to define and predict reality. In so doing, theorising imposes a conceptual structure, seemingly in direct opposition to the 'discovery of structure in experience'. How then is a 'theory of fluidity' possible?

In response to this paradox, person-centred theorists, following Rogers, have tended to generate theories that are propositional, hypothetical or suggestive rather than predictive. Nevertheless, the claim that the purpose of therapy is to facilitate the 'flowing, changing organization' of personality change (Rogers, 1989, p.143) is inevitably a theoretical statement that becomes, in its very utterance, an imposition of structure on experience.

It is, perhaps, only human to develop a certain rigidity about theoretical structures, even 'theories of discovery', so that propositional theory comes to take the form of belief. Such beliefs can become dogmatic or axiomatic. Further, they can be used to exclude people who either question the *de facto* claims of a particularly treasured theory or fail to live up to its perceived strictures, leading to the frequently raised fear among person-centred counselling trainees, 'Am I person-centred enough?' and its corollary accusation, '*You* are not person-centred enough.'

Pluralistic therapy emerged in this context as a proposal that therapists embrace *multiple* theories as potentially helpful to clients, requiring neither dogmatic adherence to theory nor its abandonment, but instead a pragmatic stance of openness to all theories. So, pluralism takes a both/and approach to theory, rather than an either/or approach (Cooper & McLeod, 2011a). In the context of therapy, this stance results in a therapy that is adaptable and fluid, in the sense of Rogers' statement above. In this chapter, I will unpack what it means to take a pluralistic attitude towards person-centred theory and practice, explore the common features that emerge from a pluralistic reading of the person-centred way of being, and consider some important implications for person-centred therapy in the current social climate.

The pluralistic framework is a trans-theoretical approach. It is meta-theory of therapy that offers a particular lens through which to view the therapeutic relationship, whatever modality is being practised. In this chapter, I won't explore pluralistic therapy as it might be practised by therapists of other orientations. For more information on this, please read the core pluralistic texts suggested at the end of this chapter. I also won't describe in detail other forms of integration in person-centred therapy, although I will occasionally refer to these by comparison. This chapter articulates a particular way of being *both* person-centred *and* pluralistic that is informed by both theoretical inheritances but is distinct in its own characteristics from pluralism *per se*, and from classical person-centred practice (Chapter 2, this volume). The model emerged from the practical application of a pluralistic lens to a core person-centred counselling training, and many of the theoretical insights in this chapter were co-created with colleagues and students on that programme. This chapter is dedicated to that generous, bright community.

Pluralistic person-centred therapy is not concerned with imposing pre-existing structures or theoretical beliefs, but in discovering structure and a unique therapeutic approach through close, interpersonal co-creativity. This promotes a person-centred therapy that is culturally attuned (Khan, 2023), richly varied in its practices, flexible, and integrative in its permission for clients and therapists to draw from a range of theories, practices and cultural resources.

As a note on language, you will notice that I refer to the approach as either 'person-centred pluralism' or 'pluralistic person-centred practice'. I am not privileging either the person-centred or pluralistic worldview, and therefore I'll vary these terms to allow for your own self-identification.

The emergence of person-centred pluralism

The pluralistic framework

In 2005, Mick Cooper and John McLeod developed what they termed a 'pluralistic framework for therapy' over the course of a series of train journeys from Edinburgh to Sheffield (Cooper & McLeod, 2007). The framework was proposed as a meta-theory in which therapists could locate their client work, challenging the notion of one superior modality. They advocated for flexible and adaptive therapeutic partnerships that are tailored to clients' explicit needs and wishes. They defined therapeutic pluralism as both a *sensibility* (the belief that there is no one best therapeutic approach) and as a *practice* (characterised by co-production with the client of the goals, tasks and methods of therapy). Applying this framework, the therapist and client collaboratively design a unique therapeutic approach that responds to the client's particular needs and preferences. As it is devised anew in each therapeutic relationship, a pluralistic therapy approach is necessarily integrative, potentially incorporating a range of diverse theories and practices that might be helpful to the client. Given that the approach is *co*-created, those resources might derive from either the client or the therapist, according to their knowledge, experience and expertise. Such resources might be termed 'cultural resources' (McLeod, 2017), encompassing any potentially useful theories, techniques and activities from the broad field of human knowledge that can be brought to bear to help the client. Providing that the therapeutic dyad has sufficient confidence and competence, these can be integrated into a unique, co-produced approach that is adapted to each therapeutic relationship.

Cooper & McLeod (2011a) described their pluralistic framework as an expression of person-centred values and practices, and as one reading of what it means to be person-centred. Their reading draws heavily on the dialogical turn in the person-centred approaches, in which theorists promoted a mutual and dialogical understanding of therapy, as opposed to an approach where therapists are seen primarily to facilitate clients' independent emotional processing (Mearns & Schmid, 2006; Mearns & Cooper, 2018; Rennie, 2010; Tickle & Murphy, 2014; Wilkins, 2015; Chapter 3, this volume). Pursuing this dialogical emphasis and incorporating the work of philosopher Emmanuel Levinas, they argued that the basis of ethics in therapy is to recognise and respond to the uniqueness of the client as an *Other*. This agential Other is 'infinitely foreign' and 'irreducibly strange', and therefore cannot be known in advance through reference to any pre-derived theoretical structure (Cooper, 2009). It follows from the inherent irreducibility of the client that what they need and want is beyond prediction. The client's Otherness therefore demands from the therapist a unique, in-the-moment response. Their suffering, furthermore, is a particular call for help to which the therapist is required to respond, not in a pre-conceived way but in a new, person-to-person encounter. For Cooper and McLeod, this is not merely a pragmatic stance, it is a moral principle. From this principle, it follows that dogmatic adherence to a particular therapeutic framework, centred in the belief system of the therapist, is unethical. An 'ethic of care' (Cooper & McLeod, 2011b) instead requires the therapist to be prepared to release their most dearly held assumptions, potentially including the theories of the person-centred approach, that might be taken otherwise for granted.

Person-centred challenges to the pluralistic framework

Perhaps in part as a reaction to this challenge, Cooper and McLeod's pluralistic framework has received reproachful criticism from some person-centred theorists. Ong and colleagues (2020) describe the framework as 'unnecessary and incompatible' with the person-centred approach, which they claim has a 'distinct anthropological, epistemological, developmental psychological position which cannot be combined with any other orientation' (p.174).

They pose three main challenges to the pluralistic approach. The first is their claim that the unique person-centred ontology – founded on a belief in the actualising tendency – is incompatible with a pluralistic ontology. Second, they argue that the person-centred approach is already adaptable and responsive to the actualising tendency of the client, rendering pluralistic flexibility unnecessary. Finally, they challenge the centrality of clients' goals in Cooper and McLeod's framework.

To address the first point, it would seem likely that an absolutist 'ontology' (i.e. theory of being) is inherently incompatible with a pluralistic one. However, it is not obvious that person-centred theories make such absolutist claims about ontology: in other words, that there is only one reality and that it has already been sufficiently articulated. Such a position would seem inherently to contradict Rogers' many exhortations to fluidity with regard to beliefs and concepts. It is also not obviously the case that the pluralistic framework makes the ontological claim that multiple realities exist. However, pluralists do assert that multiple *ways of describing reality* exist (Smith et al., 2021), and that none of these should take precedence over the unique needs of the client. This is a pluralistic 'epistemology' (i.e. theory of knowledge), and it takes a more pragmatic view than ontology, concerning itself more with the practical and ethical requirements of the therapeutic relationship. It is not clear from Ong and colleagues (2020) whether they would see a pluralistic epistemology as inherently incompatible with a person-centred ontology, but given the phenomenological perspective of Rogers himself and many writers since, it follows that person-centred theory is comfortably compatible with the possibility and validity of multiple ways of describing reality.

To address Ong and colleagues' second point (2020), while it is true that person-centred theory indeed supports and advocates for adaptability and responsiveness to the unique world of the client – as can be seen in Rogers' quote at the start of this chapter – the pluralistic approach does present that adaptability in more intersubjective and co-productive terms. Because the pluralistic framework is a meta-theory that can encompass a range of perspectives and worldviews, it does not exclude a classical reading of the person-centred way of being, which might indeed represent the most useful and meaningful response to the client's 'call for help'. Pluralism also offers a new lens through which to view the more contemporary approaches, as well as practical possibilities for integrating them into a co-created approach.

In their third critique, Ong and colleagues (2020) argue paradoxically that clients should be self-directing in regard to therapeutic goals, and also that clients do not have the ability to choose goals, especially at the outset of therapy. This incapacity of the client to set aims for therapy is, in their view, due to the 'axiomatic' person-centred belief that the client is in a state of incongruence. As I will explore later, applying a pluralistic lens to the idea of client incongruence does not in itself exclude the idea that clients' choices in therapy are intelligible and trustworthy, given that client directionality is also in play. Both processes can be true.

Person-centred pluralism in action

Schmid (2002) noted that Rogers consistently asserted that there is only one axiom inherent to person-centred theory. Far from being a belief in client incongruence, this axiom is the presence of the client's actualising tendency. In this section, I will explore how the concept of the tendency to actualise underscores a distinctively person-centred reading of the pluralistic framework. From this reading, several characteristics of person-centred pluralistic therapy will emerge, beginning with the foundation of pluralistic practice: the ethic of care.

The primary intention – an ethic of care

As we have seen, pluralistic therapy is primarily an ethical and dialogical response to the uniqueness of the client (Cooper & McLeod, 2007). In the context of person-centred therapy, this translates to a primary therapeutic intention. This intention is to respond to the unique 'call of the client' in such a way that their suffering will be alleviated, or that their flourishing will unfold, without the need to impose a pre-existing structure. This establishes from the outset a certain resolve – *to discover how to be helpful*. This means in practice not assuming that our usual theories are going to help *this* client at *this* time, because each person is fundamentally beyond prediction. So, the primary intention leads the therapist to work explicitly with the client to find a therapeutic approach that is helpful. This co-creation, happening in real time, has the quality of discovery, as described by Rogers in our opening quote. In the classical person-centred approach (Chapter 2, this volume), the client's discovery of structure is implicit and contingent on the therapist's application of their private theoretical framework. In pluralistic person-centred practice, therapist and client deconstruct and reconstruct therapy explicitly, discovering together how to be helpful in this unique circumstance in the absence of a pre-determined, pre-eminent theoretical structure.

Although each iteration of person-centred pluralistic practice is unique, a set of common practices or features tends to emerge from this dialogical context.

The features of person-centred pluralistic therapy

To discover how to be helpful to the client in their uniqueness, the therapist and client begin by forming an emergent understanding of the *client's directionality*, sense of agency and tendency to actualise. They refine this shared understanding by offering *mutual transparency* to each other, not only about the purpose of therapy but about its processes and structure. Their mutuality is supported by a concurrent process of *metatherapeutic communication*. Together, the therapist and client evolve a therapy structure that is responsive to the client's needs and wishes, *co-designing a unique therapeutic approach*. This approach might incorporate or *integrate other resources*, such as knowledge from other domains, therapeutic techniques, or culturally diverse activities. This co-creative process leads to deepening, reciprocal *co-reflexivity* between the dyad, prompting ongoing discovery and an increasingly specific and personalised therapeutic response.

To illustrate how each of these features might appear in practice, I will use a fictional example. You may find it useful to try to identify the features of person-centred pluralistic practice, as described above, in this illustrative dialogue.

Marcus

Marcus, the client, has come for therapy because he has not been sleeping well for several months. He is exhausted, irritable and has persistent feelings of nausea and disorientation.

He spends his nights trying everything possible to overcome his insomnia and spends his waking hours in foggy anxiety about the coming night-time ordeal. Feeling hopeless, he consulted his doctor, who recommended that he try talk therapy before using medication. Marcus found Melissa, a person-centred pluralistic therapist, online. We meet them during their fourth session. Marcus has not been sleeping better, and he is expressing frustration and hopelessness.

Marcus: I've done all the sleep hygiene things. I've done the lavender baths and the no-screens after dinner, and the night-time routine, and cutting caffeine. Nothing works.

Melissa: Nothing has worked – you've tried everything…

Marcus: I'm just lost. I've run out of tricks. [*Silence*]

Melissa: I'm… I'm wondering about what we should do. I'm feeling lost too. I don't know any more tricks to try, and I'm not sure if...

Marcus: [*Interrupting wearily*] I don't know. I worry I'm wasting your time. Maybe I should just put up with it.

Melissa: With not sleeping?

Marcus: Yeah. What's the point? Nothing works.

Melissa: Well… I don't feel that you're wasting my time at all, but I do want these sessions to be helpful to you. Is there something else that we could be doing, at least for now, that might be more useful?

Marcus: … How do you mean?

Melissa: Well, I'm wondering, beyond finally being able to sleep, what is it that you want or… what do you need?

Marcus: Honestly? I don't know. I've been so tired for so long. I don't really think about anything else anymore. Maybe… it would be nice just to be able to relax. Like, if I just accept that I'm not going to sleep, is there some way to live with it better? Not just counting the hours, feeling like crap. If I'm going to be awake anyway… I'd like to be awake and alright. Or, better than alright. I don't feel I'm alive really. I'd like to find a way to feel alive again.

Commentary – Marcus and Melissa have come to an impasse. He had originally come to therapy to try to overcome his insomnia, but he feels he has made no progress, and has finally run out of ideas. Melissa shares his feeling of being lost and stuck. She wonders if this would be a good time for them to try to align to a 'deeper' objective for the therapy, and she is curious about what vision he might have for the work, beyond the immediate goal of sleeping better. When she poses this question, Marcus is initially thrown, but when he searches within himself for an answer, the question seems to release a deeper, existential awareness within him: that he is searching for a way to live with his sleeplessness, and somehow to live well. We will return to Marcus and Melissa later in the chapter.

The actualising tendency, non-directivity and goals

All approaches that come under the person-centred umbrella maintain that human flourishing is an expression of the natural tendency to actualise (Brodley, 1999; Wilkins, 2003, Ch. 7). Clients are conceived as directional, future-oriented organisms (Cooper, 2019, 2021). This directionality includes agency, hope, aspiration, motivation and readiness, goals, preferences, expectations and vision (Oddli et al., 2021). The intention of person-centred therapists is to facilitate a relationship aligned to that self-determined orientation.

A corollary to the belief in the actualising tendency is the ethical stance of non-directivity in the person-centred approach (Sommerbeck, 2003). It stems from a belief in the client's right and inherent capacity to pursue their own direction. A trust in this immutable capacity of clients to direct themselves is not a belief that all clients know at all times what is best for them. But it is a recognition that it is only the client who can orient themselves towards or away from their own flourishing, by reference to their own feelings, in the moment. Deliberate, intentional movement towards flourishing, in a future-oriented way, might be termed in the most prosaic fashion 'goal setting'.

On the topic of therapeutic goals, a person-centred therapist, as with Ong and colleagues (2020), once asked me with frustration, 'Why on earth would I ask the client what he wants? How could he possibly know? The client is *incongruent*.' From this therapist's perspective, client incongruence – the second of Rogers' (1957) six conditions of personality change – is a fact, leading to a tricky implication: it suggests that clients cannot know what is best for them, by definition. On this basis, a person-centred therapist can potentially dismiss clients' accounts of themselves, as well as their needs and wishes, despite the obvious contradiction with the belief that clients are the best experts on themselves. Further, as the dialogical theorists have claimed, client change is not merely an intra-psychic phenomenon that occurs in the dichotomous condition of client-incongruence versus therapist-congruence. It arises out of mutual encounter (Schmid & Mearns, 2006), requiring conscious and deliberate alignment between the therapist's and client's intentions for the therapy (Oddli et al., 2021).

A classical person-centred therapist might claim that, in the absence of directing the client, they are implicitly aligned to the client's directionality and tendency to actualise, regardless of whether either party consciously knows the client's intentions. However, there exist some important objections to this view. It is now widely accepted that all therapists exert influence, whether intentional or not (Kahn, 2012). Despite their best intentions, if the therapist tries deliberately to be non-directive, they come up against the paradox of theory: because, in terms of behaviour, non-directivity is construed as inactivity, this instrumentalisation becomes influential in its own right (Grant, 1990). Perhaps because of the inherent difficulty of defining an absent quality in positive terms, the theory of non-directivity, according to Schmid (2005), has lost all meaning. For instance, it does not mean avoiding techniques, opinions or suggestions (Grant, 1990); nor does it mean refraining from therapist-frame responses (Kahn, 2012). It is none of these things, because it is attitudinal, not behavioural. Yet, it is frequently assumed that, if a therapist intervenes in any way, they have become 'directive'.

Given the unequal context of therapy, it is unlikely that person-centred therapists can ever avoid being directive. For instance, Paul Wilkins (2003) highlighted that there is a powerful directive ('Talk to me') in classical person-centred therapy that is essentially identical to the explicit directions that might be made by a person-centred creative therapist (Chapter 10, this volume). In many ways, from a pluralistic standpoint, implicit directives may be more insidiously powerful than explicit ones, because they are beyond challenge. The implicit and powerful direction 'Talk to me' constitutes a pre-existing structure that is imposed on clients by talk-therapists of all orientations.

In pluralistic person-centred therapy, assumptions such as these are deconstructed by both client and therapist. The primary ethical intention (to discover how *in this case, with this person* to be helpful) leads the pluralistic person-centred therapist to want to understand and align to the client's direction, rather than inadvertently impose our own. Client directionality encompasses everything within their phenomenal world, including the structure and processes of therapy. Following Bohart (2004), then, pluralistic person-centred practitioners might define therapist non-directiveness more accurately as getting alongside *client-directiveness.*

Client-directiveness

Client-directiveness involves more than mere goal setting. It is an expression of the client's agency. In person-centred terms, this is expressed through their organismic valuing, which is a privileged form of knowing that belongs to the person themselves. This valuing orients them in space and time and is an 'ongoing psycho-physiological flow' (Rogers, 1980, p.141), manifested through the 'felt sense' (Gendlin, 1994; see Chapter 4, this volume). This inner referent allows individuals to verify the accuracy of their symbolisations of experience. Trust in this embodied, self-organising process differs from simply accepting a client's opinions – it is the recognition that the client's moment-by-moment evaluations are the sole means for both parties to assess whether the therapeutic process aligns with or against the client's self-orienting direction.

For this reason, person-centred pluralistic therapists work with client directionality not in order to establish rigid outcomes or extrinsic goals but to deliberately foster a space where the process of self-orientation can organically unfold and explicitly inform the therapeutic approach. Clients might well find it difficult to pinpoint a meaningful, intrinsically motivated goal straight away. But the symbolisation of a goal (or, alternatively, an intention, purpose, or vision) is an evolving process that can be initiated from the beginning of therapy, if the therapist does not assume that the client's perspective is hopelessly flawed. Making the client's inner valuing process salient from the outset of therapy deliberately establishes a basis for how therapy will be evaluated: by the client's reference to themself. It also enables the dyad to align to the client's tendency to actualise and deconstruct any pre-existing structures that are working against that tendency. This leads to a further process in person-centred pluralistic therapy: the process of demystification through mutual transparency.

So let's return now, to Marcus and Melissa. To recap, Marcus has begun to articulate his immediate intention – to live with his insomnia; indeed, to begin living meaningfully again. Melissa responds empathically, trying to align to this emergent vision for the future.

Melissa: You wonder if maybe there's a way of living with the lack of sleep. Not just living with it but living *well*. Really living again.

Marcus: Yeah. Being happy again. Being *healthy* again, somehow. I don't know how.

Melissa: Being happy and being healthy in some way you don't understand yet, but you can kind of sense…

Marcus: [*Quietly*] It's about going slowly. Just not rushing. Just being quiet and not feeling I always have to be productive. Just enjoying being quiet. Like, just lying in the field and resting and closing my eyes.

Melissa: Mm-hm. Just the quiet satisfaction of…

Marcus: [*Eyes closed, interrupting*] Like, in here as well, not feeling that I have to fix the problem at all…

Melissa: Not having to be productive in here either.

Marcus: Yeah. Not having to leave here today totally fixed. [*Opening his eyes and looking at Melissa*] Not having to be efficient.

Melissa: … You not having to be efficient in here. And perhaps, me not having to be efficient either.

Marcus: Do you want to be efficient?

Melissa: Well… I haven't thought about it until now but think perhaps I have wanted to be efficient. I want you to be helped in the easiest way possible, and maybe the fastest way? But… maybe that's not what you need, and maybe it doesn't help you if I am trying to be efficient as well.

Marcus: [*Closing his eyes again and sighing*] Yeah. What if we just didn't rush at all…

Melissa: Hmm. [*Softly*] Not rushing at all…

Commentary – Tuning in to this new sense of direction, it emerges that Marcus is searching for a new way of being that is 'not about efficiency and rushing'. Even in the therapeutic relationship, he senses these conditions of worth at play. Melissa responds empathically to this and involves herself, realising out loud that she has been pursuing a goal of efficiency too, and that this might have been unhelpful. Melissa knows that this response could distract Marcus from his inner experiencing, given that it comes from her own frame of reference, but she chooses to take this opportunity to share accountability for their therapeutic approach, affirming his perception that they have indeed been 'rushing'. Marcus accepts this, and goes inward, sensing the satisfaction that arises from the idea of both of them 'not rushing'.

Melissa has communicated to Marcus that the therapy is, in an essential way, constructed by them both, and that she is interested in understanding her own part in that construction, and willing to adapt in order to be helpful. This conveys a further message, that the therapy structure is not fixed, and that it is being discovered by them both simultaneously.

Mutual transparency

The power imbalance in therapy is, in part, due to mystique (Wilkins, 2003). Clients assume, often correctly, that the therapist already privately 'knows' what should happen in therapy, while they themselves are in the position of having to work out what the structure entails. Clients' confusion about therapeutic processes can lead them to mistaken, unhelpful assumptions and feelings of failing, or of being failed by, the therapist (Rennie, 1998, 2010; Cook & Monk, 2020). Worse, because of deference, clients usually don't voice these misapprehensions and concerns, amplifying confusion (Rennie, 2010). When the therapist is experienced as passive, this unhelpful mystique can thrive, leading to more unequal power dynamics and a range of potential harms to clients, such as feelings of shame and abandonment (Cook & Monk, 2020; Ladmanová et al., 2022).

By contrast, when the therapist is proactive in eliciting clients' views, clients are more likely to lose their deferential inhibitions and share their thoughts and feelings about therapy, strengthening the therapeutic relationship, reducing dropout and improving outcomes (Cooper, 2023). When the therapist defencelessly receives feedback and adapts accordingly, they show that they take seriously the client's capacity to be objective about the therapy (Rennie, 2000), modelling openness, reciprocity and mutual accountability.

Mutual transparency in person-centred pluralistic therapy is influenced by Rennie's (1998) theory of metacommunication, which he described as 'a matter of purposes and impacts' (p.91). Rennie (2010) felt that both the therapist and client are intentional and agential in contributing to the structure of therapy and reasoned that 'if each could learn what the other's intentions are, it would be easier for them to get along with each other' (1998, p.49). Rennie's work, like the pluralistic approach, sits within the dialogical understanding of person-centred therapy. In dialogical terms, therapy is not only mutually generated but also mutually impactful, involving both therapist and client in a shared vulnerability and reciprocity that Knox (2008) called a 'bi-directional encounter' (p.182). This reciprocal transparency destabilises the power hierarchy inherent to therapy. It is maintained through the process of meta-therapeutic communication.

Marcus has identified that it would feel good to rush less and not seek to be so efficiently productive, both in his life and in his therapy. Given that he is exploring the structure of therapy, Melissa takes the opportunity to ask for more detail, in order to align to his intention more accurately, and help co-create this particular therapy approach.

Melissa: If we were rushing less, and relaxing more in these sessions, how would that look to you?

Marcus: Um… well it would be less pressured. Like, I wouldn't be telling myself I have to do x, y and z by the end of the session. And… maybe I would talk about different things, to be honest.

Melissa: Mm-hm. Less pressure, and more space for you to talk about different things…

Marcus: This is going to sound stupid but, I might even tell you about a book I'm reading or an album I've heard. I haven't read a book in so long.

Melissa: It doesn't sound stupid to me. It sounds like part of... being really alive, as you said.

Marcus: Yeah, because it wouldn't be small talk. It would be... sharing what I'm enjoying. I'd feel guilty doing that, though.

Melissa: Guilty, sharing with me what you are enjoying...

Marcus: As if I should be telling you something more important.

Melissa: As if what you're enjoying isn't important enough to tell me...

Marcus: Yeah, as if I should only be telling you what I'm miserable about... I spend a lot of time working hard and struggling. I never feel I can just stop and do something just for the fun of it. This could be one thing that I do where I don't have to struggle.

Melissa: This could be a space for you to be free... not to struggle...

Marcus: And not feel guilty about it.

Melissa: I would love to hear about what you're enjoying in your life. I can see how that would be helpful because you could be more yourself here and... just do that for enjoyment's sake... without having to justify it.

Commentary – Marcus is surfacing here what he has assumed therapy 'should be' – an exploration of his difficulties. Somehow, this has made it feel wrong for him to bring his satisfactions in life. He also connects this to his more universal feeling of having to earn his own happiness through 'struggling'. Melissa largely facilitates the exploration of his phenomenal experience, empathising and prizing him throughout. But she also aligns throughout to his suggested approach – redefining the therapy as a space to be free of struggle and to explore his enjoyment in life. Their open and transparent conversation about what this therapy can include, has mobilised a new feeling of hopefulness in Marcus and closer contact between the two of them.

Metatherapeutic communication

Discussions *about* the therapeutic process are termed *metacommunication* or *metatherapeutic communication*. This dialogue takes place alongside the therapeutic space, in a concurrent stream of reflective and creative conversation in which the client and therapist discuss the therapy approach they are engaged in. Either the client or therapist can initiate a conversation about the therapy approach, whenever it feels appropriate to do so. During these conversations, therapist and client employ a range of metatherapeutic processes such as agreeing the use of new techniques; offering or eliciting feedback; reviewing and modifying goals or intentions; assessing risks; negotiating boundaries, and establishing informed consent for new ways of working (Papayianni & Cooper, 2018).

Metatherapeutic conversations are somewhat different from 'therapeutic' conversations. During therapeutic conversation – in person-centred terms – clients process their feelings and experiences while the therapist offers facilitative responses. During metatherapeutic discussion, the therapist and client mutually reflect on and adapt their therapeutic approach. While metatherapeutic communications may still have therapeutic effects – such as communicating empathy, congruence or prizing, generating insight and equalising power dynamics – these are not their primary purpose. Through metatherapeutic conversation, the client and therapist foster a unique collaborative style and approach that we might call the 'metatherapeutic relationship'. This metatherapeutic relationship is the dialogical space that protects and contains the evolving therapeutic approach. A strong metatherapeutic relationship is crucial in pluralistic person-centred therapy because it is the space in which the client and therapist co-design and refine their unique therapy structure.

Co-design of a person-centred pluralistic therapy approach

The co-design of a person-centred pluralistic approach is essentially to discover the therapy structure that is most needed by the client. As we have seen, this discovery happens mutually when the therapist and client consciously relinquish pre-existing, assumed models and work closely to deconstruct and then reconstruct the therapeutic process. This creative deconstruction-and-reconstruction process can be thought of as design (McLeod, 2017) or, in pluralistic terms, co-design. Human conversation is a creative, improvisatory process, in which meaning is collaboratively constructed in real-time. And therapy is a particular form of improvised conversation during which, in addition to meaning, other forms of making occur (Blunden, 2023; McLeod & Sundet, 2022). These include 'making a meaningful experience, making a new life, remaking oneself' (McLeod, 2017, p.37). In classical person-centred therapy, this implicit creative process is regarded as happening intra-psychically, within the client. In pluralistic person-centred therapy, the process is made explicit and shared between therapist and client. It is deliberate co-design.

In their pluralistic framework, Cooper & McLeod (2011a) advocate a structure of three domains (goals, tasks and methods) to conceptualise this design process. Once the therapeutic goal is set, it can be broken down into more discrete tasks, and methods can be selected to achieve each task. The apparent linearity of this model might erroneously suggest that pluralistic therapy proceeds in a straightforward, pre-designed fashion. However, these domains are to be applied more as areas of discussion than as uni-directional stages. Rather than adopt a strict 'goals-tasks-methods' framework, person-centred pluralists tend to emphasise the process of mutual, moment-by-moment alignment towards client-directionality. In design terms, person-centred pluralists might therefore be more concerned with how to make the next immediate choice in the therapeutic process (Oddli et al., 2023) than with devising a longer-term therapy design.

Either way, co-design requires that both the client and the therapist symbolise in increasingly accurate ways both *what* they are creating together (the purpose of the therapy) and *how* they are creating it (the process of therapy). Because this co-design is mutual and reciprocal, it incorporates the cultural knowledge and resources of at least two people, meaning that it is inherently integrative in nature in the sense of incorporating multiple resources and worldviews. The pre-existing framework of the therapist would not take a pre-eminent position but would sit alongside the client's own framework. The interaction of both perspectives will lead inevitably to a novel therapeutic design. In practice therefore, pluralistic forms of person-centred therapy can potentially incorporate a diverse variety of theories and practices into their structure.

Marcus and Melissa have been applying their evolving therapy design, which now includes 'space to talk about enjoyment, and to be free of struggle'. Marcus has spent the past 10 minutes or so recounting what gives his life meaning and value, while Melissa has closely listened, facilitating the therapeutic space. Then Marcus initiates a shift towards a metatherapeutic conversation. He has a suggestion.

Marcus: So, I have had an idea, but I'm not sure if it's possible. It crossed my mind earlier.

Melissa: [*Nodding*] Okay.

Marcus: I'm wondering if we could do these sessions somewhere else.

Melissa: … I…

Marcus: I've read that some therapists do walking therapy. Walk and talk. Outside.

Melissa: Oh, yes. That's true.

Marcus: Is that something we can do?

[*Melissa hesitates. She has offered outdoor therapy before, but not in this location, and not recently. She also wonders if this would be too sudden a change to their approach.*]

Melissa: It's something we would have to think about first. What appeals to you about it?

Marcus: I just love being outside. I find it easier to slow down. I can imagine sitting in the sun and talking…

Melissa: I can see how that would be nice, especially now the sun is out. [*She looks out the window, briefly*]

Marcus: I don't want to just *talk* about what I enjoy, after the fact. It would be interesting to *do* something I enjoy, and really enjoy it. You know, since I'm thinking about what it would be like not to be pressured. It was the first thing that popped into my mind when you asked me what that would look like – I just had this really clear picture in my mind of being outside in the fresh air, and it felt really nice. I mean, I get if it's not possible. It's fine. It's just an idea.

Melissa: [*Nodding*] It sounds like a good idea. I'm not hesitating because I think it's not doable. I am just pondering some of the things that we would need to think about and find out first. Let's talk about it.

Commentary – Marcus's idea emerged spontaneously, when he was encouraged to consider what helpful therapy would look like, although it has taken him some time to develop enough confidence to raise this question with Melissa. When he shares the idea, Melissa takes it as an expression of his agency and his tendency to actualise. She wants to remain open and attuned to his directionality. At the same time, she does not feel confident to incorporate outdoor working into their therapy approach without carefully considering both her own competence in this area and the potential consequences of this change to their way of working. She suggests that they explore the idea at more depth.

Co-productive integration in person-centred pluralistic therapy

When the client and therapist incorporate new knowledge or practices into their therapy design, this can be viewed as an integrative process. Pluralistic integration begins as a dialogical response to the unique needs and wishes of the client, not as a pre-existing framework. To differentiate it from other forms of therapeutic integration, I will refer to it as 'co-productive integration'. Co-productive integration is achieved through 'sustained engagement with the client's view of what will be helpful for them' (Cooper & McLeod, 2011b, p.6). For this reason, pluralism offers a more 'client-directed' means of integration, making it of specific utility and interest to person-centred practitioners.

In the previous, second edition of this book, Worsley (2012) suggested that person-centred therapists could integrate knowledge and practices drawn from other modalities and still maintain their person-centred integrity. Employing a continuum from purism to liberalism, he offered a range of theories that he felt person-centred therapists could comfortably integrate into their understanding and practice without compromising their core person-centred beliefs. He also briefly introduced the then nascent pluralistic approach, hoping that it would provoke controversy and a growing edge in our thinking. In my view, these hopes have been fulfilled.

In that chapter, Worsley raised an important critical question about pluralistic integration: namely, that it needed to be differentiated from technical eclecticism. To respond to this point, it is useful to distinguish pluralistic co-productive integration from two forms of therapeutic integration: the 'synthesising form' and the 'eclectic form'. In synthesising integrative approaches, the therapist attempts to achieve a coherent fusion of more than one modality into a new framework. This synthesis can be likened to a merging or blending of theories, and it can be achieved in a number of ways. One approach involves looking for common factors or theoretical ideas that are shared across modalities. Alternatively, a practitioner who has been trained in one modality may assimilate other theories and practices over the course of their career (Cooper & McLeod, 2011a), likewise aiming for an internally coherent framework over time. This synthesis effectively creates a new integrative model intra-psychically within the therapist. Within the person-centred communities, this practice has enabled the development of several integrative person-centred approaches, such as emotion-focused therapy (Chapter 5, this volume), expressive arts person-centred therapy (Chapter 10, this volume), and existential person-centred therapy (Chapter 8, this volume). Outside the person-centred community, synthesising integration has also enabled the person-centred approach to be combined with a range of other modalities, some of which align smoothly with its precepts and some of which have proved more difficult to combine. The question of whether it is possible systematically to integrate other therapeutic modalities into a person-centred worldview and retain one's person-centred credentials has been somewhat contentious, but many have maintained that it is possible (e.g. Bohart, 2012).

By contrast, the eclectic approach to integration requires the therapist to learn a range of methods and theories detached from substantive theory, drawing from these in an ad hoc, flexible way, session by session. This approach might be seen as a 'toolbox' approach, varying according to the therapist's particular choices about what they suppose will be helpful. 'Technical eclecticism' is one of the best-known examples of this approach (Lazarus, 1981), and is sometimes criticised for its potential to confuse and disorient clients by employing inconsistent, sudden changes of practice (Lazarus & Beutler, 1993).

Both the synthesising and eclectic forms of integration effectively place the design of the therapeutic approach into the hands of the therapist, who is responsible for devising the integrative therapeutic structure. Pluralistic integration, by contrast, places responsibility for the integrative design of therapy on the co-productive therapeutic relationship. For this reason, it avoids the trap of imposing a pre-existing framework (as is implied in synthesising forms of integration), because the structure of therapy is mutually discovered by the therapist and client in real time. Pluralistic integration also avoids the second trap of confusing clients with unexpected changes in approach (which is the risk in eclectic forms of integration) by carefully and systematically sharing the integrative design process with clients, according to their needs and inclinations. Because it is co-productive and rooted in the dialogical encounter, pluralistic integration is therefore able to be both responsive to the moment and coherently predictable to clients.

Integrative possibilities

As we have seen, the co-created pluralistic person-centred approach discovers structure as it proceeds. Each time that structural decisions are taken, the client and therapist must carefully examine the potential benefits and risks that may ensue. The integration of additional practices and knowledge can present a complex design challenge for the therapist and client. It may help here to discuss briefly how such integration might look in practice, and to name some important ethical considerations.

In some ways, the biggest challenge facing person-centred pluralistic therapy dyads is the sheer enormity of potential material for integration. There exists in the modern social context a dizzying array of potentially helpful knowledge and practice from which clients and therapists can draw. Such knowledge might be scientific, philosophical, spiritual, professional, political, cultural or technological. It can derive from Western, non-Western, and Indigenous epistemologies, and can also include knowledge gained from lived experience. Depending on their experience and knowledge, person-centred pluralistic therapists and clients can incorporate into the structure of therapy:

- stand-alone practices, such as techniques and methods
- contemporary person-centred theory and practices
- different therapeutic modalities
- cultural resources of all kinds.

Incorporating stand-alone methods

To meet a particular need or preference of the client, a therapeutic dyad might decide to integrate into their therapy design one or more stand-alone practices, such as sand-tray work, journalling, outdoor therapy, relaxation or grounding techniques, graded exposure exercises, two-chair techniques, thought records, creative visualisation, letter-writing, mood-tracking, meditation and many other methods. Therapists can develop, if they so choose, a diverse menu of therapeutic activities for clients to choose from, either to meet their specific needs or to enhance the therapeutic approach more generally. Some clients enjoy and benefit from well-defined exercises. However, it is crucial that integration of techniques is explicitly *co*-created, that it results from a client's expressed need or desire, and that it is carefully incorporated into the approach.

Incorporating contemporary person-centred theory

A therapeutic dyad might also integrate knowledge and/or practices from one or more of the approaches discussed in this book. Person-centred pluralism can be understood as a meta-approach, encompassing diverse ways of being person-centred. This might take the form of using process identification or direction as part of person-centred experiential practice, exploring the client's self-plurality through the lens of configurations theory, or incorporating creative/expressive work to facilitate the symbolisation of their experience without words.

Incorporating different therapeutic modalities

A therapist and client might also choose to integrate an additional therapeutic theory or model. This might be incorporating cognitive-behavioural theory and techniques to manage panic attacks or drawing from attachment theory to explore the resonances between the client's formative and current relationships. To incorporate theory in this way, most therapists will have either received an integrative training or will have completed enough subsequent training in another modality. All therapeutic theories can be seen as cultural narrative structures that clients and therapists can draw from if helpful, to construct a way of working that resonates with their particular experiences and needs (McLeod, 2017). This perspective broadens the scope of therapeutic theories and practices that can be tailored to your collaborative work with clients.

This approach might overlap with a more synthesising integrative approach, in that the therapist might have previously assimilated more than one core modality into their everyday practice. Alternatively, the co-designed approach might be flexible enough to integrate other modalities in a ring-fenced way, incorporating several explicitly contracted sessions within a longer person-centred relationship. For example, a therapist with training in eye movement desensitisation and reprocessing (EMDR) might agree to offer their client a defined number of EMDR sessions to reduce the intensity of post-traumatic distress, before continuing with their usual process-led approach. It is important, when integrating theories and practices from other modalities, to consider carefully if doing so might destabilise the person-centred foundation of the shared therapeutic approach. The therapist and client might spend considerable time exploring the risks of integrating practices that are potentially directive or that see clients in very analytic terms, for example. Transparency about these risks will enable the client to take informed decisions, and to reflect meaningfully on the effects of integrating in this way, enabling the dyad to re-orient their work if needed.

Incorporating cultural resources

Finally, a therapist and client might incorporate knowledge from other professional fields, such as political theory, the social sciences, the arts, Indigenous knowledge or neuroscience to enrich and inform therapeutic practice. For example, numerous therapists have incorporated the theory of intersectionality into their thinking and practice, to understand the cumulative and complex effect of oppressions on people who are multiply marginalised by society (Crenshaw, 2017). Similarly, many person-centred therapists have also incorporated knowledge from neuroscience to better understand the particular needs of clients who have a neuro-difference, such as autism or ADHD. Many therapists also draw from interdisciplinary knowledge, such as their experience of being an artist, a social worker or a teacher. Co-productive integration provides a framework for person-centred therapists to understand when and how to bring such knowledge into the therapeutic space, in response to the particular wishes and needs of the client.

Confidence and competence in pluralistic integration

Within the person-centred pluralistic approach, both therapists and clients can draw freely from any of the above resources and more, if this integration emerges from a dialogical understanding and agreement. However, before integrating any new knowledge or practice, the therapist must know their own limitations, and must develop both confidence and competence in the new technique or approach (Norcross & Cooper, 2021). Confidence includes detailed clarity about the potential risks involved and how these will be managed. Competence includes a depth of personal and professional experience that makes the application of the practice safe and relaxed. The principles of confidence and competence also apply to clients, to the extent that any proposed adaptation to the design of therapy must not over-stretch the client's capacities.

Achieving both confidence and competence is likely to involve the therapist doing additional training, incorporating the practice into their own therapy or supervision, reading relevant research, and proceeding at a pace that allows for feeling secure while incorporating the new element of practice. In some cases, a therapist may already possess both confidence and competence in a certain activity, such as mindfulness. Before offering that resource to a client who expresses an interest, it is likely that the therapist will still need carefully to consider how to transition a personal familiarity into a safe and useful therapeutic activity.

Checklist for pluralistic integration

Before you incorporate additional knowledge or practices to the therapy design, consider the following:

1. **Confidence and competence**: Are you both *competent* (trained to the level that you need to be and aware of the latest relevant research) and *confident* (experienced in the method or approach, clear about how to manage any risks involved) enough to be able to manage any bumps in the road for you and your client?
2. **Client consent**: Have you either responded to an explicit desire or idea that has been offered by the client? Have you ensured that your client is fully informed and consenting to the use of the technique or approach?
3. **Client feedback**: Are you asking for regular feedback and discussion about the integration process? Are you continuously refining and adapting your co-created approach in response to this feedback?
4. **Ethical considerations**: Are you following relevant ethical frameworks and guidance? In addition, are you carefully discussing the risks and potential ethical considerations with your clients as you co-create your integrative approach?
5. **Supervision and consultation**: Have you discussed this potential integration in supervision? Is your supervisor qualified and experienced (confident and competent enough) to supervise this work? Alternatively, could you work with a different supervisor who has the right knowledge and experience?
6. **Cultural attunement**: Have both you and the client included your client's cultural background and beliefs in your co-creation? Have you considered what barriers they may have in freely accessing or using this approach or information?

Having explored the possibilities and limitations of integration in person-centred pluralistic therapy, let us return to the therapy illustration to consider the final characteristic of this practice: mutual reflexivity.

Since the last session, Melissa and Marcus have carefully explored the possibility of incorporating outdoor therapy into their approach. They have discussed potential risks (being observed or overheard) and benefits (incorporating 'enjoyment' directly into the sessions as well as the mental health benefits of being in nature), locations (assessing them for suitability and safety), and contracting (where and when to meet, what to do in the event of a cancellation). Melissa has also discussed the issue in supervision, and has completed a brief, online CPD training in outdoor therapy. She enjoyed two outdoor therapy sessions with her own therapist. Eventually, she and Marcus embark on their first outdoor therapy session together. We join them now that the session is almost over and they are walking back to the therapy room, reflecting on the experience.

Marcus: It's weird how different it's been, but how much it's the same. I'm feeling so relaxed, and it's been so beautiful today, but also, it's very different to being in the room.

Melissa: Mm-hm. I feel that too. How is it different for you?

Marcus: Well, I think it's something to do with being side by side. I don't feel you are looking at me. So, it feels more social? But less intense.

Melissa: Mm-hm, it's more social. It's a different frame, side by side. And somehow… is it that I am not offering you the same visual attention?

Marcus: I mean, I know you are listening. And I know you're paying attention to what I'm saying.

Melissa: But something about not having eye contact is different?

Marcus: I feel quite liberated by you not observing me face-on. I feel I am just looking into the distance. And you are next to me, so I don't feel alone. It's less pressured.

Melissa: Ah, okay. Yes, it's that freedom you spoke of before.

Marcus: How is it different for you?

Melissa: I guess I was worrying about whether the contact between us would feel less, but hearing you say that you feel liberated reassures me.

Marcus: [*Thoughtful silence*] I don't know why but not having to look at you, being able to just look into the distance, really takes the pressure off. I want to be, kind of, left to my own devices?

Melissa: You want to be able to look where you like, and maybe think what you like, without being observed face-on.

Marcus: Yes, I want to be free-range. [*Laughs*] That's the whole point, really. Being watched makes me want to… be good. In the sense of well-behaved. If you aren't watching me, I can maybe relax.

Melissa: So, my attending to you closely, by looking at you, has been a kind of pressure… to be good.

Marcus: Yeah, I guess it has.

Melissa: But my being next to you is a kind of permission to…

Marcus: [*Interrupting*] Be free. Yes.

Commentary – While researching and planning the outdoor sessions together, Marcus and Melissa have developed their meta-therapeutic relationship, and they move seamlessly into a reflective meta-therapeutic discussion about the session, initiated by Marcus. He is exploring the difference in his experience of outdoor therapy, and Melissa, perhaps because she is somewhat anxious about the new change in approach, initially assumes that his statement about the lack of intensity is negative. But, as he processes his feeling, Marcus clarifies that this lack of intensity feels like a lack of pressure and a liberation. He is curious about her experience in turn, and she responds with a short but transparent account of her worry and its reassurance by his sense of freedom. Marcus goes on to symbolise this freedom more accurately, making an association between his experience of 'being watched' and 'being good'. Melissa has now learnt that Marcus needs freedom and 'being-

alongside' more than he needs her steady eye contact. Over time, this optimal feeling of being 'unwatched-but-alongside' will become an important theme for Marcus, not only for the therapy structure, but in his pursuit of a 'free-range life'.

Mutual reflexivity

The development of client self-awareness is a central feature of person-centred therapy. In addition to self-awareness, clients develop the meta-skill of reflexivity, in which they are 'aware of their self-awareness, and are agential in terms of this capacity' (Rennie, 2010). In other words, clients not only come to an understanding of themselves; they are also able to reflect on their process of understanding, making use of this awareness to inspire further change. This 'radical reflexivity' (Rennie, 2010) creates a refining process of client self-attunement, leading to their deepening capacity to engage in self-reflection. Because their therapeutic approach is co-designed, the client and therapist develop a complex phenomenon of self-awareness, self-reflexivity, mutual awareness and co-reflexivity, in and on the process of therapy. This is emergent from the dialogic process of reflection, in an iterative cycle of expressing and receiving awareness (Mearns & Cooper, 2018).

Just as with other forms of co-creation, such as improvised play or music-making, the pair are likely to develop a culture and set of ground rules that is unique to their relationship, encompassing a distinctive style, a shared vocabulary, interpersonal familiarity and a sense of shared purpose. To maximise these qualities, both the therapist and client develop mutually reflexive capacities and habits, learning from each other and from their experiences, individually and as a team. Reflecting in and on experience, the therapist and client are free to explore mis-steps and mistakes, which become opportunities to refine the therapeutic approach, reducing shame and anxiety about performance for both the therapist and the client. This co-reflexive practice over time creates a shared expertise with regard to their uniquely designed and created approach.

Mutual reflexivity represents a new way of understanding expertise in pluralistic person-centred therapy. In the view of Schmid (2005), there are three possible positions on expertise in therapy. In the first, the therapist can be seen as the deciding expert for both content and process (such as in cognitive-behavioural therapy). In the second, the client is seen as the expert on content, and the therapist is regarded as the expert on process (such as in experiential therapies). In the third, the client is seen as the expert on both content and process, which Schmid (2005) describes as 'a stance only to be found in genuine person-centred therapy' (p.11). Pluralism offers a fourth position: in person-centred pluralistic therapy, both client and therapist share in a co-created, evolving, mutual expertise and craftsmanship about their tailored structure of therapy, which can include its process (the how of therapy) and its content (the what of therapy). This expertise is developmental, becoming stronger over time. Because this expertise is not solely possessed by either party, but is collectively owned, its power is shared. Being shared, it can be freely exchanged. In other words, when the therapist and client are developing a unique framework for therapy, through discussion and design, they not only have permission to make suggestions and contribute ideas, but in doing so they increase their collective resource of expertise.

Mutual reflexivity in pluralistic person-centred therapy is both the culmination of the approach and its foundation. It underpins the co-productive process of the therapy in dialogically meeting the client, finding and aligning to the client's direction, demystifying the process through meta-therapeutic communication, co-designing the approach, and integrating the client and therapist's cultural resources, with the intention of discovering a structure that responds meaningfully to the client in their uniqueness. Mutual reflexivity *is* the experience of discovery, together, in the emergent moment of therapeutic encounter.

Person-centred pluralistic therapy: A decolonial imaginary

One of the consequences of taking a pluralistic stance towards therapy is that it quickly emerges as a creative practice. Creativity is not a matter of dichotomies (art *or* science, mind *or* body, container *or* space) – it is a way of being that encompasses all binaries. For Rogers, creativity was closely aligned to flourishing. His 'fully functioning person' interacts in fluid, self-trusting ways with material reality: 'He is creatively realistic, and realistically creative' (Rogers, 1961, p.181). The creative process for Rogers was 'the emergence in action of a novel relational product, growing out of the uniqueness of the individual on one hand, and the materials, events, people, or circumstances of his life on the other' (1961, p.350; see Chapter 10, this volume). For Rogers this creativity is individual: a 'feel' of being 'me in action' (1961, p.354). But Rogers' examples of creative practice are consistently solitary practices such as 'painting a picture' and 'composing a symphony' (p.349). Pluralistic person-centred therapy is conceived dialogically as a *co*-creative process (such as improvising music, dance or conversation) involving the active, intentional, intimate and reflexive participation of both persons.

But co-creativity in therapy, while mutual in many ways, is not identical to the more social relationships experienced in co-creating music or dance. As Buber pointed out to Rogers, during their famous debate, 'He comes for help to you. You do not come for help to him' (Buber & Rogers, 1997, p.15). The client brings a specific ethical demand and a particular vulnerability to therapy, and the therapist's primary role is to respond meaningfully to this request. But in a colonial and patriarchal society such as ours, convivial and natural human relationships are replaced with dehumanising, power-laden interactions. The therapeutic relationship is inescapably trapped within this social framework, at present.

In resonance with the Black Lives Matter movement, the call for the decolonisation of therapy has gathered momentum, challenging the systemic oppressive assumptions at the heart of the psychological professions (Canham et al., 2021). European colonisers attempted to displace and replace diverse ways of knowing and being with a normative racial and sexist hierarchy that excludes, divides, dehumanises and exploits human beings. This was violently presented to the world as a universal ontology (Mignolo, 2011). Despite the beautiful variety and complexity of human experience, this colonial worldview has dominated culture (including therapy culture), resulting in a homogeneity that positions itself as central, while marginalising other ways of understanding the world and human experience (Khan, 2023). In response, liberation, decolonial and Indigenous psychologies have begun to reclaim the social, practical and intellectual space to create new imaginaries of the therapeutic frame (Beshara, 2021; Fanon & Philcox, 2021; Martín-Baró et al., 1994).

We might say that 'modality separatism' is itself an expression of colonial thinking that we can overcome. A pluralistic imaginary of therapy would embrace multiple accounts of what it is to be human. It would not attempt to invade and erase a client's account of their experience by imposing a pre-designed structure of therapy – no matter how subtle – that is founded on axiomatic beliefs or models of incompatibility. Therapists, because of their power, can *choose* whether to co-produce therapy with clients. This is the therapist's essential privilege. By contrast, clients have no choice but to co-produce with therapists, because, as Buber pointed out, they are in a position of vulnerability, needing help. The client welcomes the therapist into their space and hopes that they do no harm. So, to co-produce therapy with clients constitutes radical political action. It is a refusal to impose the therapist's worldview on the client as if it were universally true. Co-production makes space for the client to re-imagine a therapeutic frame that is constructed on their own terms, beyond the colonial frame of existing models.

One of the consequences of my attempt to decolonise my thinking as a therapist, teacher and writer is my increasing scepticism about borders. Borders between countries are arbitrary lines of possession and exclusion, and they are a central defining feature of the colonising project of oppression, theft and violence. Borders around ideas are part of a Western Enlightenment project to define, categorise and monetise reality: 'If we can put a border around it, we can own it, use it, and sell it'; 'If we can place a border between us, we can exclude people we consider "other" to ourselves.' Borders legitimise one class of people and delegitimise another, dehumanising them and putting them 'on the other side of an abyss' (Andreotti et al., 2011). So too, disciplinary, modality and professional borders obscure the freedom at the heart of being human. In offering you the theoretical model outlined in this chapter, I do not want to erect a border that keeps you out – or, indeed, one that keeps you in.

When I describe the features of person-centred and pluralistic practice to students, instead of borders, I use the metaphor of *pleasure paths*. I would like to share this metaphor with you, as a small contribution to decolonising our collective theory. Unlike borders, which are barriers, pleasure paths are those inviting natural paths that appear in landscapes when countless people have trodden the same natural track, maybe as a short cut to a town across a field or a gentle route to a stream for their dog to swim in. Pleasure paths head towards reliable features in the landscape and they help us to locate and direct ourselves according to our own satisfactions and expedience. They denote familiarity and a community of habitual or repeated practice.

Many of the features that you have seen described here should be regarded as pleasure paths, rather than borders around practice. You are free, just as your client is free, to take a completely new path if it is more appropriate or desirable. I invite you to be politically radical, courageous and convivial in your person-centred pluralistic therapy, sharing in its co-creation and power with your client and discovering new, exciting paths together. Pluralistic therapy is profoundly about compatibility, inclusion, conviviality and celebration of difference. My hope is that, in the future, person-centred pluralism will re-imagine ever more radical and emancipating ways to re-construct a therapy without borders.

Suggested reading

Pluralistic therapy

- Pluralistic Practice is a website for counsellors and psychotherapists, with a range of regularly updated resources, blogs and events, such as the annual pluralistic practice conference. You can access it at www.pluralisticpractice.com
- See, for example, my blog on meta-therapeutic communication:
  Blunden, N. (2022). *The metatherapeutic current in pluralism*. Pluralistic Practice. https://pluralisticpractice.com/main-blog/training/the-metatherapeutic-current-in-pluralism/
- For an early perspective on pluralism and being person-centred: Cooper, M. & McLeod, J. (2011). Person-centered therapy: A pluralistic perspective. *Person-Centered & Experiential Psychotherapies, 10*(3), 210-223.
- For more detail on the pluralistic framework as a trans-theoretical therapeutic approach: Cooper, M., & McLeod, J. (2011). *Pluralistic counselling and psychotherapy*. Sage Publications.

  McLeod, J. (2017). *Pluralistic therapy: Distinctive features*. Routledge.
- For a simple introduction to pluralistic therapy, with a focus on practice:

  Smith, K. & de la Prida, A. (2021). *The pluralistic therapy primer*. PCCS Books.

Co-production

- For an accessible overview of co-production across health and social care:
  Social Care Institute for Excellence (SCIE). (2022, July). Co-production: what is it and how to do it. www.scie.org.uk/co-production/what-how

Decolonising therapy

- To explore the decolonising potential in therapy:
  Charura, D. & Lago, C. (2021). *Black identities and white therapies: Race, respect and diversity*. PCCS Books.
- For a general overview of colonial thought and its harms, as well as the possibilities for re-imagining society:
  Mignolo, W.D. (2011). *The darker side of Western modernity*. Duke University Press.

References

Andreotti, V., Ahenakew, C., & Cooper, G. (2011). Epistemological pluralism: Ethical and pedagogical challenges in higher education. *AlterNative: An International Journal of Indigenous Peoples, 7*(1), 40–50. 10.1177/117718011100700104

Beshara, R.K. (2021). *Critical psychology praxis*. Taylor & Francis. 10.4324/9781003119678

Blunden, N. (2023). A grounded theory of improvisation in therapy: Lessons from decoloniality. *Counselling and Psychotherapy Research, 23*(4), 882–892. https://doi.org/10.1002/capr.12634

Bohart, A.C. (2004). How do clients make empathy work? *Person-Centered & Experiential Psychotherapies, 3*(2), 102–116. 10.1080/14779757.2004.9688336

Bohart, A.C. (2012). Can you be integrative and a person-centered therapist at the same time? *Person-Centered & Experiential Psychotherapies, 11*(1), 1–13. 10.1080/14779757.2011.639461

Brodley, B.T. (1999). About the nondirective attitude. *Person-Centred Practice, 7*(2), 79–82.

Buber, M. & Rogers, C. (1997). *Martin Buber–Carl Rogers dialogue: A new transcript with commentary.* State University of New York Press.

Canham, H., Baloyi, L. & Segalo, P. (2021). Disrupting the psychology canon? Exploring African-centered decolonial pedagogy. In G. Stevens, C.C. Sonn (Eds.), *Decoloniality and epistemic justice in contemporary community psychology* (pp.193–212). Springer International Publishing.

Cook, D. & Monk, L. (2020). 'Being able to take that mask off': Adolescent client experiences of power in person-centered therapy relationships. *Person-Centered & Experiential Psychotherapies, 19*(2), 95–111. 10.1080/14779757.2020.1717982

Cooper, M. (2009). Welcoming the Other: Actualising the humanistic ethic at the core of counselling psychology practice. *Counselling Psychology Review, 24*(3&4), 119–129.

Cooper, M. (2021). Directionality: Unifying psychological and social understandings of well-being and distress through an existential ontology. *Journal of Humanistic Counseling, 60*(1), 6–25. 10.1002/johc.12148 Cooper, M. (2019). *Integrating counselling and psychotherapy*. Sage Publications Ltd.

Cooper, M. (2023). *Psychology at the heart of social change*. Policy Press.

Cooper, M., & McLeod, J. (2007). A pluralistic framework for counselling and psychotherapy: Implications for research. *Counselling and Psychotherapy Research, 7*(3), 135–143. 10.1080/14733140701566282

Cooper, M. & McLeod, J. (2011a). Pluralistic counselling and psychotherapy. Sage.

Cooper, M. & McLeod, J. (2011b). Person-centered therapy: A pluralistic perspective. *Person-Centered & Experiential Psychotherapies, 10*(3), 210–223. 10.1080/14779757.2011.599517

Crenshaw, K. (2017). *On intersectionality*. The New Press.

Fanon, F. & Philcox, R. (2021). *Black skin, white masks*. Penguin Books.

Gendlin, E.T. (1994). Response. *Human Studies, 17*(3), 381–400. 10.1007/BF01322978

Grant, B. (1990). Principled and instrumental nondirectiveness in person-centered and client-centered therapy. *Person-Centered Review, 7*(8), 77–88.

Kahn, E. (2012). On being 'up to other things': The nondirective attitude and therapist-frame responses in client-centered therapy and contemporary psychoanalysis. *Person-Centered & Experiential Psychotherapies, 11*(3), 240–254. 10.1080/14779757.2012.700285

Khan, M. (2023). *Working within diversity*. Jessica Kingsley Publishers.

Kirschenbaum, H. & Henderson, V.L. (Eds.). (1989). *The Carl Rogers reader*. Houghton Mifflin.

Knox, R. (2008). Clients' experiences of relational depth in person-centred counselling. *Counselling and Psychotherapy Research, 8*(3), 182–188. 10.1080/14733140802035005

Ladmanová, M., Řiháček, T. & Timulak, L. (2022). Client-identified impacts of helpful and hindering events in psychotherapy: A qualitative meta-analysis. *Psychotherapy Research, 32*(6), 723–735. 10.1080/10503307.2021.2003885

Lazarus, A.A. (1981). *The practice of multimodal therapy.* McGraw-Hill.

Lazarus, A.A. & Beutler, L.E. (1993). On technical eclecticism. *Journal of Counseling and Development, 71*(4), 381–385. 10.1002/j.1556-6676.1993.tb02652.x

Martín-Baró, I., Aron, A. & Corne, S. (1994). *Writings for a liberation psychology.* Harvard University Press.

McLeod, J. (2017). *Pluralistic therapy: Distinctive features.* Routledge. 10.4324/9781315398266

McLeod, J. & Sundet, R. (2022). Psychotherapy as making. *Frontiers in Psychology, 13*, 1048665. 10.3389/fpsyg.2022.1048665

Mearns, D. & Cooper, M. (2018). *Working at relational depth in counselling and psychotherapy* (2nd ed.). Sage.

Mearns, D. & Schmid, P.F. (2006). Being-with and being-counter: Relational depth – the challenge of fully meeting the client. *Person-Centered & Experiential Psychotherapies, 5*(4), 255–265. 10.1080/14779757.2006.9688417.

Mignolo, W.D. (2011). *The darker side of Western modernity.* Duke University Press. 10.1515/9780822394501

Norcross, J.C. & Cooper, M. (2021). *Personalizing psychotherapy.* American Psychological Association. 10.1037/0000221-000

Oddli, H.W., McLeod, J., Nissen-Lie, H.A., Rønnestad, M.H. & Halvorsen, M.S. (2021). Future orientation in successful therapies: Expanding the concept of goal in the working alliance. *Journal of Clinical Psychology, 77*(6), 1307–1329. 10.1002/jclp.23108

Oddli, H.W., Stänicke, E., Halvorsen, M.S. & Lindstad, T.G. (2023). Causality in psychotherapy research: Towards evidential pluralism. *Psychotherapy Research, 33*(8), 1004–1018. 10.1080/10503307.2022.2161433

Ong, W.T., Murphy, D. & Joseph, S. (2020). Unnecessary and incompatible: A critical response to Cooper and McLeod's conceptualization of a pluralistic framework for person-centered therapy. *Person-Centered & Experiential Psychotherapies, 19*(2), 168–182. 10.1080/14779757.2020.1717987

Papayianni, F. & Cooper, M. (2018). Metatherapeutic communication: An exploratory analysis of therapist-reported moments of dialogue regarding the nature of the therapeutic work. *British Journal of Guidance & Counselling, 46*(2), 173–184. https://doi.org/10.1080/03069885.2017.1305098

Rennie, D.L. (1998). *Person-centred counselling.* Sage.

Rennie, D.L. (2000). Aspects of the client's conscious control of the psychotherapeutic process. *Journal of Psychotherapy Integration, 10*(2), 151–167. 10.1023/A:1009496116174

Rennie, D.L. (2010). Humanistic psychology at York University. Retrospective: Focus on client experiencing in psychotherapy: Emphasis of radical reflexivity. *The Humanistic Psychologist, 38*(1), 40–56. 10.1080/08873261003635856

Rogers, C.R. (1957). The necessary and sufficient conditions of therapeutic personality change. *Journal of Consulting Psychology, 21*(2), 95–103.

Rogers, C.R. (1961). *On becoming a person.* Houghton Mifflin.

Rogers, C.R. (1980). *A way of being.* Houghton Mifflin.

Rogers, C.R. (1989). A client-centered/person-centered approach to therapy. In H. Kirschenbaum, & V. L. Henderson (Eds.), *The Carl Rogers reader* (pp.135-152). Houghton Mifflin.

Schmid, P.F. (2002). Presence – Im-media-te co-experiencing and co-responding: Phenomenological, dialogical and ethical perspectives on contact and perception in person-centred therapy. And beyond. In G. Wyatt & P. Sanders (Eds.), *Rogers' therapeutic conditions: Evolution, theory and practice. Vol. 4: Contact and perception* (pp.182–203). PCCS Books.

Schmid, P.F. (2005). Facilitative responsiveness: Non-directiveness from an anthropological, epistemological and ethical perspective. In B. Levitt (Ed.), *Embracing non-directivity* (pp.74–94). PCCS Books.

Schmid, P.F. & Mearns, D. (2006). Being-with and being-counter: Person-centered psychotherapy as an in-depth co-creative process of personalization. *Person-Centered & Experiential Psychotherapies, 5*(3), 174–190. 10.1080/14779757.2006.9688408

Smith, K. & de la Prida, A. (2021). *The pluralistic therapy primer.* PCCS Books.

Smith, K., McLeod, J., Blunden, N., Cooper, M., Gabriel, L., Kupfer, C., Murphie, M., Oddli, H., Thurston, M. & Winter, L.A. (2021). A pluralistic perspective on research in psychotherapy: Harnessing passion, difference and dialogue to promote justice and relevance. *Frontiers in Psychology, 12*, 742676. 10.3389/fpsyg.2021.742676

Sommerbeck, L. (2003). *The client-centred therapist in psychiatric contexts: A therapist's guide to the psychiatric landscape and its inhabitants.* PCCS Books.

Tickle, E. & Murphy, D. (2014). A journey to client and therapist mutuality in person-centered psychotherapy: A case study. *Person-Centered & Experiential Psychotherapies, 13*(4), 337–351. 10.1080/14779757.2014.927390

Wilkins, P. (2003). 'Non-directivity': A fiction and an irresponsible denial of power? In P. Wilkins, *Person-centred therapy in focus* (pp.85–89). Sage. 10.4135/9781446219560.n7

Wilkins, P. (2015). *Person-centred therapy.* Routledge.

Worsley, R. (2012). Integrating with integrity. In P. Sanders (Ed.), *The tribes of the person-centred nation* (2nd ed.) (pp.161–186). PCCS Books.

10. Person-centred creative arts therapies

Ani de la Prida

Creativity is at the heart of the person-centred approach, and there are many person-centred therapists who integrate creative media and methods in their practice in their own, idiosyncratic way (Walshaw, 2015). There are also four distinct models situated within the 'fuzzy circle' (Bohart, 2012, p.3) of the person-centred approach, each with their own training and distinctive features. They all focus on creating a therapeutic space where a client feels able to express feelings freely by using creative mediums.

In this chapter, I explore how these four models relate to each other, what differentiates them from person-centred therapy (Chapter 2, this volume), and what makes them a valid 'tribe of the person-centred nation'. I then go on to outline a contemporary perspective that encompasses theory and practices from the key models. I also introduce some new ideas to bring the approach into a contemporary digital context.

The chapter starts by briefly introducing the models and their development and highlights key features. It then defines a contemporary person-centred creative arts approach and explores its credentials for inclusion as a tribe of the person-centred nation. I re-vision the six necessary and sufficient conditions to develop a theoretical context for engaging creativity, imagination and the unconscious in the therapeutic process, and I outline a series of stages to describe different levels of engagement and ways of working with the fluid creative process.

Most importantly, I then explore practice, using key theoretical concepts that are distinctive to the approach, and offer a range of examples to show the approach in action. I am very grateful to my clients and students for allowing me share examples of their artwork and experience to help to illustrate this approach.

I hope this chapter will help develop understanding of the approach and bring a fresh contemporary perspective to this colourful, creative tribe of the person-centred nation. I also hope that it inspires you to bring more creativity into your practice.

The development of person-centred creative arts therapies

There are four pioneers who developed person-centred models using creative media and methods, and a full description of each can be found in their key publications: Virginia Axline (1964/1990), Laury Rappaport (2009), Natalie Rogers (1993) and Liesl Silverstone (1997). Each rejects diagnosis and interpretation and aims to provide a climate of empathy, congruence and non-judgemental attitude, but they also have key differentiating features.

Virginia Axline – Child-centred play therapy (CCPT)

Virginia Axline was a pioneer of applying person-centred principles to play therapy (Chapter 12, this volume). She saw play as the external, symbolic expression of an internal process, and believed that the skill of the therapist was in their ability to respond to verbal and non-verbal processes, moving between reflecting the external play process and responding empathically to a child's internal process and feelings. The approach is very clearly illustrated in her book *Dibs in Search of Self* (Axline, 1964/1990). In this moving account, she shows how a deep trust in the actualising tendency can foster growth and healing. She describes how, through symbolic play, Dibs 'poured out his hurt, bruised feelings, and... emerged with feelings of strength and security… achieving personal integration' (Axline, 1964/1990, p.177).

Axline illustrates how to work non-directively with play, with imagination, and with materials such as sand tray, miniatures, puppets and visual art. Although developed with children, the approach is applicable to working with creative media with adults.

Natalie Rogers – Person-centred expressive arts therapy (PCEAT)

Natalie Rogers was an artist, a person-centred therapist and daughter of Carl Rogers. She became frustrated with the limitations of verbal expression and expanded the person-centred approach in the 1980s to develop an expressive arts model she called Creative Connection (N. Rogers, 1993). It prioritises expression and process and can be defined as a classically non-directive approach (Bohart, 2012). It is comparable in many ways to CCPT – for example, it uses a range of media to establish a feeling of freedom of expression and reflect back what is expressed. Natalie Rogers considered the person-centred core conditions as necessary in therapy but was explicit that something more was needed – the extra quality of creative expression. She saw creative expression as providing a bridge between our inner and outer realities, bringing messages from the unconscious. But, she argued, while the art product 'supplies important messages to the individual… it is the process of creation that is profoundly transformative' (1993, p.7). She expanded on the connection between art and the unconscious, seeing the unconscious as the source of creativity, intuition, feelings and insight. The approach integrates elements from Gestalt and Jungian psychology, and is distinctive in how it uses various expressive arts in sequence to generate synergy in a multi-modal, free-flow approach (Brown, 2012).

Liesl Silverstone – Person-centred art therapy (PCAT)

Liesl Silverstone came to London in 1940, fleeing Prague when her family were sent to Theresienstadt, the ghetto that served as a Nazi transit camp for Czechoslavakian Jews. She was a social worker, person-centred counsellor and art therapist. In adulthood, she visited the camp and was significantly impacted by the art created by the children incarcerated there, and she describes how this sowed the seeds of her work with art therapy (Silverstone, 1997).

Silverstone developed her person-centred art therapy (PCAT) approach in 1980s in London. PCAT shares the fundamental concepts of PCEAT but tends to focus mainly, although not exclusively, on visual art. She believed that images tap into the unconscious world of spontaneous knowing, a non-verbal wisdom accessed through right-brain processing rather than the left-brained thinking mode (Silverstone, 1997). She also saw art as containing a message, an internal truth, and some aspect of the self that wants to be known and can be made visible in art form. She saw this communication as unconsciously intentional, arising from the human desire to self-actualise. An image can contain suppressed material, 'hopes or fears, diverse aspects of self, expressed symbolically, come up from the subconscious, to be known, to be integrated… a kind of aura of the as-yet-unknown, requiring our respect' (p.121).

Where PCEAT tends to focus on the healing value of expression, PCAT takes the approach further. It prioritises engaging the imagination and working with the art object with a distinctive, dynamic style of facilitation. The key skills of *reflection* and *bridging* help to bring unconscious aspects into conscious awareness, communicated via the image. When using these skills, the process can be quick, often with an instant cognitive recognition of meaning.

Laury Rappaport – Focusing-oriented art therapy (FOAT)

Laury Rappaport developed her approach in the 1990s (Rappaport, 2009) using Gendlin's six-step focusing method (Chapter 4, this volume) to connect to the inner bodily felt sense and provide a means to express this externally with art. She describes focusing as providing an inner direction and art therapy as providing an outer expression, fitting together 'like a pair of matching gloves' (Rappaport, 2016, p.89). In FOAT, attention is paid to the therapeutic relationship and creative process to enable clients to access their internal source of creativity and wisdom. It engages the imagination to help clients dis-identify and gain emotional distance from overwhelming feelings (Rappaport, 2009). Clients are invited to find a symbol called the *handle* that matches an inner felt sense, which is then expressed in art form to foster connection with the internal authentic self.

Current context

Person-centred therapy has sometimes struggled to maintain its identity in a landscape where it is marginalised in favour of psychodynamic or cognitive behavioural therapy (Cooper et al., 2013). This struggle is even more evident for person-centred creative arts therapies as, while play therapy has developed as a profession with a visible person-centred presence (Ayling et al., 2019; Chapter 12, this volume), art therapy has not. In the UK, art therapy is a psychodynamically dominated profession, with a legally protected title (Health & Care Professions Council, 2018), where the person-centred art approach seems to have no visible place. Generally, art therapy focuses on materials and the creative process from an interpretive perspective, and while it recognises the value of the therapeutic relationship, it isn't grounded in person-centred theory to inform non-directivity.

The person-centred creative arts approaches have struggled to find a place within the person-centred family too, not being considered a fully-fledged tribe of the person-centred nation (Sanders, 2012; Wilkins, 2015), and with some person-centred therapists questioning whether it is directive to integrate creative methods (Davis, 2000; N. Rogers, 1993; Silverstone, 1997). The current climate of regulation, standardisation and competency frameworks adds confusion, with some counsellors feeling unsure whether it is ethical to integrate creative arts methods and how to define it when they do (Rosen & Atkins, 2014). All of this has contributed to fragmentation and a lack of awareness and understanding of the approaches, and without a clear identity there is a danger that they may become side-lined or regulated out of existence.

To begin to meet this challenge, the Association for Person-Centred Creative Arts (APCCA) was created in 2020. The term 'person-centred creative arts' is inclusive of key models and idiosyncratic creative practice and avoids using the protected title. It aims to develop the approach and provide opportunities for practice and funding for community-based person-centred creative arts projects. APCCA had its first conference in 2022, has developed a specialised training pathway, and currently has around 200 members (see Resources for more information).

The creative arts approaches are a valid and vibrant expression of the actualising tendency of the person-centred approach, but the key models were developed several decades ago, long before digital media and online working. To ensure a place in counselling, psychotherapy and art therapy, it is crucial not only to develop contemporary theory and practice but also to do so within our current landscape and digital context.

A contemporary person-centred creative arts approach

Broadly speaking, the three main processes of the approach I will describe here are art-making, reflecting on the art product, and eliciting meaning and insight. The view that the creative process and expression in art-making can be therapeutic can be referred to as 'art *as* therapy'. Simply engaging in art-making can create physiological changes, reduce stress levels, increase cortisol and 'can quite literally rewire your brain… a secret sauce that helps build new synaptic connections' (Magsamen & Ross, 2023, p.309).

But Silverstone (1997) declares that 'to "become an I, I need a thou" (Buber), and so it is with images. A client can get further, talking about the picture with a counsellor' (p.5). By using the creative process intentionally with 'art *in* therapy', the counsellor fosters the development of insight through reflection on the art-making process and product. The counsellor sees the art product as an externalised symbolic representation of the client's inner world: understanding, for example, that a drawing of a cat can represent a sibling, or a feeling, or both. It is a non-interpretative approach where metaphors are seen as unique to each person. This approach focuses on the client in the moment and on what is symbolised in art form by the client, which is seen as arising from the organismic self.

To work with art in therapy, it is advisable to have further training to develop understanding of psychological processes in 'the making of art, the creative process, the attributes of different media, the power of imagery' (Rappaport, 2009, p.71). Self-awareness is essential when working with unconscious material as the tendency to identify with or interpret the symbolic language of art can be greater than with verbal therapy (Silverstone, 1997).

A wide range of materials and methods can be used, such as visual art, dance, story, drama, sand, play, music, movement, digital media, and even food (de la Prida, 2016) to provide a variety of ways to promote, enhance and contain the therapeutic process. In this chapter, I primarily focus on visual art, but it is important to remember that many other media can be used in a similar way.

A valid tribe of the person-centred nation

To argue that the person-centred creative arts approach is a valid 'tribe of the person-centred nation', it is essential to show a theoretical base that both distinguishes it from and shows its relationship to classical person-centred therapy (Sanders, 2012; Chapter 2, this volume).

Whether the six conditions are necessary and sufficient is a central debate within the person-centred approach (Gillon, 2007). For the creative approaches, the focus tends to be not on sufficiency but on what can enhance therapy. For example, we can survive on bread and butter; it is sufficient. But… maybe some jam or marmite would be nice? Jam doesn't stop the bread being bread, but it can enhance it. However not everyone wants jam, and not everyone will want to work with creative materials. A client may prefer to talk, and as a person-centred counsellor I can equally support that choice. What suits one client may not suit another, and what is helpful for a client at one time might not continue to be so (Smith & de la Prida, 2021; see Chapter 9, this volume).

The creative arts approach is curious about what might enhance the therapeutic process –perhaps paint, or journalling or movement might foster the expression of a long-buried experience. It actively explores what materials or methods might make *this* therapy with *this* client more effective (Smith & de la Prida, 2021). Curiosity and flexibility are key principles of both pluralistic practice and the person-centred creative arts approach, engaging the client and therapist in a shared creative process of learning to discover what is helpful and what is not. A therapeutic rationale for the approach is to draw on a range of ideas and theories, deconstructing and integrating any method or activity that is helpful. By providing a route for expression without influencing what is being expressed, the therapist invites the client to collaboratively shape and direct the therapeutic encounter, while maintaining a non-directive attitude at the level of content and a deep trust in a client's capacity for self-direction. This is what characterises it as person-centred (Gillon, 2007).

Offering a range of methods and materials provides concrete opportunities for a client to learn 'to trust their own thoughts and feelings and to make decisions in accordance with their own perceptions and desires' (Mearns et al., 2013, p.9). For a client whose trust in their organismic valuing process has been damaged, the art-making process can be a potent antidote that can help reconnect them to their inner locus of evaluation (see Chapter 2, this volume). To illustrate how a contemporary approach to person-centred creative arts may use methods and materials in a flexible way in response to the needs and preferences of the client, I will draw on my work with a client, Asha.

Asha: (*Quiet and passive*) I'm not sure what I want to do today.

Ani: So right now, you aren't sure what you want to do. I'm wondering how you are feeling right now.

Asha: I feel sad and heavy, but not sure why.

Ani: As you notice that feeling, do you feel drawn to any of the materials, or would you prefer to talk today?

Asha: (*Becomes animated*) Yes, I think I'll paint, the dark colours match my mood.

Asha moves from not knowing what to do to locating a feeling of sadness. As she connects with her inner locus of evaluation, there is a perceptible shift in her energy. Asha goes on to externalise her feelings using paint, but is then motivated to explore further, so I invite her to work with movement. She moves around the room with slow, heavy steps, and I move too, mirroring her, which can deepen levels of empathy through embodied experience (McGarry & Russo, 2011). Asha angrily punches the air, then holds herself in a hug. She says, 'My sadness was covering up hurt and anger. As I punched the air, I felt the anger leave my body.' Asha's movements, contained and reflected within an empathic relationship, help her to access and process her deeper feelings of hurt and releasing anger.

The facilitative conditions

The person-centred creative approach argues that an extra quality of creative expression can enhance therapy. Therefore, it is essential to reconsider the necessary and sufficient conditions and process of therapy as it applies to the person-centred creative arts approach. By adapting Rogers' six necessary and sufficient conditions for therapeutic change

Table 10.1: Facilitative conditions for a contemporary person-centred creative arts approach

Facilitative conditions for a contemporary person-centred creative arts approach
1. The counsellor and client are in psychological contact.
2. The client is curious and motivated.
3. The counsellor offers stimulating experiences with materials and methods that provide an opportunity to explore, experiment and engage the creative process.
4. The counsellor is congruent, curious and integrated into the relationship and the process of exploration, creative expression and art-making.
5. The counsellor experiences unconditional positive regard and is a witness for the client's creative and expressive process.
6. The counsellor experiences an empathic understanding of the client's internal world, for what is and what isn't yet in conscious awareness, and aims to communicate this experience to the client.
7. The communication of curiosity, empathy and unconditional positive regard is received at conscious or unconscious levels of awareness.

(C.R. Rogers, 1957; see Chapter 1, this volume), we can propose the following conditions for a contemporary person-centred creative arts approach.

1. The counsellor and client are in psychological contact

Creating 'an environment where people feel safe enough to open up and make psychological contact with themselves and each other' (Davis, 2000, p.208) is central to the art-making process. It sees art as promoting depth of contact with self and others rather than seeing contact as a precondition (Davis, 2000).

2. The client is curious and motivated

Here 'incongruence' can be translated as 'curiosity' (Embleton-Tudor et al., 2004) to describe the gap between a client's current experience and their desired level of understanding of their internal experience. Curiosity generates motivation to explore the creative process and, while a client may be incongruent and experiencing anxiety, it isn't a requirement: for example, they might engage for reasons of personal development.

3. The counsellor offers stimulating experiences with materials and methods that provide an opportunity to explore, experiment and engage the creative process

This additional condition provides the basis for stimulating creativity (N. Rogers, 1993). Often working 'with an image can be safer than talking about me – I am talking about me via an image, a gentler process' (Silverstone, 1997, p.121). This gentleness and perceptual distance may help to promote depth of self-exploration, which is central to client change (Elliott et al., 2016).

4. The counsellor is congruent, curious and integrated into the relationship and the process of exploration, creative expression and art-making

Counsellor curiosity is central, as each mark, movement and gesture is potentially meaningful, expressing some aspect of the client's world even when a client doesn't recognise meaning. Conditions of worth (see Chapter 2, this volume) may inhibit expression, and congruent integration in the process and relationship supports the creative process, which enables the client to take the risk of 'abandoning of safe familiar thoughts, facing the unknown, where anything may emerge' (Silverstone, 1997, p.120).

5. The counsellor experiences unconditional positive regard and is a witness for the client's creative and expressive process

Unconditional positive regard for the client and the process is necessary so that, when the client 'knows that all of her is accepted unconditionally, she may in turn accept all of herself, and move on to discover what she may become' (Silverstone, 1997, p.3). Witnessing is closely related to *presence* and *relational depth* (Geller, 2012; see Chapter 3, this volume), and involves the therapist being in contact with themselves and their client, noticing, attending, attuning, caring, holding and responding to the creative process and the client in-the-moment, being affirming of whatever emerges.

6. The counsellor experiences an empathic understanding of the client's internal world, for what is and what isn't yet in conscious awareness, and aims to communicate this experience to the client
Being empathic to all elements of the process – a mark, a gesture, the force with which paint is splashed on paper – offers an opportunity to the counsellor to empathise with what has been made visible consciously and unconsciously in art form.

7. The communication of curiosity, empathy and unconditional positive regard is received at conscious or unconscious levels of awareness
Communicating the conditions when working with art is distinct from verbal therapy in the way it engages with the creative process. For example, the therapist might observe, 'I am wondering about this mark here,' or physically reflect a movement, affirming the pace of a client's art-making. Witnessing and reflecting what has been expressed symbolically in art form may help a client receive empathy even when they aren't ready to allow the material into conscious awareness.

The stages of the therapeutic process

The seven facilitative conditions provide the context for engaging creativity, imagination and the unconscious in the therapeutic process. The process can be broken down into six stages, for clarity of explanation. However, there is no therapeutic hierarchy; each stage can be deeply therapeutic. They can occur in sequence, or not, and clients may engage at one or two, or all of the stages at different times in a fluid, kaleidoscopic Gestalt of creative process.

Table 10.2: Stages of therapeutic process in a contemporary person-centred creative arts approach

Person-centred creative arts approach: Stages of therapeutic process
Stage 1: Symbolisation
Stage 2: Externalising
Stage 3: Witnessing
Stage 4: Cognition
Stage 5: Exploration and facilitation of meaning
Stage 6: Integration and actualisation

Stage 1: Symbolisation

This stage describes when an aspect of a client's internal world comes to mind, represented in imagination as a visual image, a symbol. Symbols can represent 'something deeper – the experience of larger and more complex concepts' (Morrell, 2011, p.2). Carl Rogers' client (C.R. Rogers, 2003) describes this spontaneous process of symbolisation:

> Whenever I felt or experienced anything, whenever I felt anything 'happened' I could find no way of expressing the feelings or understanding I had either to you or to

> myself, except through these images. The only times I can remember, and the only times which seem important to me, are those in which I experienced the feelings expressed by these images. (p.169)

Symbolisation describes the internal process; it can be instant and spontaneous, as in the example above, or a counsellor can offer a theme or visualisation to promote symbolisation. The formation of visual images in imagination can activate sensory pathways and promote healing (Lusebrink, 2004). However, a client may engage in art-making without symbolising, and some clients may not be able to symbolise – they may have aphantasia, for example, which is an inability to create mental imagery (Fox-Muraton, 2021).

Stage 2: Externalising

This stage allows material that might be available to conscious awareness to be expressed and made visible to both client and counsellor, creating an external representation of a client's internal world in art form. A client can externalise without internal symbolisation – for example, by working spontaneously with dance, music, play or also with visual art.

Stage 3: Witnessing

Witnessing describes a quality of 'being' deeply empathically observant and fully engaged in the client's creative process with mind, body, ears, eyes and heart (Silverstone, 1997). It is a relational process that communicates to a client that they are being truly seen and valued. When an empathic observer holds a safe space for the creative process, and both therapist and client witness the art product, it can be transformational (Rappaport, 2016; N. Rogers, 1993).

Stage 4: Cognition

This is where a client develops awareness and insight through engaging intentionally with the art object, recognising or intuiting meaning cognitively. Verbalisation is important, although it isn't always necessary. For example, you can bury a doll in sand without needing to know who or what this represents, as witnessing and processing can occur non-verbally and at an unconscious level (Lusebrink, 2004). Exploration with a counsellor can promote cognition, although insight can be gained from reflection on the art object on one's own, such as in a journal. For example, on the APCCA certificate course I offered the following creative prompt online:

> Take a moment to close your eyes and focus on how you feel as you are sitting here in this room. Now imagine if you were a flower right now, what flower would you be? See if you can allow an image of a flower to come to mind. Notice the colour, the size, the shape. Where is the flower situated? Now open your eyes perhaps draw or paint the shape.

One student, Yana, a refugee from Ukraine drew a flower (Figure 10.1) and wrote in her journal:

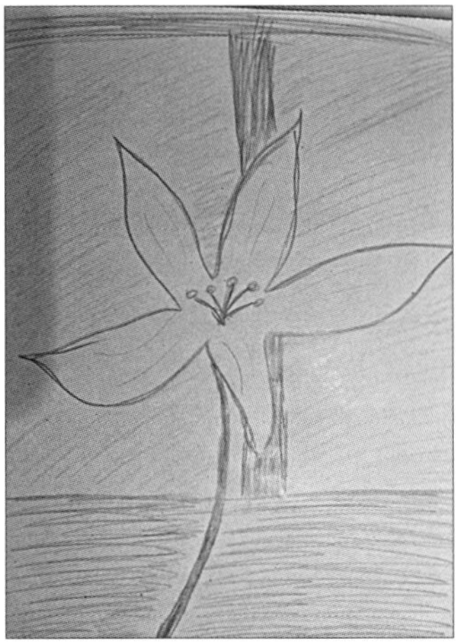

Figure 10.1: Yana's flower

> I drew this flower when I had to leave home for Germany once again. This is a flower which symbolised myself then. It is not the image of a real flower. I created it in my imagination as a very strong flower which can bloom everywhere. I drew it staying 'on the real window of my home'. It recreates the image of myself, a person who lives in two countries and has two homes. The flower has no pot and can grow in every place and every soil it is put to. When I look at this image now, it gives me a sense of empowerment. Imagining it every time in my head helps me to feel myself stronger and more capable.

By reflecting on the drawing and writing in her journal, Yana was able to bring her inner qualities into awareness and the drawing became a resource and touchstone, reminding her of her strength and resourcefulness.

Stage 5: Exploration and facilitation of meaning

At this level a counsellor and client engage in active dialogue with the art process or product. The marks on paper, the position of elements, the movements and the play process all contain symbolised meaning. The aim here is to help bring symbolised meaning to conscious awareness. Facilitation styles can vary: for example, PCAT employs a dynamic style of facilitation, using reflecting and bridging to help bring material to awareness. Facilitation fosters cognition, often resulting in 'moments of "Aha!"' (Silverstone, 1997, p.1) when the image or art product 'gives up' its message and its meaning is recognised.

Stage 6: Integration and actualisation

As material comes into conscious awareness through the creative arts process, a person becomes more aware of their feelings, ideas and physiological reactions in a process of actualisation. As self-awareness grows, the structure of self changes to assimilate this information. Art-making can serve as a container and testing ground for this process, where clients can try new things in an abstract form. The changes that occur in art form on paper or in play or movement can represent and promote change in the client's external life. For example, a client who becomes bolder in their art may find they become bolder in their life.

As clients gain access to inner resources and undistorted aspects of self, they can feel energised as they move towards greater authenticity and actualisation. The example of Daisy illustrates this experience of her growing congruence and of her connection to an internal non-verbal understanding and experience.

Daisy came to the session feeling happy. I invited her to symbolise her feeling – to imagine its shape, size and colour. She said it was huge, red and orange and bursting out, and externalised it on paper (Figure 10.2). I witnessed her process, and we explored her drawing.

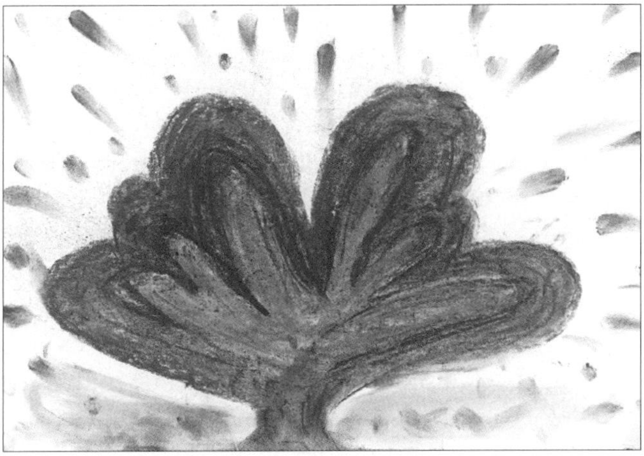

Figure 10.2: Daisy's feeling of happiness

Daisy said:

> This really feels significant, it represents me, exactly! What is inside and what is on the outside match – in sync. I can see it, and you can see it too. Words can't really convey how it feels. I know even if I don't talk about it, it means something, and I sort of know what that is without words. Lately I'm more unapologetically me, more of the real me. Authentic.

The creative arts process helped Daisy to cognitively connect with her internal experience, expanding her awareness as she expressed her excitement at living more authentically.

The conditions, materials and stages are flexible elements in the creative therapeutic process. To use the analogy of a cake, the seven facilitative conditions are the ingredients, the creative methods and materials bring different flavours, and the six stages are slices of the process that allow us to see inside the therapy cake.

Key concepts

Three concepts that distinguish a creative arts approach from a classical approach to person-centred therapy (Chapter 2, this volume) are the 'unconscious', the 'triangular relationship' and the 'perceptual distance' created by the art-making process (Morrell, 2011).

1. The unconscious

Carl Rogers (1979) described consciousness as a 'peak of awareness of symbolising capacity topping a vast pyramid on nonconscious, organismic functioning' (p.102). Because we are limited to knowing what is experienced in consciousness, 'This means that the greater the area of experience not in consciousness' (p.495).

There has been a lack exploration of the 'unconscious' in person-centred theory (Conradi, 2000; Coulson, 2000; Thorne, 2003; Wilkins, 2000). However, person-centred theory does use terms like the 'nonconscious mind', 'out of awareness', 'edge of awareness', 'intuitive knowing', and 'transpersonal self' (Coulson, 2000; Wilkins, 2000). The concept of 'subception' indicates that Rogers believed experience could be denied or distorted in awareness, but in classical person-centred theory (in contrast, say, to classical Freudian notions of the 'unconscious'), such subceived experiences can still potentially become available to awareness. In other words, use of the term 'unconscious' – as widely takes place in the creative arts approaches – refers to a model of the mind in which greater levels of suppression and unknowability can be conceived than would be typical in a classical person-centred approach (see Chapter 2, this volume).

We can hypothesise that the unconscious contains experience that is denied to conscious awareness, but Carl Rogers also saw our unconscious as being more than simply a container for denied experiences – rather, it encompasses a 'wisdom and purposiveness which goes well beyond our conscious thought' (Coulson, 2000, p.209). This idea underpins non-directivity in the creative arts approach, which sees art as being presented with unconscious intention within the therapeutic encounter, and as containing some message or aspect that wants to be known (Silverstone, 1997).

Natalie Rogers (1979) described a transcendent phenomenon, a spiritual experience of feeling connected with something greater than the individual self, a 'broader, universal consciousness' (p.103). This transpersonal aspect has also been somewhat neglected in person-centred theory, although Natalie Rogers describes the creative arts process as a spiritual and transpersonal process of actualisation where, when 'we reach our inner core, we find our connection to all beings… our inner source… the world, and the universe' (N. Rogers, 1993, p.4). Along with Jung, we can consider this a 'universal unconscious'.

While there are many conceptualisations of the unconscious we can draw on – both inside and outside of the person-centred approach – with creative arts practice, it is important this does not lead towards interpretation of unconscious processes. It is crucial to ensure that insight and meaning arise from the frame of reference of the client and not the counsellor. A simple four-level model of the unconscious conveys fundamental aspects relevant to this perspective and can be used to illustrate the creative arts process and its role in expanding self-awareness (Figure 10.3).

In this model, material can rise from unconscious levels to the edge of awareness and is filtered through internalised conditions of worth, which may deny, distort, suppress or in some other way censor the material before allowing it into conscious awareness (see (a) in Figure 10.3). With the creative arts process, material is externalised directly from the unconscious, unfiltered and expressed in symbolic form. It becomes more readily available to conscious awareness, and as assimilation occurs the area of consciousness expands. The flow of internal communication between the levels becomes more fluid, and as awareness expands it can promote internal connection, helping to bring awareness of deeper levels and 'universal' unconscious into conscious awareness (see (b)). The role of the creative arts counsellor is to facilitate this process, helping the client translate the meaning expressed in symbols into words and into conscious awareness.

If a client isn't ready to integrate what has been expressed, it is still possible that the therapist's empathy may be received or subceived at some unconscious level. As Carl Rogers writes, the therapist's inner self may be 'in contact with the inner self of the client in a way that my conscious mind wouldn't recognise it' (Coulson, 2000, p.211).

Figure 10.3: A four-level model of consciousness

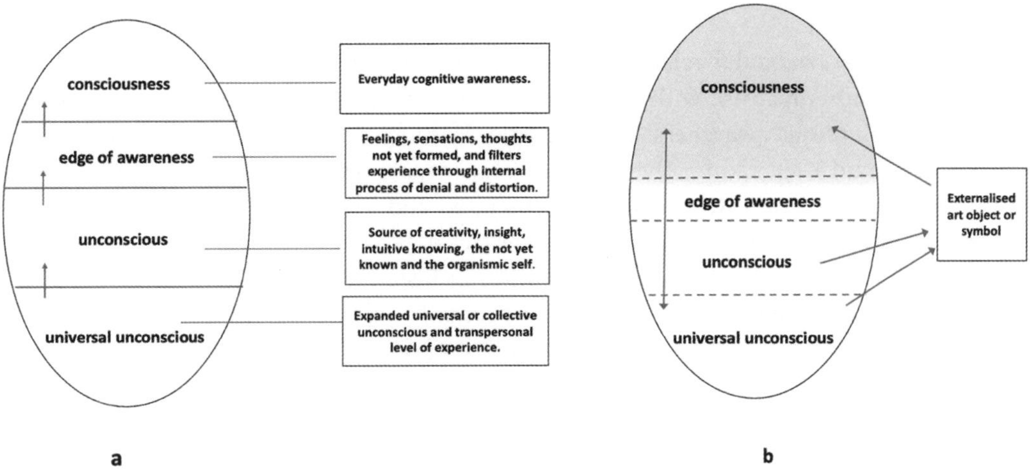

2. The triangular relationship

The art product, whether visual art, dance or play, has a literal existence separate from either therapist or client. This adds a third dimension to the relationship, creating a triangular dynamic (Figure 10.4)) where the client and therapist 'can talk about it, to it, or through it' (Morrell, 2011, p.5).

Figure 10.4: The triangular relationship

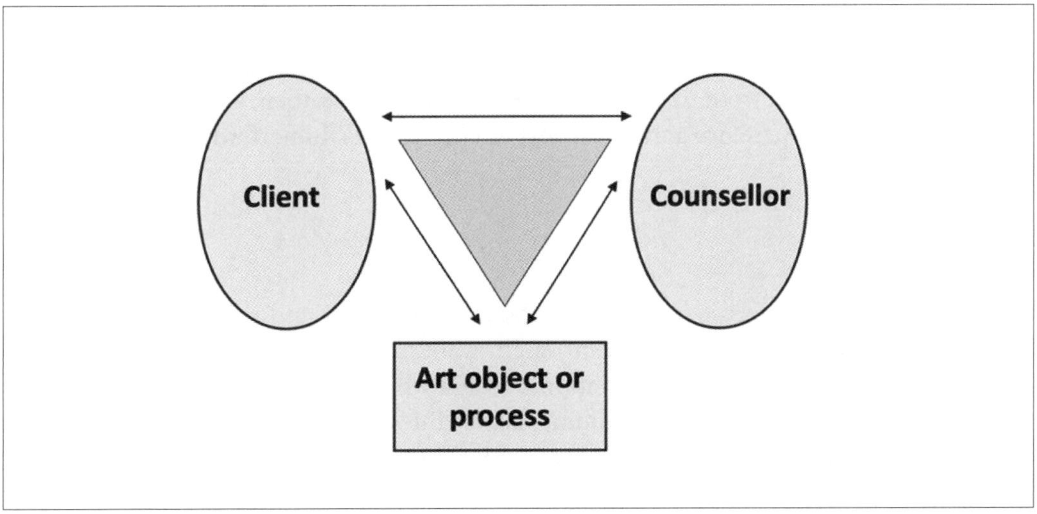

The symbolised, externalised expression of a client's inner landscape is brought directly into view within the triangular relationship. Carl Rogers (1979) saw focused conscious attention as helping to bring our nonconscious organismic functioning into the light of consciousness. Looking with intentionality at the art-making process and object can help a client to intuit meaning, bringing the unconscious to conscious awareness (Betensky, 1995). This may help to account for awareness to develop through reflecting on an art object on one's own.

Through the triangular relationship, the counsellor can empathise with the client in the moment and empathise with deeper and more complex aspects that may not yet be available to conscious awareness. For example, Hamish drew himself as a giraffe with a short neck. I said I felt sad for the giraffe because it couldn't reach its food. Hamish said he also felt sad for the giraffe, which was frustrated and hungry. He said the solution was for the giraffe to move to an area with shorter trees. The triangular dynamic provided an opportunity for Hamish to look with intention at his artwork and develop insight. This prompted him to leave his job and start a new career.

The triangular dynamic creates a relational synergy between the client, the therapist, and the art product. As a greater proportion of the client becomes available to receive empathy within the therapeutic encounter, this may help to promote relational depth (see Chapter 3, this volume).

3. Perceptual distance

The triangular dynamic creates a *perceptual sense of distance* from internal experience, allowing a client to engage intentionally, or not, with the art object. This distance can help promote feelings of emotional safety and facilitate the processing of difficult feelings. For example, a child who is afraid of thunder can depict this fear, and explore, process and contain it in art form (Silverstone, 1997).

When overwhelming or traumatic experiences cannot be processed and integrated, they are stored in memory as fragments of sensory experience, visual images and intense feelings that may only be accessible through non-verbal means (Malchiodi, 2020; van der Kolk et al., 2001). Providing a route for the expression of these experiences in art form, with perceptual distance, frees the client from threat in the present reality. Here, then, a client can choose to engage with and re-experience a traumatic experience or not (Rutherford, 2007).

Practice

Contracting

Contracting involves offering information about art materials and methods available and is an opportunity to explore how a client might want to work. It is also an opportunity to explore the client's curiosity and motivation. A client who feels intimidated by art materials might prefer a less structured art medium, such as the sand tray. It is also an opportunity to invite the client's creativity into the process. For example, I might say something along the lines of:

> I have a range of art and play materials and an iPad available which you are free to use or not. I sometimes offer guided visualisations, or I might invite you to engage in movement to help you explore and process feelings. Feel free to bring anything to

> sessions that you'd like to work with. Or if there is some way of working you like to try that isn't on show, just ask. While I might invite you to work creatively, it's always okay to say 'no'. How does that sound?

Inviting clients to collaboratively design their therapy ('metatherapeutic communication', see Chapter 9, this volume) invites greater creativity into the process. Clients may believe they are not creative or that they cannot draw, which is an opportunity to talk about the process. For example, I might say to a client:

> There's no pressure, you can't get it wrong, working creatively isn't about being good at art. The process itself can be healing. It can shift things. Exploring what you create can help you connect with your unconscious and may help you understand yourself in more depth. For example, if you feel depressed and don't know why, it can sometimes help to bring new information into awareness. Or we can talk, there's no pressure.

Creative wounding

Our creativity can become wounded and hidden under layers of psychological defences, (C.R. Rogers, 1954). Clients can find it difficult to engage when their creativity is wounded. Criticisms, expectations, even indifference to creative work can all cause psychological wounding that blocks the creative process – anything 'that makes us feel ashamed of our work or ourselves can render us incapable of the self-expression we yearn for' (Pierce, 2019, p.3).

Believing 'I can't draw', or 'I'm not creative' are examples of a creative wound. Conversely, being a trained artist can also wound a person's innate creativity because training to meet an aesthetic standard is in effect a set of conditions of worth: 'This is how you should draw this'; 'Your art is acceptable if…'

An understanding of the qualities of different materials and methods can help a therapist to offer suggestions to help a client reconnect to their creativity and promote psychological healing. For example, themes and guided visualisations can be offered to engage the imagination and creative process. It is crucial to ensure a visualisation is not prescriptive or directing content. For example, telling the client: 'You are walking along the shore, it is sunny, you are relaxed' is prescriptive; it is telling the client how to feel. However, inviting the client: 'Imagine you are walking along a shore. Notice the weather. How do you feel?' allows a client to freely symbolise unconscious material. Curiosity can stimulate exploration: Is the weather stormy or sunny? Perhaps the client likes storms, or perhaps the storm represents a stormy argument. A theme can act as a container for the process, and the imagined scene can then be externalised in a sand tray, or explored verbally if a client is too inhibited to draw.

When using sand, stones or finger painting, a client is less likely to have an internalised expectation or aesthetic standard to meet, which can help them to engage more freely in the creative process. For example, Li-Mei was a high-achiever who had introjected demanding expectations around the standards of art. She would draw but would immediately criticise her artwork and throw it in the bin. I invited her to work with finger paints, starting with her eyes closed. Not seeing what she was painting helped her engage in the process and stimulated her creativity. She worked spontaneously, playfully making patterns on the paper and exclaimed, 'I feel free, and I love my painting!' After this session, Li-Mei engaged creatively with a wider range of materials. Using finger paints helped her bypass her introjected standards and engage in the process and unblock her creativity. Over the following weeks, she reported feeling more relaxed and less anxious in her life.

Key skills

The relational aspects set out earlier in this chapter are key to fostering creativity and freedom of creative expression within the person-centred creative arts approach. But there are also three key skills, originally developed by Liesl Silverstone (1997), that can promote exploration, facilitation and cognition: reflecting, bridging and facilitating insight.

1. Reflecting

Reflecting involves mirroring movements, emotions or words, which can promote self-awareness and empathy (McGarry & Russo, 2011) . When working with symbols in visual art, the aim is to reflect what the client says, without interpretation or distortion, so as to mirror their exact words and intonation. Reflecting exactly what is said is crucial, as a small change can entirely distort the meaning (Silverstone, 1997). The symbols are seen as a metaphor; meaning is personal, contextualised, cultural and specific to each individual, and can only be understood from the frame of reference of the client.

2. Bridging

Flattening objects in a sand tray or punching the air in dance are physical symbols that may represent frustration. Externalised symbols may represent more than one thing – for example, a car can represent a relationship, a job or both. Bridging helps to elicit meaning by connecting the symbolic expression that is externalised 'out there' to the client's inner world. For example, a drawing of a house for one person may represent safety, while for someone who is experiencing abuse, it may represent imprisonment or danger. This can be explored by asking 'What does "house" mean to you?' Each element may be significant: for example, a house with a doorway but no door might represent an absence of boundaries, or it might represent escape. Bridging can help bring meaning into awareness and avoid the therapist imposing their interpretation.

3. Facilitating insight

This is where a client intuits and accurately perceives the meaning or message that is being expressed – its *essence*. Silverstone believed this to be an essential element of the creative arts therapeutic process, and it is often incredibly enlightening for both client and counsellor when insight occurs. Facilitating insight can be used as a way to bring the exploration to an end by simply asking, 'If this has a message for you today, what is it saying?', or 'What do you think this telling you?' If this is done too soon, too late, or is missed out entirely, the client may not be able to connect to the essence, and the meaning may remain unconscious. Insight doesn't always occur, or it may occur spontaneously, as it is dependent on a client's readiness to allow unconscious material into conscious awareness, as well being influenced by the skill of the counsellor.

The example of Matt (Figure 10.5) illustrates these skills in practice.

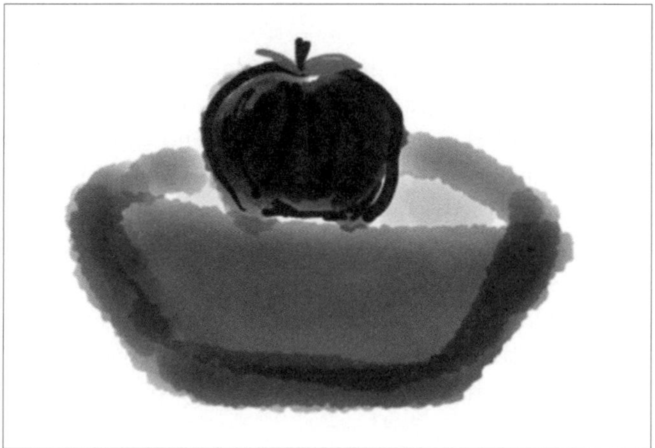

Figure 10.5: Matt's drawing

Ani: Can you tell me what you have drawn.

Matt: I've drawn a red apple.

Ani: You've drawn a red apple. Red, what does red mean to you? [*Reflecting and bridging*]

Matt: Red is love.

Ani: Red is love. And apple, what do you associate with apple? [*Reflecting and bridging*]

Matt: My daughter – she loves apples.

Ani: … and where is the apple situated? [*Exploration*]

Matt: In a blue bowl.

Ani: Blue, what does blue mean to you? [*Reflecting and bridging*]

Matt: Blue is sadness.

Ani: And bowl?

Matt: Bowl is something that holds, and a barrier. It is holding the apple.

Ani: So, this drawing represents love and your daughter, and also sadness, holding and a barrier… I'm wondering if that makes sense to you? [*Reflecting and bridging*]

Matt: Yes! I love my daughter, but she said some hurtful things and I am feeling sad about our argument.

Ani: So, if this has a message for you today, what do you think it is saying? [*Facilitating insight*]

Matt: That I need to let go of some of the hurt I'm holding, let down my barriers and connect with her. I think perhaps she is hurting too. [*The essence*]

Integrating skills into practice

The example of Matt shows how the three key skills of reflecting, bridging and facilitating insight can be used. But the person-centred creative arts approach is more than a set of skills; it is a relational practice. The example of Harry illustrates this by showing how the three skills can be integrated into the relationship, and how the relationship, the skills and the art process combine to foster change and growth.

When Harry was little, he wanted to be a musician, but his parents laughed at his attempts to play the violin. His creativity was wounded, and he stopped playing the violin. His parents wanted Harry to become a doctor. Harry denied his desire to be a musician. He had become incongruent. He had developed an outer locus of evaluation, valuing his parents' opinion over his own. To gain approval, his self-concept had changed, and he now believed he wanted to be a doctor.

At our first session Harry said he felt sad and depressed but didn't know why. He was curious about his feelings and motivated to explore them. I invited Harry to engage with art. He said he wasn't artistic, so I offered a guided visualisation, explaining that he could work creatively without drawing. I could see Harry relax.

I invited Harry to imagine he was on a magic carpet that took off and landed somewhere. This engaged his imagination in a playful, non-threatening way. He imagined he landed in a concert hall and watched a concert. He felt excited, which confused Harry, who believed he wasn't musical. The imaginary trip provided a route for his unconscious to communicate his congruent feelings towards music in the imagined scene, but his conscious mind wasn't yet ready to allow this into awareness. His incongruence was revealed by his confusion. Harry's conscious and unconscious experience became available to us both in the therapeutic relationship. I responded by empathising with feelings of both excitement and confusion.

At the next session, Harry said he had been feeling confused since the visualisation. I invited him to draw his feelings, to express his confusion creatively. He painted patterns using vibrant colours on one half of the paper and a black square on the other (Figure 10.6). I used key skills to explore the painting with Harry.

Ani: Can you tell me what you have painted? [*Exploration*]

Harry: A black box.

Ani: A box. What does that represent for you? [*Reflecting and bridging*]

Harry: Trapped, no escape.

Ani: The box is black – what comes to mind when you think of black? [*Reflecting and bridging*]

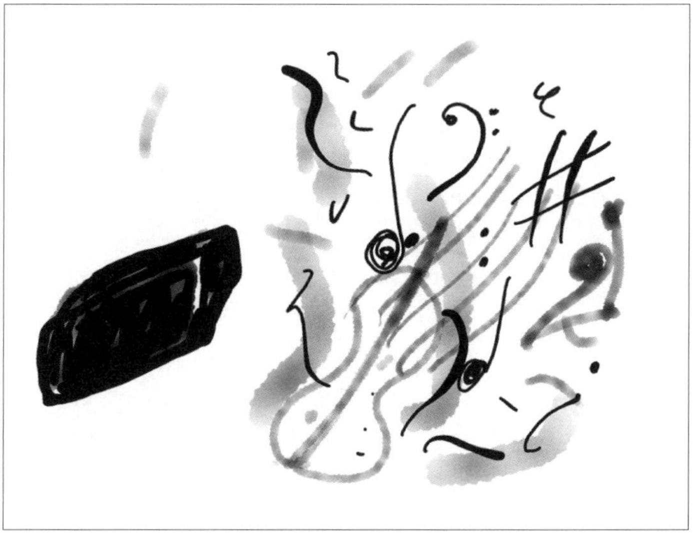

Figure 10.6: Harry's painting

Harry: Darkness. It's heavy and sad. It reminds me of a doctor's bag.

Ani: The box represents a doctor's bag. Can you connect to feeling heavy and sad? [*Reflecting and bridging*]

Harry: Yes, I don't like it. I want to be over here with the bright colours.

Ani: You don't want to stay here with the black, heavy and sad feeling, you want to be over here. What do you see as you look at the bright colours? [*Reflecting and exploration*]

Harry: It's vibrant, happy; the shapes remind me of musical notes, and I can see a violin.

Ani: You can see a violin and music, and it's vibrant and happy – what comes to mind as you look at the violin? [*Reflecting and bridging*]

Harry: When I was little, I used to love playing the violin, I wanted to be a musician, but stopped playing because I wasn't any good. I am training to be a doctor, but I don't really enjoy it. I guess I feel trapped. [*Insight*]

The structure of a visualisation helped Harry feel relaxed and able to engage in the creative process. The visualisation engaged his imagination and provided an opportunity for his denied feelings about playing the violin to be expressed symbolically. Harry wasn't initially ready to allow this information into conscious awareness and empathising with his organismic excitement might have helped him feel understood at an unconscious level. Harry's curiosity and motivation, along with the development of trust at the first session, helped Harry to engage with art at the second session. Reflecting and bridging the elements of the artwork helped Harry connect with his unconscious feelings and bring them to conscious awareness. He could integrate his feelings for the violin and his feelings about becoming a doctor into his self-concept. As a consequence, there was less discrepancy between his inner and outer experience.

Over the next weeks, Harry bought a violin and began to play again. He decided to continue to train as a doctor, but he now enjoyed playing violin as a hobby. Resolving his incongruence opened new opportunities and enabled him to make decisions from a more internal locus of evaluation. Harry said he no longer felt depressed and that he was excited about the future.

Materials

Bringing creative media into the therapy actively invites creativity into the therapeutic process. This involves making space for co-creation, inviting clients to explore creative ways of working they might not have considered. A specialised kit is not always necessary: a guided visualisation that engages the imagination, a set of stones, a pencil and paper or whatever is available can provide a medium for creative expression. However, having a range of materials and ways of working on offer fosters client choice, and making paints, pastels, clay, music, a sand tray, small objects and figures or an iPad available can be helpful. Different media have distinct qualities that can foster the process: for example, abstract art such as squiggle drawing or sponge painting can promote unconscious symbolic formation, while movement can help a client to break through physical and psychological numbing (Hinz, 2015).

The tactile qualities of media can also be helpful. For instance, working with sand can help clients to relax and engage. It can stimulate right-brain limbic processes, helping to process painful experiences and enable clients to talk about their experiences (Fleet et al., 2023). For example, Mustafa was a refugee who had experienced war but was unable to talk about his experiences. He used the sand tray silently to create scenes that expressed the horror he had witnessed. At first, he positioned a small figure face down in the sand within the scene, but after several sessions he changed its position to standing, facing the scene, and he began to talk about his ordeal. Working silently with figures in sand helped Mustafa begin to process and integrate his experiences.

Clients may choose to bring something new to the session themselves to stimulate their creativity: for example, a selection of fabric or leaves and twigs to create a collage, or their own objects to use in the sand tray.

Counsellor creativity is also part of the therapeutic process and can help to generate new ways of working that may be individualised to each client. For example, Jacob had experienced significant sexual and emotional abuse. He felt a deep sense of shame and struggled to talk about his experience. He had had therapy before but said talking did not help and was curious about working with art. He described how he felt:

> It's like the abuse is imprinted on me, on my skin. Like it stained me. I feel dirty. I can't see *me,* only the stains are visible. I feel like other people see it too. I wish I could wash it off, but I don't think it will ever wash off.

After the session, an idea came to my mind. I bought a large white shirt and showed it to Jacob at the following session, and said to him:

> I thought about how you feel the abuse is imprinted on you, like a stain. I have a shirt here and wondered if you might find it helpful to express that externally – put the stains directly on the shirt?

Jacob spent two sessions painting and drawing on the shirt, externalising the emotional 'stains' he perceived and using the shirt as an external metaphor for his 'skin'. I witnessed his process, which was filled with pain and emotion. When he was finished, we sat together on the floor and explored what he had created. He said:

> Now that I have put the stains on the shirt, I feel lighter. The stains aren't on me, somehow; they are now on the shirt. Weird, but I feel cleaner. I still have stains, but they are lighter. I think maybe they are part of me, but not all of me anymore.

He decided he might wash the shirt at some point, but for the moment it was enough to have externalised his abuse. Doing so had changed how he felt inside. The shirt became a safe container and created a perceptual distance from his abuse. He became able to see his abuse as something separate – part of his experience, rather than the entirety of his being.

This illustrates how a counsellor's creativity can be used within the therapeutic process, arising 'out of the unique qualities of the individual in his interactions with the materials of experience' (C.R. Rogers, 1954, p.250). I offered a way of working tailored to *this* therapy with *this* client, which fostered Jacob's process in a creative and personalised way.

Digital media

Whilst there is not scope for a full exploration of digital media in this chapter, it is important to address this new and rapidly developing context. Working with creative arts online can be complex. For example clients may have limited access to art materials, and the absence of shared physical presence can limit the counsellor's ability to view the art-making process. But the online environment can also positively influence the process (Walters, 2022). For example, Jamal, one of my child clients, found working online less intimidating. He told me, 'It's better seeing you online, you are smaller on my iPad screen, and I can use my own toys.' Online disinhibition can also influence clients to feel able to express themselves more freely (Suler, 2015) and may contribute to exploration and facilitation of meaning of the art object.

Digital tools such as an iPad can contribute positively to the therapeutic process (de la Prida, 2014). For example, Ben has arthritis and could not hold a pencil, so he used an iPad to draw and added photos and a voice recording to create a digital multimedia collage that he felt accurately depicted his internal symbolisation.

The creative process can be harnessed online even when art materials are not available. For example, one week Jenny joined the session via zoom from her parked car.

Jenny: I'm so angry.

Ani: Close your eyes… see if you can get in touch with that anger… Where in your body is it located…? What colour is it…? What shape…? How big is it…? What would it feel like to touch?

Jenny: It is huge, a large hot lump that fills in my throat and stomach, red and blue, like a bruise.

Ani: Your anger is huge, and hot, and is like a bruise. Red, what do you associate with red?

Jenny: Anger.

Ani: … and blue?

Jenny: Sadness.

Ani: … and it's a bruise inside. Can you connect to that at all?

Jenny: Something happened at work today. I am angry but didn't realise I was hurt and sad too.

If Jenny had been in my therapy room, she might have painted her angry bruise, which could have offered greater potential for exploration. However, even when working online without art materials, Jenny could symbolise and externalise verbally and bring her deeper feelings into conscious awareness.

Groups

Creative arts can be used as a whole-group process, with everyone contributing to the same image. Drawing the outline of a *group island* and inviting members to fill the island with what they need can bring unconscious dynamics to light so they can be explored – by noticing who is in the centre, or who has built a wall, for example (Silverstone, 1997).

Participants can also be invited to work on their own within a group setting. In groups, I often start by inviting participants to close their eyes and listen to music and allow their body to move, and then to make marks on paper. Listening to music 'allows us to move into a deep sensory state of feeling' (N. Rogers, 1993, p.87), which can then be symbolised and illustrated using creative media.

Offering a theme to a group can engage all the participants in a shared experience. For example, at an online workshop, I invited participants to introduce themselves. Khalila said, 'I am a trainee therapist, and a mother of two children. I'm excited to be here.' I then invited participants to imagine they were a vegetable and to depict that externally. I invited them to introduce themselves using their artwork. Khalila said:

> I've drawn myself as a carrot. A carrot is bright orange, strong and sturdy. I can associate with being quite strong, and I try to be bright and cheerful. The top is green and fluffy, and that's me exactly – a bit fluffy headed. I like the green colour, it's peaceful.

You can see in the second introduction Khalila was able to connect more deeply with herself. She was curious and motivated to explore, and she communicated openly and authentically. It's also important to note that Khalila didn't think to herself, 'I'm strong and bright, I'll represent myself as a carrot'. First came the image, then came insight.

Next, I invited Khalila to describe the carrot. She said: 'It's been pulled out of the ground and is lying dead on the ground.' I empathically reflected her exact words. She started to cry and said, 'I am from Syria, a refugee, I was pulled away from my roots, like this carrot. My old life is dead. I miss it.'

This example shows how Khalila quickly gained insight into the deeper meaning of her symbolic representation of the carrot and expressed her distress. The shared experience within the group generated a greater depth of encounter for participants. The group witnessed her process and Khalila perhaps experienced a greater depth of empathy as a result.

Couples

The creative arts approach can quickly make underlying issues and dynamics visible when working with couples in therapy. The art object can serve as a mirror, bringing incongruence into view and helping a couple gain a new perspective. For example, Jane and Michelle came to therapy after Jane had had an affair. Both said they were equally committed to working on repairing their relationship. I offered a prompt of drawing a house together (Silverstone, 1997). Michelle drew food, a sofa, and herself holding a bunch of flowers for Jane. Jane drew herself in a room with no door. This seemed to symbolise how Jane was unconsciously closed off from the relationship, and how Michelle felt she was making all the effort to rebuild their relationship. Bringing this to awareness meant that Jane's underlying emotional disconnection and Michelle's hurt and resentment could now be explored more openly in therapy.

Research

Research that focuses on understanding the mechanisms of change in creative arts therapies is only beginning to emerge, and research specifically from a person-centred perspective is even more sparse.

A recent scoping review of 67 studies and articles examined the therapeutic factors and mechanisms of change of a range of expressive media, documenting the impact on a wide range of psychological and physiological outcomes (de Witte et al., 2021). The study is not specific to person-centred approaches but does seem to support the notions outlined in PCEAT of the way in which different media can foster different therapeutic processes.

A qualitative study in Japan with three participants who had completed PCEAT training examined the influence of expressive arts on psychological growth during training. It suggested that non-verbal expressive arts within a safe and supportive person-centred environment can promote the development of self-awareness and connection to self and others (Ono, 2018). The scoping review (de Witte et al., 2021) indicated that deepening connection with one's internal self through creative arts can promote change. Ono's study

(2018) indicated that the congruence and depth of awareness of whole-body experiencing is crucial. This view is consistent with the outcome of a study using grounded theory methods to analyse the experience of 14 art therapists (Schwarz et al., 2018). Its findings also highlight how the therapist's personal development can have a positive impact on the therapeutic arts process.

The view that online disinhibition may foster the therapeutic process when working with creative arts online was identified in a recent study (Jo, 2022). The study employed constructivist grounded theory to explore online working with art therapy students. It found the online classroom created a feeling of safety and deeper reflections on the artwork, and that greater openness seemed to occur. It acknowledged that more research was needed in this area, and that therapists who have facilitated working online have adapted their practice in new ways that may help to meet the needs of a wider range of clients.

Summary

In this chapter I have set out a theoretical foundation that anchors the creative arts approach within person-centred theory and defines it as a person-centred and pluralistic approach (Chapter 9, this volume). The chapter integrates some new ideas and outlines a framework of conditions and stages to illustrate the creative process and its relation to unconscious processes. My aim has been to present a contemporary perspective on the theory and practice of this colourful and creative tribe of the person-centred nation, which I hope will inspire greater integration of creative methods and practice in counselling and psychotherapy.

Resources

Websites

- Association for Person-Centred Creative Arts: www.apcca.org.uk
- Person-Centred Expressive Arts: https://personcenteredexpressivearts.com
- Focusing-Oriented Expressive Arts: https://www.focusingarts.com

Key texts

- This book provides a detailed description of the experience of students on a PCAT training course to illustrate the philosophy and practice of PCAT:
  Silverstone, L. (1997). *Art therapy: The person-centred way. Art and the development of the person* (2nd ed.). Jessica Kingsley.
- This book offers a vibrant account of the philosophy and practice of the PCEAT model, which focuses on using a range of creative media:
  Rogers, N. (1993). *The creative connection: Expressive arts as healing*. Science and Behavior Books.
- This text is a comprehensive description of the theory and practice of the FOAT model:
  Rappaport, L. (2009). *Focusing-oriented art therapy: Accessing the body's wisdom and creative intelligence*. Jessica Kingsley Publishers.

References

Axline, V.M. (1964/1990). *Dibs in search of self: Personality development in play therapy*. Penguin.

Ayling, P., Armstrong, H. & Clark, L.G. (2019). *Becoming and being a play therapist: Play therapy in practice*. Routledge.

Betensky, M. (1995). *What do you see?: Phenomenology of therapeutic art expression*. Jessica Kingsley.

Bohart, A.C. (2012). Can you be integrative and a person-centered therapist at the same time? *Person-Centered & Experiential Psychotherapies, 11*(1), 1–13. https://doi.org/10.1080/14779757.2011.639461

Brown, D. (2012). New developments: Person-centred expressive arts therapies. In P. Sanders (Ed.), *The tribes of the person-centred nation: An introduction to the schools of therapy related to the person-centred approach* (2nd ed.) (pp.1878–200). PCCS Books.

Conradi, P. (2000). Dreams, the unconscious and the person-centred approach: Re-visioning practice. In T. Merry (Ed.), *Person-centred practice: The BAPCA reader* (pp.218–231). PCCS Books.

Cooper, M., O'Hara, M., Schmid, P. F. & Bohart, A. (2013). *The handbook of person-centred psychotherapy and counselling*. Macmillan International Higher Education.

Coulson, A. (2000). The person-centred approach and the re-instatement of the unconscious. In T. Merry (Ed.), *Person-centred practice: The BAPCA reader* (pp. 208–217). PCCS Books.

Davis, S. (2000). Psychological contact through person-centred expressive arts. In G. Wyatt & P. Sanders (Eds.), *Rogers' therapeutic conditions: Evolution, theory and practice. Vol. 4: Contact and perception* (pp.204–220). PCCS Books.

de la Prida, A. (2014). *A qualitative study of experiences of digital technology through using an iPad in therapy.* Unpublished master's dissertation. University of East London. https://repository.uel.ac.uk/item/8q35x

de la Prida, A. (2016, October 1). Let food be thy medicine... *Counsellors Café Magazine.* www.thecounsellorscafe.co.uk/single-post/2016/09/30/let-food-be-thy-medicine

de Witte, M., Orkibi, H., Zarate, R., Karkou, V., Sajnani, N., Malhotra, B., Ho, R.T.H., Kaimal, G., Baker, F.A. & Koch, S.C. (2021). From therapeutic factors to mechanisms of change in the creative arts therapies: A scoping review. *Frontiers in Psychology, 12.* https://www.frontiersin.org/article/10.3389/fpsyg.2021.678397

Elliott, R., Lago, C. & Charura, D. (2016). Research on person-centred/experiential psychotherapy and counselling: Summary of the main findings. In C. Lago & D. Charura (Eds.), *The person-centred counselling and psychotherapy handbook: Origins, developments and current applications* (pp.223–232). McGraw-Hill/Open University Press.

Embleton-Tudor, L., Keemar, K., Tudor, K., Valentine, J. & Worrall, M. (2004). *The person-centred approach: A contemporary introduction.* Palgrave.

Fleet, D., Reeves, A., Burton, A. & DasGupta, M.P. (2023). Transformation hidden in the sand: A pluralistic theoretical framework using sand-tray with adult clients. *Journal of Creativity in Mental Health, 18*(1), 73–91. https://doi.org/10.1080/15401383.2021.1936738

Fox-Muraton, M. (2021). A world without imagination? Consequences of aphantasia for an existential account of self. *History of European Ideas, 47*(3), 414–428. https://doi.org/10.1080/01916599.2020.1799553

Geller, S.M. (Ed.). (2012). Therapeutic presence as a foundation for relational depth. In R. Knox, D. Murphy, S. Wiggins, & M. Cooper (Eds.), *Relational depth: New perspectives and developments* (pp.175–184). Palgrave Macmillan/Springer Nature.

Gillon, E. (2007). *Person-centred counselling psychology: An introduction.* Sage.

Health & Care Professions Council. (2018, November 6). *Professions and protected titles.* HCPC. www.hcpc-uk.org/about-us/who-we-regulate/the-professions

Hinz, L. (2015). Expressive therapies continuum: Use and value demonstrated with case study (Le continuum des thérapies par l'expression?: Etude de cas démontrant leur utilité et valeur). *Canadian Art Therapy Association Journal, 28*, 43–50. https://doi.org/10.1080/08322473.2015.1100581

Jo, P.S. (2022). Online art therapy classroom in Thailand. In M. Winkel (Ed.), *Virtual art therapy: Research and practice* (pp.167–173). Routledge.

Lusebrink, V.B. (2004). Art therapy and the brain: An attempt to understand the underlying processes of art expression in therapy. *Art Therapy, 21*(3), 125–135. https://doi.org/10.1080/07421656.2004.10129496

Magsamen, S. & Ross, I. (2023). *Your brain on art: How the arts transform us.* Canongate Books.

Malchiodi, C.A. (2020). *Trauma and expressive arts therapy: Brain, body and imagination in the healing process*. Guilford Press.

McGarry, L.M. & Russo, F.A. (2011). Mirroring in dance/movement therapy: Potential mechanisms behind empathy enhancement. *The Arts in Psychotherapy, 38*(3), 178–184. https://doi.org/10.1016/j.aip.2011.04.005

Mearns, D., Thorne, B. & McLeod, J. (2013). *Person-centred counselling in action*. Sage.

Morrell, M. (2011). Signs and symbols: Art and language in art therapy. *Journal of Clinical Art Therapy, 1*(1), 25–32,

Ono, K. (2018). Psychological growth through person-centered expressive arts therapy training in Japan. *Person-Centered & Experiential Psychotherapies, 17*(2), 91–110. https://doi.org/10.1080/14779757.2018.1440623

Pierce, M. (2019). *The creative wound: Heal your broken art*. Mark Pierce.

Rappaport, L. (2009). *Focusing-oriented art therapy: Accessing the body's wisdom and creative intelligence*. Jessica Kingsley Publishers.

Rappaport, L. (2016). Focusing-oriented art therapy. In J.A. Rubin (Ed.), *Approaches to art therapy* (3rd ed.) (pp.286–307). Routledge. https://doi.org/10.4324/9781315716015-25

Rogers, C.R. (1954). Toward a theory of creativity. *ETC: A Review of General Semantics, 11*(4), 249–260.

Rogers, C.R. (1957). The necessary and sufficient conditions of therapeutic personality change. *Journal of Consulting Psychology, 21*, 95–103.

Rogers, C. R. (1979). The foundations of the person-centred approach. *Education, 100*(2), 98–107.

Rogers, C.R. (2003). *Client-centred therapy: Its current practice, implications and theory*. Constable.

Rogers, N. (1993). *The creative connection: Expressive arts as healing*. Science and Behavior Books.

Rosen, C.M. & Atkins, S.S. (2014). Am I doing expressive arts therapy or creativity in counseling? *Journal of Creativity in Mental Health, 9*(2), 292–303. https://doi.org/10.1080/15401383.2014.906874

Rutherford, M.C. (2007). Bearing witness: Working with clients who have experienced trauma. Considerations for a person-centered approach to counseling. *Person-Centered & Experiential Psychotherapies, 6*, 153–168. https://doi.org/10.1080/14779757.2007.9688439

Sanders, P. (Ed.) (2012). *The tribes of the person-centred nation: An introduction to the schools of therapy related to the person-centred approach* (2nd ed.). PCCS Books.

Schwarz, N., Snir, S. & Regev, D. (2018). The therapeutic presence of the art therapist. *Art Therapy, 35*(1), 11–18. https://doi.org/10.1080/07421656.2018.1459115

Silverstone, L. (1997). *Art therapy: The person-centred way. Art and the development of the person* (2nd ed.). Jessica Kingsley.

Smith, K. & de la Prida, A. (2021). *The pluralistic therapy primer: A concise introduction*. PCCS Books.

Suler, J.R. (2015). *Psychology of the digital age: Humans become electric*. Cambridge University Press.

Thorne, B. (2003). *Carl Rogers*. Sage.

van der Kolk, B.A., Hopper, J.W. & Osterman, J.E. (2001). Exploring the nature of traumatic memory. *Journal of Aggression, Maltreatment & Trauma, 4*(2), 9–31. https://doi.org/10.1300/J146v04n02_02

Walshaw, T. (2015). Creativity in private practice. In P. Wilkins (Ed.), *Person-centred and experiential therapies: Contemporary approaches and issues in practice* (pp.104–114). Sage.

Walters, J.A. (2022). Experiences of art therapists during the COVID -19 pandemic. In M. Winkel (Ed.), *Virtual art therapy: Research and practice* (pp.26–34). Routledge.

Wilkins, P. (2000). Towards a person-centred understanding of consciousness and the unconscious. In T. Merry (Ed.), *Person-centred practice: The BAPCA reader* (pp.200–207). PCCS Books.

Wilkins, P. (2015). *Person-centred and experiential therapies: Contemporary approaches and issues in practice.* Sage.

11. Pre-therapy and contact work

Dion Van Werde and Pete Sanders

For this chapter for the third edition of *The Tribes of the Person-Centred Nation*, I (DVW, the first author) have taken as its starting point Pete Sanders' short chapter on pre-therapy and contact work in the second edition (Sanders, 2012), which was included under the heading of 'New Developments'. Needless to say, Pete's death is not only a personal loss but a loss for the Pre-Therapy International Network and for the person-centred community as a whole.

Garry Prouty and the origins of pre-therapy

American psychologist Garry Prouty worked for several years with clients in persistent vegetative, regressed states and/or suffering from psychotic experiencing. He had a natural talent for reaching out and making contact with these clients. More often than not, people in these persistently uncommunicative states were believed to be unsuitable for psychotherapy and consigned to the back wards of long-stay psychiatric institutions. Prouty's work turned the spotlight on Carl Rogers' first therapeutic condition, namely *psychological contact* (Rogers, 1957). In his original work, in which he identified six 'necessary and sufficient' conditions for therapeutic change, Rogers proposed that psychological contact is a prerequisite for all the other therapeutic conditions. Prouty's work reiterated Rogers' position that, in order for psychotherapy to take place, psychological contact must be established, and drew our attention to the fact that, in some circumstances, for some people, psychological contact appears, to the casual observer, difficult, if not impossible.

Carl Rogers, listening to Garry Prouty's lecture at the celebration of the 15th anniversary of the Chicago Counseling Center in 1986, explicitly acknowledged his innovative and historically important professional work (Prouty et al., 2002).

Prouty's contribution to psychological helping was ground-breaking in the following respects:

- Practitioners were reminded that psychological contact cannot be taken for granted.
- A theory of psychological contact allowed for a more sophisticated understanding of therapeutic relationships and theories of change.
- Proper engagement with psychological contact through disciplined practice can help clients who were previously thought to be beyond help and unable to engage with therapy or everyday care activities – namely, those clients who have an impaired ability to establish and maintain psychological contact with another human being due to illness or injury, organic or psychological.

Pre-therapy is a person-centred, deeply respectful approach that is dedicated to restoring the essential psychological contact necessary for all people to engage in reciprocal relationships (Van Werde & Prouty, 2024).

Garry Prouty's work thus can be considered a theoretical evolution of person-centred therapy (Prouty, 1994). However, when starting his clinical work, Prouty discovered that the clients he worked with in those days – people tragically suffering psychosis, with an average admission duration in long-stay hospital of about 30 years and no proper care offered – were not able to engage in therapeutic relationships, since contact in itself was problematic. Hence, a kind of pre-relationship activity was necessary before they could enter Rogerian psychotherapy. The clients that Prouty worked with seemed unable to 'touch' their experiences; indeed, some appeared completely frozen. This echoes Eugene Gendlin's (1968) consideration of the concrete and bodily-felt process of experiencing as the key issue in psychotherapy (see Chapter 4, this volume). Prouty consequently proposed that 'pre-experiencing activity' was needed to unfreeze their active functioning, so that such people could access their inner life again. Pre-therapy thus can be defined as pre-relationship and pre-experiencing activity.

Prouty called his approach 'pre-therapy' because it prepared otherwise unresponsive, out-of-contact people for therapy. It is a set of processes that needs to be completed before therapy is possible with this client group. Prouty initially believed that, while pre-therapy actively establishes psychological contact, it is not in itself therapeutic. However, experience of working with out-of-contact clients revealed that, for some people, pre-therapy was intrinsically therapeutic, for two possible reasons.

First, some of the behaviours observed in a number of groups of clients, from agitation to chronic withdrawal, may not be a symptom of an underlying disorder but a secondary symptom of social isolation and the associated interpersonal disengagement that can accompany disturbing behaviour. When psychological contact is restored, the isolation is bridged and the symptoms 'spontaneously' dissolve.

Second, many theorists asserted that interpersonal contact, meeting or connection is the pivot of human psychology. As John Shlien (1961) put it:

> The mind emerges through a process of communication. This involves social interaction through what Mead [1934/1967] calls 'significant symbols' (usually words). A significant symbol is one that is 'reflexive', i.e. when it is used, *it presupposes another*

> *person… Acknowledging the other is essential to the existence of mind, from beginning to end.* (p.296; emphasis in original)

Thus, it could be said that an absence of connection is, *per se*, pathological, and so a restoration of contact must be therapeutic.

From its beginnings in Prouty's experience and practice in long-stay psychiatric institutions, pre-therapy was enthusiastically embraced in Northern Europe following a workshop led by Garry Prouty in the Netherlands city of Breda, organised by psychotherapist Bart Santen. The approach soon extended into other fields where clients' and service users' daily lives were limited by problems with psychological contact (see Pörtner, 2002, for a summary of the history).

Although he had been developing his ideas for more than 10 years, Garry Prouty published the first integrated account of theory, method and the research possibilities implicit in his work in his 1994 book *Theoretical Evolutions in Person-Centred/Experiential Therapy: Applications to schizophrenic and retarded psychoses.* Further books on pre-therapy (e.g. Sanders, 2007; Prouty et al., 2002; Prouty, 2008) were published by PCCS (see Resources, at the end of this chapter).

Pre-therapy continues to be well-represented and/or known in Northern Europe – for example, in Belgium, France, UK, Scotland, Germany, Austria and the Netherlands, with interest also in Brazil and, more recently, Switzerland.

Pre-therapy versus contact work

The title of this chapter, 'Pre-therapy and Contact Work', introduces a qualitative difference in the uses of pre-therapy interventions (called *contact reflections*, see below):

- *Pre-therapy* is the systematic and intensive use of contact reflections in relationships where therapy is the prime objective, but 'normal' therapy is impaired by the client's sustained lack or temporary loss of psychological contact. It is practised by psychiatrists, psychologists, psychotherapists, and counsellors.

- *Contact work* is the occasional use of a more limited set of contact reflections with the aim of restoring psychological contact to facilitate everyday care, such as personal hygiene and toileting, eating and drinking, pain relief, and so on. It can be practised by all staff intermittently to make better-informed decisions about everyday care, or constantly as part of a pervasive 'contact milieu' (see below).

The terms have developed to delineate the different professional uses of contact reflections so that staff not involved in explicitly therapeutic relationships can implement Prouty's insights without the connotations and expectations normally attached to therapeutic interactions.

Contact work should be part of good, effective communication in care settings, *per se*. It calls on all staff to think how they actually engage with people – that is, it requires all staff to deliberately consider how to approach people who are in an altered or 'pre-expressive' state ('pre-expressive' functioning is explained below). Finally, contact work teaches all staff to be explicit about something that was, and is still perhaps, taken for granted.

A contact milieu

Pre-therapy and contact work are more effective when the principle of contact and the use of contact reflections permanently permeate a social or institutional milieu. Here the term 'milieu' can mean 'family,' just as much as it can mean 'hospital ward', 'care home', 'school', or indeed any institutional or social environment where people who struggle with maintaining psychological contact might find themselves. Most often, though, the term 'contact milieu' is applied to an institutional care setting where all staff – professional, care and support, and ancillary – are trained in using contact reflections in their everyday work in order to establish a better social environment and more useful relationships with out-of-contact people.

This method of working was first developed in a psychiatric ward setting by the first author (Van Werde, 2002a, 2007, 2014), and then by Swiss psychologist Marlis Pörtner in institutions caring for older people and people with learning and other mental disabilities (e.g. Pörtner, 2007). When an all-embracing contact milieu is established, all aspects of care are made easier, more effective and, importantly, more rewarding for residents and staff alike.

Contact milieus are often effective with the most challenging people in situations where high levels of agitation, confusion and distress are debilitating for staff and other residents and contribute to a high-stress environment. Furthermore, contact milieu do not interfere with other psychological or medical interventions. If implemented properly, a contact milieu will enhance the effectiveness of these other interventions, since all therapeutic interactions benefit from full, mindful, interpersonal contact in a fully experienced social setting.

Pre-expressive functioning, the pre-expressive self and pre-expressive process

Prouty developed Rogers' ideas from a uni-dimensional notion of psychological contact to the pre-therapy theory of three types of contact:

a. contact with self

b. contact with the environment

c. social contact (or contact with others).

Sanders and Wyatt (2002) described this as a 'cascade of contact', arguing that the process of contact that is recognised by most people as 'normal' may be critically impaired if any element is missing. This means that the 'internal economy' of contact between self and experience (or environment) is as important as contact between self and others and the world in order for therapy or everyday meaningful conversation to be possible.

Prouty and his associates explained how contact can break down (and can be re-established) in the presence of psychotic symptoms, such as hallucination (Prouty et al.,

2002; Prouty, 2008). They postulated that, under certain circumstances, a combination of internal and external experiential isolation causes pathological withdrawal. The person becomes *pre-expressive* – by which Prouty means that, beneath the symptoms of autism, psychosis, brain damage or whatever, 'there is somebody in there' (Prouty, 1998, p.82). In this respect, the notion of *pre-expressive functioning* is highly important. It is an intuitive and heuristic concept derived from Prouty's personal experience as well as from clinical and quantitative case studies of pre-therapy. It suggests that disorganised and incoherent experiencing is capable of being transformed into a meaningful pattern. In that respect, Prouty considers all symptomatic behaviour as implicitly carrying relationship content as well as experiential content, even if it is not yet at an expressive level. If the therapist is able to work with these forms of functioning, the person might be able to develop into expressiveness, and thus form relationships and function experientially. The use of the word 'pre-' indicates a highly therapeutic vision, since it underlines the 'teleological capacity of symptomatology': symptoms carry in themselves the key to understanding and meaning.

If, for example, a man is standing in the hospital corridor, face anxious, looking at the ceiling, and asks you as you pass, 'Do you hear them?', this can be seen as somebody trying to relate by asking a question and trying to pre-experientially 'express' his fear by his facial expression, the tone of his voice and his physical closeness to you. Even when he is not conscious of how he looks and how he gives away his inner world by his appearance and behaviour, it is obvious that this man is trying to deal with the strange experiences he has and the feelings he is consequently struggling with. His contacting you is a significant moment in a possible process of disclosure of everything that is locked up in the alienating symptomatology of experiencing auditory hallucinations.

Prouty has long recognised the influence of his brother, who has learning disabilities and has been diagnosed with schizophrenia, on the development of pre-therapy. He says:

> One day when I was 11 or 12 years old, I invited a friend to visit my home. While we were talking, I said 'I wonder if he [brother] understands what we are saying?' To my intense surprise, my brother responded by saying, 'You know I do, Garry', and then he relapsed back into his autistic-regressed state. This 'episode of lucidity' 'haunted' me for many years, often giving the feeling 'there was someone in there'. My brother and other cases express 'episodes of lucidity' which indicate the presence of *the pre-expressive self* embedded in autism, regression, psychosis, brain-damage, learning difficulties and dementia and so on (Dodds et al., 2004). The 'episodes of lucidity' manifest the pre-expressive self. (Prouty, personal communication to the first author)

This pre-expressive self is also revealed in other signs too. First is the fact that all case histories and quantitative studies on pre-therapy illustrate movement from fragmented, incomplete, bizarre, incoherent expression ('pre-expressive functioning') to fuller cogency and self-congruence ('expressive functioning'). Signs of the pre-expressive self are also observed in the verbal process of psychotic expression. The semiotic structure of initial psychotic expression can be characterised as follows. These pre-expressive forms have no general context to derive meaning from and they have no referent to complete their symbolic function. This means the expression lacks reality sense and appears to be void of a reality source. Hence their dismissal by psychiatry (see, for example, Laing, 1969). For instance, a young man diagnosed with catatonia expressed himself by repeatedly saying 'Priests are devils'. By carefully using 'word-for-word' reflections, this eventually processed into the reality of a homosexual overture by a local priest. The highly condensed metaphor contained 'latent-reality' content.

The movement from a highly condensed metaphor to latent reality is called *pre-expressive process*. If there is no understanding that latent reality is 'packaged' in a pre-expressive way, the therapeutic potential of psychotic expression is not considered. Later in the chapter, we will situate Prouty as a classical and experiential psychotherapist, as well as existentially informed. What stands out is his radical practice of the values and theory represented in these approaches, even and precisely when working with clients thought unreachable for psychotherapy as such.

The therapeutic method of pre-therapy

Prouty described pre-therapy as 'applied phenomenology' and explained its action as 'pointing at the concrete', re-establishing the connection between sensation, experience and self: isolation is reduced, and a bridge is built across the gulf of contact impairment. This essentially goes a step further than Rogers (Chapter 2, this volume) and Gendlin (Chapter 4, this volume), who did not elaborate on the pre-conditions for psychotherapy being 'contact' and did not concentrate on working with severely contact-impaired clients.

The therapeutic method of pre-therapy is deceptively simple. In practical terms, it is a continual re-presentation of elements of shared reality (see the case descriptions below). This encourages contact with self, reality and others.

In pre-therapy, the therapist uses five kinds of reflections through which the client is invited to (re)contact reality, affect and other people. Contact reflections are attuned to the low level of contact functioning of the client, and thus have to be extraordinarily literal and concrete if they are to reach the severely withdrawn or regressed client. Through this technique, the realities of world, self and others are offered in a non-directive yet very concrete, non-judgemental, non-evaluative and non-interpretive way. As a result, the client is enabled to give the caregiver and reality a bridge into their idiosyncratic world. If the client permits themselves to contact the reality that is mentioned in a reflection ('You are standing in the corridor,' 'You look scared,' 'You look into my eyes and ask whether I hear them'), this means that they have already come out of their idiosyncratic, sheltered position a little bit, and have let the world and the person who verbalises it come in. They have recognised that they are in the hospital corridor, that they are addressing the nurse/carer, and that, in doing so, they have been showing and sharing some of their psychotic functioning for maybe the first time. This is individual pre-therapy. Basically, the client now can freely choose to stay in their reality or engage in a shared reality. This latter reality can be about outer and 'objective' realities, such as people, places, events and things, or it can be about communication with others, but it can also be about contacting their own inner feelings.

Integrating what pre-therapy has to offer has significant implications for daily therapeutic practice:

- Therapists should not gratuitously assume that psychological contact is a 'given'.
- Therapists are reminded to use all their senses – shifting the emphasis to looking as well as listening – to accurately sense when a client moves in and out of psychological contact.
- Psychological contact should be viewed as existing in a range of degrees, although there is a logical cut-off point where a person is out of contact and pre-expressive.
- Therapists must be ready to work in different ways when clients move between expressive (in contact) and pre-expressive (out of contact) states.
- Therapists now have a strategy for being with a wide range of contact-impaired clients (for specific references see below), including those with:
  - psychotic symptoms, severe psychotic withdrawal or regression
  - catatonia, dissociation and depersonalisation
  - dementia and other degenerative brain diseases, brain injury or damage
  - temporary contact impairment due to an organic condition
  - learning disabilities, from mild to severe and enduring
  - autistic spectrum disorders
  - terminal or degenerative illness that impairs communication or contact, including where palliative care reduces contact
  - coma
  - double or multiple diagnosis (as, for example, in a combination of learning disabilities, physical disability and psychotic experiencing).

Prouty describes pre-therapy as a theory of psychological contact, encompassing three constituting elements. He talks about *contact functions* (functions that make awareness possible; that show what happens psychologically 'inside' the client), *contact behaviours* (the client's behaviour that shows that the client is in touch with what is happening, that they are aware of who and where they are), and *contact reflections* (the therapist's responses; what the therapist says or does to invite the client to become aware again, to come out of their isolation, to anchor in the here and now, and stop being disconnected). Contact reflections (what the therapist does) facilitate contact functions (client process), which result in the emergence of contact behaviours (which can be measured; for a review of the research, see Dekeyser et al., 2008).

We will now say something more about these three elements, knowing that contact functions and contact behaviours are more abstract concepts that help us understand what happens within the client and how we can see change, whereas contact reflections are more related to the practice of how to do pre-therapy.

Contact functions

Prouty describes three functions/dimensions of awareness:

- you can be aware of yourself – *intrapersonal or affective contact*
- you can be aware of the people, places, events and things in the world surrounding you – *reality contact*
- you can communicate in a socially understandable way about how you feel and how you perceive the world – *contact with others* or *communicative contact.*

What we understand as normal psychological functioning consists of full awareness in these three domains.

It is now clear where and how psychological contact can break down (see, for example, Langner, 2017; Peters, 2014). Individuals might have impaired contact in any one of these domains or in any combination of these domains. Indeed, therapy literature is replete with attempts to understand partial breakdowns in contact. Prouty systematises this in pre-therapy along with a method of working with the client's fractured contact.

Contact behaviours

Contact behaviour is anything that the person does, and in so doing shows that they are in psychological contact. Helpers should be particularly interested when the client:

- talks about events, places, things and people verifiable by the helper – indicating (shared) reality contact
- talks about or makes facial expressions or bodily postures showing emotional or feeling content – indicating affective contact
- uses words indicating social or any interpersonal/relational awareness – indicating communicative contact.

While this might seem arbitrary, readers are invited to think for a moment about what they would consider to be behaviour signalling psychological contact. There is a surprising convergence of views. In short, every behaviour is potentially contact behaviour. It is important to approach every person in every setting with this in mind. The helper has to have their antennae and sensitivity set to 'high' to pick up expressive signs and behaviours.

Contact reflections

Contact reflections are what the therapist does. They are the contact-oriented responses of the therapist, contact worker or anybody reaching out to meet the client/person at their level of functioning. Contact reflections 'point' to the most concrete elements of the shared world, behaviour and experiences of the client. They look like stripped-down empathic reflections, but with the distinction that contact reflections only reflect what is there. The pre-therapy practitioner does not ever go beyond the concrete expression or behaviour of the client or a verifiable aspect of the shared reality. Prouty says that therapists as a discipline must learn to stop listening and start looking, in order to curb their more creative, idiosyncratic reaching for empathic alignment. A contact reflection is irreducible.

In practice, the therapist has to choose which kind of contact reflection is to be used, how often, and at what pace. There is no hierarchy among the contact reflections, and no pre-set order. In the case illustrations that follow below, you will get an idea what this might look like. Prouty says about using contact reflections: 'The technique is easy, but the art is difficult' (Personal communication to the first author).

There are five types of contact reflections, as follows:

- *situational reflections* (SR) reflecting aspects of the shared environment, naming people, places, events and/or things: e.g. 'The wall is painted yellow'; 'The sun is shining'; 'The chair is made of wood'
- *facial reflections* (FR) reflecting verbally or 'mimicking' the facial expressions of the client: e.g. 'A tear is running down your cheek'; 'Your eyes are closed'; 'You are frowning'
- *body reflections* (BR) reflecting, verbally or posturally, the gestures, movement and postures of the client: e.g. 'You are standing upright'; 'You are making a fist'
- *word-for-word reflections* (WWR) repeating back what the client says word for word: e.g. 'You are asking if I hear them'; 'You say: "Everyone noticed"'
- *reiterative reflections* (RR) remaking contact by repetition of previous reflections that showed an effect: e.g. 'This morning, you asked me if I heard them'; 'You looked into my eyes and smiled'.

Classical person-centred therapy versus pre-therapy

Here is a short vignette that presents two possible outcomes in parallel to illustrate how, on the one hand, pre-therapy contact reflections might be used, and, on the other hand, how 'classical' person-centred therapy (Chapter 2, this volume) might be used with the same client.

The side-by-side vignettes are also intended to show how pre-therapy contact reflections can change the course of a therapy session. Classical person-centred therapy does not provide a method for directly intervening in such experiences as dissociative or delusional episodes. But, without contact reflections, the therapist might carry on with 'therapy- as-usual', or they might perhaps wait patiently and reassuringly until the dissociative episode passes. While such strategies may be seen as adequate, and better than trying to jolt the client back to 'reality', they do not positively engage with the out-of-contact client. During such episodes, clients might become more distressed, delusional and agitated. Pre-therapy provides a gentle reaching out, an invitation, that is likely to draw the client back into meaningful contact. You will see exactly this happening in the vignette below, where pre-therapy reflections are used. It is important to say that what happens with Dan, the client, is the result of the pre-therapeutic intervention, and was not a pre-set aim when starting the session. In other words, change was a consequence of the therapy, not the goal. In this sense, pre-therapy is consistent with 'real' classical person-centred psychotherapy, even when working with these out-of-contact clients.

Dan

Imagine a psychiatric day-care situation in which a young person (Dan) starts to behave in an unusual way during a therapy session. His therapist, Sunny, intervenes. In the left-hand column we see Sunny using classical person-centred therapy only. In the right-hand column we see Sunny using classical person-centred therapy and pre-therapy (the reflections are in bold).

Dan has been talking about being bullied at school as a teenager. Then there is silence for two minutes. Dan looks at the window and wipes his brow, as though he is hot, and smiles broadly.

Classical	**Pre-therapy**
SUNNY: Are you warm? It's a bit stuffy in here. Shall I open the window? DAN: Why hasn't anyone done anything about the notice on the kitchen door? S: You're worried because no action has been taken about a notice on the kitchen door? D: [*Getting a little agitated*] Yes, and all the other notices. S: I can see it's upsetting you. I'm not sure what notice you mean on the kitchen door, or all the other notices. *Although we can't be completely sure, it is possible that Dan has gone into a fugue state of some sort with some thought disturbances. Sunny continues with empathic responses, without commenting on the 'flavour' of the process at this stage.*	SUNNY: Are you warm? It's a bit stuffy in here. Shall I open the window? DAN: Why hasn't anyone done anything about the notice on the kitchen door? S: You're worried because no action has been taken about a notice on the kitchen door? D: [*Getting a little agitated*] Yes, and all the other notices. S: **All the other notices.** [*As a flat statement, a WWR, not a question*] *Sunny is on the alert. She sees that Dan's agitation, and his references to 'all the other notices', makes her wonder whether he is drifting out of contact. Her response, empathic, has the advantage of being a 'word-for-word' (WWR) contact reflection.*
D: I thought everyone knew about them. That's what has happened lately, the notices. S: I'm not sure I understand what you're saying about the notices. Would it help to say what it is that's upsetting about them? D: I know you know. *Now we can be more certain that Dan's thinking is becoming more unusual. Sunny has continued until now with empathic responses and letting Dan know that she is not understanding him without being judgemental or interpretative.*	D: Everyone knows about them. That's what has happened lately. I know you know. [*Stares at Sunny wide-eyed*] S: **We are sitting in Sunny's room in the hospital. (SR) Dan says 'Everyone knows about them. That's what has happened lately, I know you know.' (WWR)** *Sunny is now in 'pre-therapy' mode, responding to Dan with contact reflections: first, a situational reflection (SR), followed by another WWR.*

S: I'm not following what you're saying now, Dan. You seem to be struggling to tell me something and I'm struggling to understand. D: The notices all around, you know, what they're saying. Everyone does. [*Frowns and bites lip*] S: OK, you think that the notices here are all saying the same thing, and that I know what they're saying. It seems to be upsetting you as well, as though you think I'm holding something back from you. *Sunny is more congruent in her empathic response – honest about not understanding and noticing Dan's upset. She knows his thinking is unusual but doesn't draw attention to this or 'reality correct' his mild delusion.*	D: [*Dan looks down and then looks back at Sunny, more in focus.*] What? What them? [*Shakes his head*] S: **You are shaking your head (BR) [*Sunny shakes her head*: BR] and asking me 'What them?' (WWR)** D: Oh yes, I was thinking about the nasty messages that people put on the notice boards at school about me. I got muddled up and thought that there were notices on the kitchen door here. There aren't any, are there? *Sunny is sure that Dan is now back in contact and resumes 'usual' person-centred therapy.*
[*Silence for a minute in which Dan frowns and appears to say something under his breath, then looks directly at Sunny and smiles.*] D: What time is it? S: I'm not sure what happened then. You were talking about notices and seemed upset. Is that right? D: Errm … [*Silence and a distracted look*] S: Now you seem to have snapped out of it. Can you remember what you were telling me about the notices?	S: No, I don't think there are any notices… So you remembered the cruel messages at school and got confused, thinking they were on doors here, is that right? D: Yes, I think about those messages a lot. The bastards. They used to put *really* bad things about me. Lies. Stupid nasty things. I could kill them. Fucking bastards. S: **The bastards at school put up lies about you on the walls and you just can't get it out of your head. You want to kill them for it. (WWR).** D: I hate them, the fucking bastards. [*Dan's eyes fill with tears*]

The notion of grey zone functioning

When contact is restored, meaning the client is functioning on an expressive level, the therapist may then help the client with a range of problems, from restoring everyday personal functioning through to psychotherapy. Once a therapist becomes sensitised to the contact state of their clients, they will become aware that many clients move quite quickly between a pre-expressive state and an expressive state. This movement between contact states presents a further challenge to the therapist.

As can be seen from the two further vignettes that follow, the difference between pre-expressive and expressive functioning is not completely clear. The first author, DVW (Prouty et al., 2002), called this region of functioning *the grey zone* – where people oscillate, sometimes almost imperceptibly, between pre-expressive and expressive functioning, or where these levels of functioning may both be present at the same time.

The vignettes illustrate how, depending on the person and situation, the out-of-contact state can vary from a fleeting hallucination or delusion (as in the vignette above) to catatonia and dissociation (the vignettes that follow). These vignettes show how the helper or therapist must be on constant alert. For expressive functioning, the therapist uses regular empathic listening; for pre-expressive functioning, they use pre-therapy reflections. In the grey zone, which comprises a mixture or quick changing of pre-expressive and expressive functioning, the therapist's reaction will also be a mixture: classical empathic listening to work at the expressive level, and pre-therapy reflecting to welcome and attune to the pre-expressive level.

The pre-therapy vignettes make this much more obvious and appear easier than it is in a real-world situation.

Pre-therapy in practice

The following vignettes give you a flavour of how pre-therapy looks in practice. As well as demonstrating contact reflections, the vignettes explain the therapist's thinking that led to their choice of which reflections to use.

At the same time, they show how someone can get into a state of loss of contact, and they underline the importance and value of pre-therapy in enabling the therapist to stay with them in these states, using this very concrete and phenomenological approach. In both the examples, as a consequence, the person worked with was able to get back in touch with their own strength and re-connect with the expressive level of functioning without anyone having to take over their process – such as, for example, getting them admitted to hospital or use of prescribed medication.

The vignettes are set in everyday social care practice, rather than psychiatry or residential care. This shows that familiarity with pre-therapy can be helpful in any situation when someone is experiencing contact loss. The guiding principle is the 'meta-diagnostic' view on the level of contact functioning. Pre-therapy is indicated whenever, and for whatever reasons, the person reverts to pre-expressive functioning.

Vignette 1: Catatonia and pre-therapy

The first vignette is about a middle-aged woman participating in an outpatient occupational rehabilitation programme. What happens on the programme triggers a state of catatonia that lasts the whole day (see also Van Werde 2021). Anna, a long-time unemployed woman was participating in the programme to enhance her chances of getting a job. This involved being interviewed about herself and her life and hopes for the future. Unknown to the interviewer at that time, Anna's child had been killed in a car accident recently and Anna was suffering guilt feelings about it.

Anna had already started to become distressed when one of my (DVW's) younger colleagues, Lucie, who had been working with Anna in previous sessions, asked her for some biographical details. Anna began to look away and lost eye contact; her body tensed up and she started to breathe more heavily. Lucie, at that point, had intuitively changed the subject to less personal, lighter and more neutral subjects, which eased the situation.

The case interview on the day we are writing about here was done by Julia, another staff member who was not known to Anna. Lucie was also present. Julia was seeking information about Anna's career to date, her family situation and her hopes and dreams for the future. Questions included: 'What do you want to do differently in your life?' 'What are your strengths and weaknesses?' 'What about your current situation should you change?' 'How is your family situation?' and 'Where do you see yourself in five years?'

Anna clearly could not handle these questions and tried to avoid answering them. She said things like 'I don't know', 'I can't comment on that', 'I don't know anymore'. Her stress levels went up, her body posture became more and more rigid, and when the questions kept coming, she finally 'disconnected'. She froze, stopped speaking, and did not react to anything anymore. Contact with her had broken down completely. She appeared both present and absent at the same time, as though she was locked in a psychological bunker. Neither Julia nor Lucie knew what to do: stopping the questioning, soothing, giving advice, letting her sit there, giving her time… nothing really helped. Anna remained sitting there, like a wax statue.

Julia felt bad that she had triggered this state. By 2pm, when the situation had not changed, she decided to call me and asked me to come in and help.

When I arrived, I saw that Anna was obviously stuck in a kind of frozen state. Nevertheless, I had the impression she could hear me and was able to understand my words, although she did not make eye contact or react to me in any way. However, there was one exception when she indirectly and non-verbally answered a question of mine (see the transcript).

Matching her level of functioning, I offered various ways for her to ground herself through connecting with the outside world and her inner world, in the hope that she would be able to consciously regain her sense of agency, instead of being imprisoned in her triggered catatonic state.

Finding the right pace for my reflections was difficult. I was trying to find a way to get through to her and invite her to engage with me without being demanding or insistent, or appear imposing or invading her personal space.

The following is a shortened description of how the intervention went. During the intervention, Lucie was also sitting in the room, but not Julia. You will see that I am the only one who spoke, and much of what I said was about what was happening around us: what we were doing, that I went out to the toilet, that Lucie went for lunch, that another colleague entered the room… Anna stayed mute all the time. Late in the afternoon, I also voiced the fact that Anna could not stay alone in the building after closing time, and that we would then have to find another solution (like call an ambulance).

Anna was sitting on the couch in a very peculiar, uncomfortable-looking and probably even painful way: upright, holding the weight of her upper body on her arms, with her hands bent back (see the reflections below).

Besides reflecting what was happening around us, I sometimes asked a question. In pre-therapy, when the contact level seems to rise, it may be possible to ask a very concrete question or give a comment, so long as it stays close to the interaction and what is happening in that moment. If the client follows you by reacting or replying to your question, this means that you correctly understood that the level of functioning was rising, and your next step would be to build on this by introducing small steps to a higher level of contact functioning by asking a further question or making a suggestion. If the client does not join you in that slightly higher level, then it's best to return to the reflection(s) that you were voicing before, where contact had still been possible.

The intervention lasted about two hours. My thoughts and comments are in italics.

[SR] You are sitting on a couch.

[FR] Your eyes are closed.

...

[FR] Your eyes are a bit open.

[RS] Your feet are both on the ground.

[SR] The woman next door comes in.

...

[BR/SR] You are sitting there, I'm sitting here, on a chair.

[SR] My colleague and I are sitting on chairs.

[BR/SR] Your arms are stretched, your hands twisted, the backs of your hands resting on the sofa, your shoulders are up.

...

[SR] We are sitting here, it is 2:30.

[RR; SR] I came in, sat down and moved a little bit closer. Now I am sitting here.

...

[Comment] (*This could possibly be labelled as a facial reflection, but since 'I' is mentioned, I regard it as a comment rather than a pure reflection)*: I can see your eyes.

...

[SR] Oh, a bit of sunshine is coming in...

...

[SR] Now I am sitting here (*I had pulled back my chair, hence I wasn't sitting so close to Anna*)

...

[Comment] (by means of an interpretation) It looks like your bent hands are carrying a lot of weight.

[BR] (*I mirror the position of her hands*)

[Question] Can Lucie touch your hands? Can she move them a bit?

[Question] Can you blink your eyes if it's okay? (*She blinks!!*)

Anna's blinking is clearly an interaction, hence communicative contact. Probably, at that moment, Anna was situated in the upper grey zone. She had been listening and understood, although she was not speaking or communicating at all. Intuitively, I had understood what she might be able to do, and then made that offer for her to answer in a non-verbal way, which she did.

This kind of interaction happened only once, but it illustrates the thin line between contact and pre-expressive functioning – the grey zone functioning.

> [RR] Lucie just touched your hand.
>
> ...
>
> [SR] Your hair is hanging down.
>
> [Comment] The colours of your shoes and shawl match.
>
> [SR] You are sitting on the sofa. There is some space between your back and the sofa.
>
> [BR/FR] You are sitting upright. You are looking down.
>
> [Comment] Lucie is going out to get something to eat. She was here with you all morning.
>
> [SR] It is now 3pm.
>
> ...
>
> [SR] The place will close in 45 minutes. It is 3.15pm. (*No eye contact, no change in body position and Anna has not spoken a word for about six hours...*)

All of a sudden, and on her own volition, Anna stood up very slowly, with her eyes and head down, and walked in a rather wooden way to the door.

Lucie and I sat and wondered: 'Do we have to intervene here, or do we trust this person and her decision to leave?'; 'Will she make it home safely?' We decided not to intervene. Apparently, Anna got home safely by bus. She did not show up the next day, probably needing the time to recover. The day after, she participated in the programme as usual.

When Lucie asked Anna about what had happened two days before, she said that she might have been able to recall the details the day after, but not any longer.

When Lucie explicitly asked Anna to give some feedback about the day of the intervention, Anna did tell her that all she could remember was not feeling good for the rest of the evening, once she got home. Anna also remembered that Lucie had touched her hand and that certain things got named. She also remembered that she spent quite a few hours in the room. She said she couldn't stand up then because her back hurt. Anna then quickly changed the subject and went into 'business as usual' mode. Lucie expressed respect for how she handled her stress levels in that moment and said she wouldn't ask any more questions about the day. She let go of the subject, not wanting to cause another episode of catatonia.

The whole pre-therapeutic intervention essentially had been directed to enable Anna to get back in charge of her life again. Indeed, the intervention did bring Anna back into contact with reality and herself: she got back control over her body, stood up unaided, and left. We didn't have to use force or other means to reach her and get her out of the building before closing time. The pre-therapeutic reflections in particular, and being attuned to her level of functioning in general, made it possible to reach her where she was. Contact was established. As a consequence, she was able to take ownership of her bodily functioning again, stood up and went home. We wanted to respect her and her psychological space, did not want to take over control, and trusted that she could take care of herself and take herself home safely, even after such an intense and difficult crisis.

The non-directive approach of using pre-therapy provided maximum respect for Anna and the state she was in. Anna remained the touchstone and cornerstone of everything that happened. Using pre-therapy reflections made it possible to sit alongside her withdrawal and muteness and invite her to come out of her involuntary isolation when she was ready to do so. The work was done without being intrusive and was respectful of her psychological space and freedom. It is rare that someone in this state should receive this level of trust and respect, regardless of their strange and incomprehensible behaviour.

Vignette 2: Dissociation and pre-therapy

The second vignette describes a session in an ongoing therapy group, where one of the participants, a young man called Willy, suddenly dissociated from himself and from the situation. In this vignette, we include the perspectives both of Dennis, the man who offered the pre-therapy reflections, and Willy, the man who was dissociating. The latter testifies how he experienced the situation, what happened to him, and how the intervention helped him come out of his state of dissociation. This is the first time the client's perspective has been recorded so clearly and exhaustively in the pre-therapy literature.

Interestingly, Dennis, the man who responded when Willy suddenly lost contact, was not one of the group therapists; he was another member of the therapy group. By profession, he was a psychotherapist and familiar with pre-therapy, and he intervened because it was clear that nobody else knew how to handle the situation and he thought that pre-therapeutic reflections, as he knew them, would be the right way to respond to Willy's sudden loss of contact. The account is formatted so that both accounts run parallel.

The pre-therapy intervention brought Willy back into the here and now and the dissociated state dissolved. This relatively small intervention had a huge effect. Everyone felt very relieved and grateful. The tension had been palpable, and everybody had felt helplessness, not knowing how best to respond. After Dennis's interventions and Willy's re-engagement that brought him back into the shared reality, everyone, including Willy, could breathe a little bit more freely again, and the debriefing could continue.

Other group members told Dennis afterwards, 'It was so authentic', 'simple', 'respectful', 'accepting', 'so focused and exactly attuned to Willy', 'so effective'.

Willy's report	**Dennis's report** (Dennis's thoughts and remarks are in *italics* and his pre-therapy interventions are in **bold**)
My memories of the exact moment are no longer clear, but I will try to reconstruct it to the best of my knowledge. If I remember correctly, we had previously done an exercise in which we were asked to form pairs and sit together on a mat and communicate with each other without using speech. For me, this exercise was incredibly exhausting from the start to the end. It was an enormous challenge even to sit opposite the other person, let alone to communicate without words. I had a strong need to escape and experienced very strong emotions that I couldn't quite grasp. It was like a mixture of fear, panic, despair and also strong anger. After the exercise, we had a debriefing and everyone in the group reported on how it had been. My feelings at that time are very difficult to describe, but I've felt them before in similar situations of great stress. I felt powerful emotions surging up, and especially in my body. I wanted to allow these feelings to come out, but at the same time I didn't want to express emotions I didn't rationally understand myself. The emotions were like waves. They swelled again and again, and when I tried to let them come through, they disappeared. It went on and on like this… It's a bit like when you feel you have to sneeze, but then the feeling and the urge to give in to it suddenly disappear, then reappear, then disappear again, and so on. Of course, sneezing does not have a comparable intensity with my emotions at that time.	A group of 10 participants – me included – were sitting in a circle on cushions on the floor. Two therapists and one assistant were also sitting in the circle, approximately opposite Willy. We were having a plenary debriefing of an exercise that was done in pairs. It was an exercise to tune in to another group member and develop a kind of mutual understanding and conversation without using spoken words. The pairs had to devise an intelligible non-verbal language to communicate. Some couples made contact by using their hands; others massaged each other, or sat back-to-back and tried to communicate that way, or started to challenge each other physically, or just looked at each other, and so on. The activities people devised took various forms: tender, energetic, varied, rhythmic, slow, powerful, continuous and so forth. Everybody had been very involved. Willy was sitting cross-legged on the ground, and said that, as he had said at the beginning of the day, he was experiencing a lot of tension. *For the group, this was a familiar theme with Willy, and it was also now very apparent.* He described how the exercise had gone for him. While speaking, he seemed to be more and more absorbed in his account of how he felt and was now feeling. *His general tension was perceptible and seemed to be increasing.* Occasionally Willy grimaced during his narration (he tensed and relaxed the muscles around his mouth, or pulled up the corners of his mouth, with his mouth half open, then clamped his teeth together again and pushed his chin forward). Sometimes a big smile suddenly appeared on his face; sometimes he withdrew into himself and looked gloomy. His moods changed quickly.

Then, when the emotions receded, I really couldn't feel them anymore. It was almost as if I'd felt nothing. In the debriefing, I just couldn't get to the point where I could let my emotions come through and out. I don't remember what the therapist said or asked me to do, but looking into his eyes made the emotions surge up again and to become even stronger. Unfortunately, I don't remember anymore what the exact input of the therapist was, although I would like to know what happened. I do remember that he wanted to give me some space to express my emotions, and I remember him making eye contact with me for that purpose.	Sometimes this was accompanied by small tics – a corner of his mouth would pull downwards, and sometimes he stared around him with big eyes. *There was clearly a lot going on, but it wasn't possible to interpret his emotions.* Suddenly he looked at the floor and went silent. He sat motionless and rigid. *The tension rose... It wasn't clear what was happening to Willy. There was something uncomfortable about the whole situation, and it was impossible to know how or where it would go.* The group therapist listened and watched attentively, allowing Willy some space without intervening immediately. Probably in response to the palpable tension, and to channel it, the therapist offered him an additional cushion, with the suggestion that he hold it tightly. Willy took the cushion, grabbed it with his two hands, and tightened his grip. So, he clearly understood the suggestion about the cushion, but made no further movement or communication, and no eye contact. Except for Willy's hands, his posture remained unchanged. *It felt like stalemate – frozen, tense…*
Probably because the therapist noticed this, he came to sit one or two metres closer to me. Although he was still sitting very far away, this reducing of physical distance and keeping eye contact was too much for me. I had the feeling that everything was fading into the background. I could still register what was happening but couldn't get emotionally involved. I wasn't even sure I could still physically move. Could I find the strength to do so? It seemed so incredibly exhausting even to try that I couldn't.	After a silence – and in an attempt to support Willy – the group leader asked if Willy wanted him to sit closer to him. No response. *Meanwhile Willy bent over and laid his forehead on his right forearm, which was resting on the extra cushion. He appeared to be very closed in and inaccessible.* The group leader moved his position towards the centre of the circle, placing himself a little closer to Willy. No response from Willy. *There was no feedback from Willy. He didn't respond to the changed position of the group therapist and remained in the same rigid position.*

<table>
<tr>
<td>
On the other hand, there was also something relieving in the whole situation. A bit like 'enjoying' a light dose of morphine. But anyhow, in the circumstances, I couldn't talk anymore, couldn't move, and everything began to look fuzzy because I couldn't focus my eyes. It felt like it would have taken too much effort.

I think some people said something to me, but I don't remember what exactly. I think questions were asked, and perhaps someone suggested letting me alone in my own space… but I couldn't react.
</td>
<td>
After a while, the therapist moved back to where he was previously seated in the circle.

I was present as a participant, and reluctant to interfere. On the other hand, I did have an idea of what was going on, and what might be of help to get out of this situation, or to move it forward.

I thought, 'This man is disconnected from himself, as well as from functioning in the here-and-now. Mentally, the functioning knob is turned to "zero". His body is frozen, abandoned and ungoverned.'

The tension was, in my opinion, clearly felt by Willy, the group members, myself, and the therapists. Willy was unable to look at the situation with the necessary distance to be aware of what was happening and free himself from it.

What was missing, it seemed to me, were steps (or something like the rungs of a ladder) whereby this man could return himself to the here-and-now of his physical self, connect with it again and become aware of what was emotionally happening at the moment.

I decided to do something, given the situation.

I said to the group and to the group leaders, and actually also indirectly to Willy – without assuming that he heard and understood me – that I thought this man needed something concrete to help him 'come back'.
</td>
</tr>
<tr>
<td>
Meanwhile, my head was lying on a cushion. I don't know how this happened, since moving around seemed too difficult, but it got there anyhow.

Then you [Dennis] said something to me. In a calm voice. This encouraged me to try to become more aware of myself and my surroundings.

To give an example of what I remember – you described my (body) position. You just described me in that situation.
</td>
<td>
In this way, I created some space for myself to go further, focus exclusively on Willy, and offer him pre-therapeutic reflections.

I started with the very concrete pre-therapeutic reflections to connect with him where he was and offer him the opportunity to become aware of the situation and to connect with himself and his body, and with the surrounding reality. The reflections came out smoothly. They felt very natural to me, and extremely appropriate for the situation. It was as if I was just making a concrete and accepting phenomenological description of what was going on.
</td>
</tr>
</table>

	[SR] You're sitting on the floor. **[SR] In front of you is a pillow.** ... **[SR] Your arm is on the pillow; your right forearm is on the pillow.** ... **[BR] Your head rests on your arm, on your right arm.** ... **[BR] You sit hunched over and...** **[RR] ... your head rests on the pillow.**
What then happened was that my thoughts, which were also blurred before, became a little bit clearer, and I could follow your words. I became more aware of the situation I currently was in. It was like having a small anchor.	Willy (he was still hunched over, with his head on his forearm) blinked his eyes. **[BR] You blink your eyes.** ... He looked a bit like he was waking up. He nodded in agreement, almost imperceptibly.
Then something caused me to twist the corner of my mouth. I don't know if it was something you said, or because I suddenly realised the absurdity of the situation when my attention was drawn to it... You immediately noticed that little smile and mentioned it in a calm voice. That made me smile even more. I felt amused, and almost immediately returned from the dissociative state of numbness.	I experienced this as a step out of his frozenness, a thawing as it were, the release from his cramp. I took it as positive feedback to me and decided to offer him more of the same. However I remained cautious. I didn't want to overload the contact that had emerged. I tried to stay with him, where he was now. So I didn't ask questions, give explanations, offer advice or suggestions or do anything else. I continued to reflect further – to support his step-by-step return to the here-and-now. **[BR] You are hunched over.** ... **[RR Then you nodded.** ... **[RR] You looked at me.** ... **[SR] You're looking at me...** **[FR] ... and you smile...**

I felt present and could start speaking again.	*Willy was now clearly freed from his frozen state. He sat up and straightened his back.* He sighed, as if he'd just finished a piece of really hard work. 'Cool trick', he said. I interpreted this as a reference to what just happened, of which he probably had no real awareness, but that he nevertheless experienced as helpful. He seemed to be present again. He seemed relieved, as if a weight had fallen from his shoulders.

Research: Evaluating the effect of pre-therapy on contact behaviours

Once overall contact is (re)established, people can either shift to psychotherapy or enjoy the restored contact as it is and the possibilities it brings. Evidence for this primarily comes from case studies. Prouty (personal communication), for instance, describes the case of a young woman with special needs who lived in sheltered housing. She often had unexpected outbursts of emotion, causing repeated behaviour and management problems with her fellow residents. These outbursts also meant she couldn't go home on weekend leave as her mother, who was a lone parent, couldn't handle them.

Pre-therapy treatment restored her contact functioning, her relationships with her fellow residents improved, and she was allowed to visit her mother at weekends again as she became able to contact her feelings of anger and even express them in a manageable way. It meant the caregivers and her mother, at home, could calm her down and prevent the outbursts. In the peer group she was more accepted, and the weekends at home did her good. So, there was no need for further psychotherapy as the pre-therapy treatment had resulted in a significant gain in her quality of life.

I have described (Van Werde, 2002b, 2014) a third form of outcome, besides the above-mentioned entering psychotherapy or 'just' enjoying the restoration of contact functioning. It occurs when pre-therapy techniques are used to offer contact to someone who is losing all functioning ability – that is, someone in the process of dying. The 'being with' then becomes a 'letting go'. Such a non-intrusive and existentially empathic way of offering contact slows the loss of contact and makes the process gentler and more gradual. It may stabilise the level of functioning that is still there, or even facilitate episodes of lucidity. This is clearly illustrated in the case described in my later paper (Van Werde, 2014). We see how a mother, who is dying with a brain tumour, which is interfering with her ability to think and speak intelligibly, all of a sudden and totally unexpectedly is able to articulate the first name of her son sitting at her bedside, and a few moments later repeat it and add the family name, saying 'That it is a beautiful name'.

The Pre-Therapy Rating Scale (PTRS) (Prouty, 1994) and the Evaluation Criterion for the Pre-Therapy Interview (ECPI) (Dinacci, 2000) are the most frequently used instruments for the assessment of contact behaviours. As Dekeyser (2022) points out, these observation scales measure contact functions and contact reflections. Using these scales requires a lot of work, but results in reliable measurements, and they can also be used to measure non-verbal behaviour. However, the construct validity of these scales presents a great challenge, since reality contact and affective contact are forms of awareness, and as such, not directly measurable. Every researcher is dependent on communicative contact to deduce the presence of the other forms of awareness (reality and affective contact). Dinacci (2000) limited his observations to registering only this kind of contact behaviour.

Dekeyser and colleagues (2008) estimated the efficiency of pre-therapy treatment by aggregating the data of five studies involving long-stay psychiatric hospital inpatients diagnosed with severe and chronic symptoms of schizophrenia. The studies were all very small; some were descriptive single case studies, although one was a comparative study of 14 patients. In one case study, three patients each received pre-therapy treatment for between nine months and two years, totalling 200 sessions. The researchers found a significant improvement in social communication in these patients. Improved communication was also found in another study of two patients with severe learning disabilities and mental health problems, who had been hospitalised for some 30 years, who received seven months of pre-therapy twice weekly. In a comparative study of patients who had been in psychiatric hospital for some 20 years, 14 participants were randomly assigned to receive either pre-therapy or another form of occupational therapy once a week, for one hour, for six months. The researchers reported that a higher number of patients in the pre-therapy group showed improvement on 'communication of basic reality', but the difference was not statistically significant. And another matched study of four long-term hospital inpatients with diagnoses of schizophrenia found that those receiving pre-therapy improved in verbal articulacy and communication, although again the effects observed were not statistically significant.

Based on these data from 18 patients across all three studies, overall, Dekeyser and colleagues concluded that the average effect size was large, and that, 'after six to seven months of pre-therapy treatment, the average inpatient with severe and chronic symptoms of schizophrenia can be expected to score higher on measures of contact behaviour than 74% of similar patients who did not receive this treatment'. These evaluations are promising but are based on studies with only a small number of patients involved, and the results are sometimes not statistically significant. An increase in contact behaviour, however, always coincided with increased social contact and a decrease in symptoms or problematic behaviour, as reported by patients' caregivers. Psychotherapists who report successful treatments mention the same phenomena (Traynor et al., 2011).

Recent research has explored the effects of introducing pre-therapy in dementia care and the subjective response from caregivers (Ashcroft, 2019; Courcha, 2015; Dodds, 2007, 2008a, 2008b). Caregivers welcomed the changes it made to their working practice (Pfeifer-Schaupp, 2007, 2008). Brooks and Paterson (2011), Carrick and McKenzie (2011) and Štěpánková (2015) have researched what pre-therapy has to offer to people presenting with autistic spectrum disorder. Brenner (2006) explores the use of pre-therapy with people with special needs. Traynor (2019) has researched practitioner and client perceptions of helpful and unhelpful practice and perceived client changes when using pre-therapy with people who hear voices or have unusual experiences or psychotic processes.

Conclusion

From personal and professional experiences, Garry Prouty knew that much mental suffering is avoidable. His life can be seen as a quest to bring people the care they need to live to their fullest potential. In the person-centred nation of psychotherapy, pre-therapy is a tribe on its own. In my (DVW) opinion, this has to do with the fact that, even though they have much in common with other tribes, pre-therapy and contact work are their own body of knowledge and practice. Prouty was always very committed to classical person-centred therapy as formulated by Rogers (Chapter 2, this volume), but when confronted with his patients' specific needs, he took it a step further and created pre-therapy. In doing so, he opened up new territory for the person-centred approach, by taking care of people for whom nobody believed psychotherapy was indicated or even possible.

In the title of his 1994 book, Prouty explicitly presented his work as a 'theoretical evolution in person-centred/experiential psychotherapy'. This means that his work integrates and is compatible with everything that Rogers and Gendlin (Chapter 4, this volume) stood for. So, yes, Prouty is a classical person-centred therapist, and yes, his work is experiential. Prouty saw Rogers as being concerned with the relationship between therapist and client, whereas Gendlin looks at what happens inside the client. In Prouty's opinion, these are two perspectives that can be combined perfectly, and do not need to exclude or contradict each other. However, Prouty was absolutely against reducing the client purely to their experiencing. The practitioner needs to stay empathic to the whole person, and not exclusively and only focus on their experiencing. Therapeutic change is seen as the result of therapy, not as its aim (Prouty, 1999). In that sense, Prouty's position differs from that of the process-experiential tribe. He stays very 'classical and non-directive'. Non-directivity, as described by Merry (2012; Chapter 2, this volume), is a principled and ethical stance taken towards the complex processes involved in human growth and development, most of which are poorly or incompletely understood.

Prouty can also be seen as an existentially informed therapist, as described by Vanhooren and Cooper (Chapter 8, this volume). Prouty himself wrote an essay on philosophical psychology (2002) in which his existential inspiration is very explicit. He states: 'Pre-therapy, in existential-phenomenological terms, is the movement of consciousness from existential autism to existential contact' (pp.51–53).

Prouty's view also has similarities with that of the existential psychiatrist R.D. Laing. They both – as did Rogers – tried to understand the 'mentally ill' in terms of their subjective experiences, rather than in terms of any 'objective' diagnosis or categorisation (see Cooper, 2012). Prouty very radically saw the actualising tendency as fundamentally present in psychological distress (hence the notion of 'pre-expressive functioning'), rather than it being corrupted or damaged. He saw the client as protecting themself by seeking refuge in their own inner world. Prouty's work enables us to be with the whole person, whatever symptomatology is presented, and to offer a welcoming invitation to the person to reconnect, without taking over control of their life, even if we do not fully understand the client's inner world.

In his work, Prouty struggled against all 'added' and thus unnecessary suffering caused by such phenomena as power inequalities, lack of money, unequal social class, race discrimination, failing social networks, unfair treatment, unwanted directivity, specialists' poor decisions, moral indifference, discrimination, and so on. Pre-therapy is about how to attune to the presented level of contact functioning; it is fundamentally about trusting the person's process within the limitations of the realities they currently inhabit. It makes this possible simply by reflecting the common and concrete phenomenological reality. This form of empathy enables the person to tap into their own strength, and it fosters maximum psychological freedom despite life's challenges.

Resources

Books

- Prouty, G. (1994). *Theoretical evolutions in person-centered/experiential therapy: Applications to schizophrenic and retarded psychoses*. Praeger.
  The first book written on pre-therapy, not only presenting pre-therapy but also Prouty's revolutionary thinking about hallucinatory process. This book has been translated into Portuguese and Japanese.
- Prouty, G. (Ed.) (2008). *Emerging developments in pre-therapy: A pre-therapy reader*. PCCS Books.
  A book bringing together some previous articles of Prouty that are hard to find, combined with other contributions presenting independent approaches to divergent issues and problems, all rooted in pre-therapy.
- Prouty, G., Van Werde, D. & Pörtner, M. (2002). *Pre-therapy: Reaching contact-impaired clients*. PCCS Books.
  This is Prouty's 1994 book expanded with an extensive contribution on the translation of pre-therapy to a ward milieu approach, and with an overview of different European projects, all inspired by pre-therapy. The most complete and best introductory book on pre-therapy so far. It is also published in translation in German, Dutch, Czech and French.
- Sanders, P. (ed.) (2007). *The contact work primer: A concise, accessible and comprehensive introduction to pre-therapy and the work of Garry Prouty*. PCCS Books.
  A succinct guide to pre-therapy, contact work and the work of Garry Prouty for everyone wanting an authoritative synopsis.

Web resources

Pre-Therapy International Network – www.pre-therapy.com
The network was founded in 1985 by Jill and Garry Prouty and coordinated since by Dion Van Werde. It brings together trainers, core international members and interested others, and features an updated list of references and a discussion list, open to everybody, to take part in the sharing, study, practise and dissemination of pre-therapy.

References

Ashcroft, K. (2019). *Person-centred therapeutic practitioner perspectives on using pre-therapy.* MA thesis. University of Cumbria. https://www.pre-therapy.com/news/person-centredtherapeuticpractitionerperspectivesonusingpre-therapy

Brenner, N. (2006). *Auf der Suche nach Kontakt. Analyse der Prä-Therapie nach Garry F. Prouty bei Menschen mit einer geistigen Behinderung und Kontaktstörungen.* Unpublished doctoral dissertation. Universität Koblenz-Landau.

Brooks, S. & Paterson, G. (2011). Using contact work in interactions with adults with learning disabilities and autistic spectrum disorders. *British Journal of Learning Disabilities, 39*(1), 161–166.

Carrick, L. & McKenzie, S. (2011). A heuristic examination of the application of pre-therapy skills and the person-centred approach in the field of autism. *Person-Centered & Experiential Psychotherapies, 10*, 73–88.

Cooper, M. (2012). Existentially informed person-centred therapy. In: P. Sanders (Ed.), *The tribes of the person-centred nation* (2nd ed.) (pp.131–159). PCCS Books.

Courcha, P. (2015). 'She's talking to me!' Training home carers to use pre-therapy contact reflections: An action research study. *Person-Centered & Experiential Psychotherapies, 14*, 285–299.

Dekeyser, M. (2022). Pre-therapie met psychosegevoelige mensen. Lessen uit proces- en uitkomstenonderzoek. *Tijdschrift Persoonsgerichte experiëntiële Psychotherapie, 60*(2), 127–131.

Dekeyser, M., Prouty, G. & Elliott, R. (2008). Pre-therapy process and outcome: A review of research instruments and findings. *Person-Centered & Experiential Psychotherapies, 7*, 37–55.

Dinacci, A. (2000). E.C.P.I. – objective evaluation criteria for the pre-therapy interview. *Pre-Therapy International Review, 1*, 31–42.

Dodds, P. (2007). Pre-therapy, contact work and dementia care. In P. Sanders (Ed.), *The contact work primer* (pp.49–73). PCCS Books.

Dodds, P. (2008a). *Pre-therapy and dementia: An action research project.* Unpublished PhD thesis. University of Brighton.

Dodds, P. (2008b). Pre-Therapy and dementia care. In G. Prouty (Ed.), *Emerging developments in pre-therapy: a pre-therapy reader* (pp.15–21). PCCS-books.

Dodds, P., Morton, I. & Prouty, G. (2004). Using pre-therapy techniques in dementia care. *Journal of Dementia Care, 12*(2), 25–28.

Gendlin, E.T. (1968). The experiential response. In A. Hammer (Ed.), *Use of interpretation in treatment* (pp.208–228). Grune & Stratton.

Laing, R.D. (1969). *The divided self.* Penguin.

Langner, L. (2017). *Personzentrierte Psychotherapie bei eingeschränkten Kontaktfunktionen. Momente der Begegnung durch Prä-Therapie und Klang.* AV-Akademikerverlag.

Mead, G.H. (1934/1967). *Mind, self, and society: From the standpoint of a social behaviorist* (C.W. Morris, ed.). University of Chicago Press.

Merry, T. (2012). Classical client-centred therapy. In: G. Wyatt & P. Sanders (Eds.), *Rogers' therapeutic conditions: Evolution, theory and practice. Vol. 4: Contact and perception* (pp.21–45). PCCS Books.

Peters, H. (2014). The relation between intersubjectivity, imitation, mirror neurons, empathy and pre-therapy. In P. Pearce, L. Sommerbeck (Eds.), *Person-centered practice at the difficult edge* (pp.138–158). PCCS Books.

Pfeifer-Schaupp, U. (2007). Prä-Therapie in der Altenpflege. *Dr. med. Mabuse, 170*, 50–52.

Pfeifer-Schaupp, U. (2008). Prä-Therapie in der Altenpflege. Neue Zugänge zu Menschen mit schwerer Demenz. *Zeitschrift für Gerontologie und Geriatrie, 41*(5), 1–7.

Pörtner, M. (2002). Psychotherapy for people with special needs: A challenge for client-centered psychotherapists. In: J.C. Watson, R.N. Goldman & M.S. Warner (Eds.), *Client-centered and experiential psychotherapy in the 21st Century: Advances in theory, research and practice* (pp.380–386). PCCS Books.

Pörtner, M. (2007). *Trust and understanding: The person-centred approach to everyday care for people with special needs*. PCCS Books.

Prouty, G. (1994). *Theoretical evolutions in person-centered/experiential therapy: Applications to schizophrenic and retarded psychoses*. Praeger.

Prouty, G. (1998). Pre-therapy and the pre-expressive self. *Person-Centred Practice, 6*(2), 80–88.

Prouty, G. (1999). Carl Rogers and experiential therapies: A dissonance? *Person-Centered Practice, 6*(2), 1–8.

Prouty, G. (2002). Pre-therapy: An essay in philosophical psychology. In: G. Wyatt & P. Sanders (Eds.), *Rogers' therapeutic conditions: Evolution, theory and practice. Vol. 4: Contact and perception* (pp.51–53). PCCS Books.

Prouty, G. (Ed.) (2008). *Emerging developments in pre-therapy: A pre-therapy reader*. PCCS Books.

Prouty, G., Van Werde, D. & Portner, M. (2002). *Pre-therapy: Reaching contact impaired clients*. PCCS Books.

Rogers, C. (1957). The necessary and sufficient conditions of therapeutic personality change. *Journal of Consulting Psychology, 21*(2), 95–102.

Sanders, P. (ed.) (2007). *The contact work primer: A concise, accessible and comprehensive introduction to pre-therapy and the work of Garry Prouty*. PCCS Books.

Sanders, P. (Ed.) (2012). New developments: Pre-therapy and contact work. In P. Sanders (Ed.), *The tribes of the person-centred nation* (2nd ed.) (pp.201–210). PCCS Books.

Sanders, P. & Wyatt, G. (2002). The history of conditions one and six. In G. Wyatt & P. Sanders (Eds.), *Rogers' therapeutic conditions, evolutions and practice. Vol 4. Contact and Perception* (pp.1–24). PCCS Books.

Shlien, J.M. (1961). A client-centered approach to schizophrenia: First approximation. In A. Burton (Ed.), *Psychotherapy of the psychoses* (pp.285–317). New York: Basic Books. Reproduced in Shlien, J.M. (2003). *To live an honorable life: Invitations to think about client-centered therapy and the person-centered approach* (pp.30–59). PCCS Books.

Štěpánková, R. (2015). The experience with a person with autism. Phenomenological study of the experience with contact and contact reflections. *Person-Centered & Experiential Psychotherapies, 14*, 310–327.

Traynor, W. (2019). *Person-centred therapy and pre-therapy for people who hear voices, have unusual experiences or psychotic processes: Practitioner and client perceptions of helpful and unhelpful practice and perceived client changes.* Unpublished doctoral dissertation. University of Strathclyde. https://stax.strath.ac.uk/concern/theses/pg15bd892

Traynor, W., Elliot, R. & Cooper, M. (2011). Helpful factors and outcomes in person-centered therapy with clients who experience psychotic processes: Therapists' perspectives. *Person-Centered & Experiential Psychotherapies, 10*, 89–104.

Van Werde, D. (2002a). Pre-therapy applied on a psychiatric ward. In: G. Prouty, D. Van Werde & M. Pörtner (Eds.), *Pre-therapy: Reaching contact-impaired clients* (pp.61–120). PCCS Books.

Van Werde, D. (2002b). Prouty's pre-therapy and contact-work with a broad range of persons' pre-expressive functioning. In: G. Wyatt & P. Sanders (Eds.), *Rogers' therapeutic conditions: Evolution, theory and practice. Vol. 4: Contact and perception* (pp. 168–181). PCCS Books.

Van Werde, D. (2007). Contact work in a residential psychiatric setting: Bridging person, team and context. In P. Sanders (Ed.), *The contact work primer: A concise, accessible and comprehensive introduction to pre-therapy and the work of Garry Prouty.* (pp. 60–71). PCCS Books.

Van Werde, D. (2014). Pre-Therapy at its edges: From palliative care to exercising newly recovered contact functioning. In P. Pearce & L. Sommerbeck (Eds.), *Person-centred practice at the difficult edge* (pp.54–66). PCCS Books.

Van Werde, D. (2021). Prä-Therapie: Halt anbieten bei Kontaktverlust. *GWG-Zeitschrift, 3*, 11–17.

Van Werde, D. & Prouty, G. (2024, in press). Clients with contact-impaired functioning: Pre-therapy. In M. Cooper, M. O'Hara, S. Stephen, Y. Gololob & G. Di Malta (Eds.), *The handbook of person-centred psychotherapy and counselling* (3rd ed.). Palgrave.

12. Child-centred play therapy

Dee C. Ray

When asked by Mick Cooper to contribute to this edition of the *Tribes* book, I was delighted at the prospect of child-centred play therapy (CCPT) being invited to move to the person-centred adult table, so to speak. Since CCPT's structured formation in the 1940s (Axline, 1947a), the approach has rarely been a subject of discussion among person-centred theorists, due to a primary focus on adult psychology. However more than 26% of the world population is aged 14 years and younger,[1] so children make up a large number of people who may benefit from the application of person-centred principles. CCPT is grounded in classical person-centred therapy and, most essentially, follows a traditional person-centred therapy approach (see Chapter 2, this volume). Yet, the developmental needs of young children require person-centred therapists to adapt person-centred therapy to work within their phenomenological worlds. CCPT, first and foremost, honours the person of the child by recognising the maturation of the organismic actualising tendency within the context of the developmental journey that takes place throughout childhood.

Carl Rogers is recognised for his many contributions to psychology and therapy, and he is certainly noted for the theory of personality that he presented through his 19 propositions (Rogers, 1951; see Chapter 2, this volume). Perhaps what may be less widely celebrated is the contribution that the 19 propositions made to a greater understanding of child development. Rogers described how infants enter the world with a self-actualising propensity towards maturity, freedom and relationship. As children develop and interact with others, they gradually gather a concept of the self, made up of perceptions from relational exchanges with others and their environments. Interactions that may not be congruent with the child's self and others' values are likely to be experienced as introjections,

1. www.theglobaleconomy.com/rankings/percent_children

possibly internalised as conditions of worth. Such experiences of incongruence are likely to lead to emotions and behaviour that are developmentally beyond the ability of the child to understand or express in words (Ray et al., 2022). Just as incongruence is initiated in conditional relational interactions, congruence is facilitated through genuine relationships characterised by unconditional acceptance and empathic understanding. The 19 propositions illuminate the significance of a child's interactions with caregivers and how children are vulnerable to experiences of evaluation that can influence the formation of the self-concept. Rogers' developmental theory has been described as 'elegant' (Wilkins, 2015, p.33), and offers the CCPT therapist a deeper understanding of how children are experiencing their worlds in the moment and the potentially life-long impacts of that experiencing.

A child can be trusted to move holistically toward behaviours, thoughts and emotions that enhance the person of the child and the child's relationships. Seeking to understand the typical development markers of childhood recognises the ever-changing world of the child and deepens empathic understanding of each child as unique within the context of observed common patterns across all children. CCPT therapists consider human development as an intersectionality of human potential and environmental tasks or challenges. Holistic development involves a child's mastery of cognitive processes, motor skills, concept identity and social interactions. A child is consistently moving forward when the actualising tendency is nurtured by primary caretakers and the systemic environment. However, when external tasks overwhelm internal resources, children encounter an incongruence in their experiences, leading to the formation of a self-construct that may distort or deny incoming experiences.

Developmental knowledge is the foundation of the classical person-centred therapist's adaptation of counselling to children. Because children lack physical and systemic power, they are vulnerable to the wellness of the adults and systems in their lives. As children face continued developmental tasks, they are balancing their internal resources (e.g. organismic valuing process, self-concept, physical and cognitive abilities) with their external resources (e.g. parental nurturance, systemic support, provision of basic necessities). Vygotsky (1966) noted that the first movement toward symbolic play is inspired by a young child's inability to make the environment fit with their desires or tendencies. Children engage in the world of play to nurture their own self-actualising tendency in the context of limited verbal abilities and resources to meet their needs. A CCPT therapist is familiar with developmental tasks, stages and phases across ages in order to facilitate an environment that is empathic to each child's phenomenological experience within those markers (Ray, 2016).

CCPT is a discrete practice described in several volumes (Axline, 1947a; Cochran et al., 2022; Landreth, 2023) and specified in a recognised protocols (Ray, 2011). In CCPT, the child leads play and verbal content, just as the adult client in classical person-centred therapy leads the content of the session. Although person-centred therapists provide therapy for children, often with play as a component, variations to therapy may diverge from the CCPT approach (Behr, 2003; Behr & Cornelius-White, 2008). The British Association for Counselling and Psychotherapy (BACP) (2022) has published competences for humanistic counselling with children and young people that define the counsellor role as:

> one of helping children and young people to extend their awareness of their subjective world and supporting their natural striving toward self-awareness, self-acceptance and personally determined solutions. (p.15)

The definition of 'helping' in this sentence is often what distinguishes person-centered tribes. In CCPT, helping consists of facilitating the child's development through identified categories of verbal and non-verbal responses, a therapist's non-directive yet authentic way of being and primacy of the therapeutic relationship. Although therapist non-directivity is a hallmark of CCPT practice, structure is essential for non-directivity to thrive within the healing relationship. Hence, CCPT requires specific education and supervised practice to fully implement an effective realisation of the approach.

Play and relationship

Valuing the child's developmental journey means valuing the role of play in children's lives. Play is important throughout childhood, serving various purposes at different ages. Infants play to explore their worlds; toddlers play to build relationships and mastery and to understand adult roles; young children use symbolic play to make meaning of their worlds; older children use play to develop mastery, social skills and self-concept. At each age, play builds on earlier experiences, with the persistent themes of its use to help children understand their worlds, build relationships, construct the self and express their perceptions. Russ and colleagues (2011) found that play facilitates problem-solving, flexibility, divergent thinking, alternative coping skills, positive emotion, ability to think about themes, ability to take the perspective of another and general adjustment. In essence, play is the precursor to, instigator for and indicator of growth and development in childhood (Ray, 2023). Definitions of play abound but certain characteristics are agreed upon, including:

1. activities are free from adult direction
2. the child is actively involved
3. the child experiences a flow, with little self-consciousness
4. the child is released from literal grounding to reality (Ray, 2011).

These characteristics are particularly aligned with CCPT in that children are offered an environment in which play is considered an intrinsically motivated experience, free from adult direction yet fostered by adult relationship.

CCPT is a developmentally sensitive mental health intervention for children aged three to 10 years old who have experienced relational disruptions, emotional distress or behavioural struggles. Through engaging in the child's natural language of play, the play therapist offers a consistent and safe relationship in which the child can communicate their inner world and real-life experiences. Children intuitively use play symbols (i.e. toys) and scenes to express their thoughts and feelings in order to work through issues of concern (Ray, 2023). As children are provided a therapeutic relationship characterised by safety and acceptance, Landreth (2023) proposed that children in CCPT feel free to explore their inner experiences and engage in play to meet the objectives of building self-concept, personal responsibility, self-direction, self-acceptance, decision-making skills, sense of control, self-reliance, coping awareness and skills, internal source of evaluation and trust in self and others.

Based on classical person-centred therapy, CCPT places a high value on permissiveness within the play therapy room and relationship in order to nurture the actualising tendency of the child. The child directs the content and process of their play within the structural limits of therapy. The value for play in the CCPT relationship communicates that the therapist seeks to empathically enter the child's world, rather than expecting the child to enter the adult world of verbalisation. The therapist's trust in the child's self-direction communicates unconditional positive regard (UPR) for the child as a person and the child's abilities, thereby unleashing the child's potentialities. In addition to the theoretical relational value of play, research has shown that play in positive relationships triggers safety through neuroception, the brain's unconscious perception of safety versus threat initiated by the environment (Porges, 2021). Play with a supportive adult also supports the release of the endogenous opioids oxytocin and dopamine, which saturate the system with positive emotions and support relational connection (Badenoch, 2008, 2018).

Through this, the child–therapist relationship within CCPT serves as the therapeutic agent of change. The therapist offers the empathic attitude of vulnerably entering the child's world through play and offering an environment of UPR for the person of the child. As discussed, play in and of itself has educational and emotional healing properties, yet CCPT considers play to be the path by which the therapist may enter the child's world, not as the primary agent of change, unlike some other play therapy approaches. CCPT is aligned with the necessary and sufficient conditions noted by Rogers (1957):

1. the child and therapist are in psychological contact
2. the child is in a state of vulnerability
3. the therapist is congruent
4. therapist experiences unconditional positive regard for the child
5. the therapist experiences and communicates empathic understanding to the child
6. the child perceives some level of UPR and empathic understanding.

The therapist's attitudinal conditions (i.e. genuineness, UPR and empathic understanding (Bozarth, 1998)) are especially salient in CCPT, as they are continually working towards authenticity and genuineness in the relationship, unconditional acceptance of and belief in the child, and greater empathic understanding of the child's world, with greater ability to communicate that understanding.

History of child-centred play therapy

As with most psychological interventions, play therapy developed from within the emergence of psychoanalysis. Sigmund Freud (1909/1955) introduced the first account of therapeutic play in his report of Little Hans, a six-year-old boy who struggled with a phobia. Hans' father, a wealthy psychoanalyst, reached out to Freud for guidance. Sigmund Freud advised Hans' father to conduct play observations and the two proceeded to psychoanalyse the child through written correspondence. As would be expected, Sigmund Freud contextualised Hans' presenting phobia and play behaviours from a disturbance framework that called for interpretation. Yet, the Little Hans case also premiered the idea that children's play might be a road into understanding children's internal worlds and behaviours. Thus, Sigmund Freud is credited for ushering in the importance of play as a therapeutic tool in working with children.

The use of play in therapy continued to rise across Europe (specifically the UK) and the US through the efforts of Melanie Klein (1932/1975) and Anna Freud (1946). Klein remained consistent with a non-directive stance of using play for interpretation, while Anna Freud integrated an emphasis on the therapist–child relationship to enable more accuracy for play interpretation. Both Klein and Anna Freud solidified play therapy as a psychoanalytic therapeutic intervention characterised by recognition of children's communication as uniquely different from adults' reliance on verbalisation, and the importance of non-directed play observation in understanding children's neuroses.

In the early 1930s, play therapy, conducted mostly from a psychoanalytic stance, grew as a widely used intervention for children with problem behaviours. In the US, Anna Freud's influential stance on the therapeutic relationship as key to play interpretation was embraced above the more traditional psychoanalytic, detached-therapist approach. In their efforts to serve children who presented with very disturbing behaviours, early child guidance clinics experimented with various forms of education and therapy in their desperate search for helpful interventions. Experimentation led to the practical acknowledgement that the child's relationship with the therapist within a play context and respect for the child's autonomy appeared to be required for change to occur. Fredrick Allen, an early noted play therapist working within the child guidance movement, stated (1942/2011):

> Effective therapy with a child depends upon the changes a child can make in himself through the medium of a therapeutic relationship. The therapist has no power to do that changing. If his point of view stems from a belief that he can change a child, irrespective of the participation of the child, he will introduce a real barrier to therapy. (p.244)

Allen's writings and presentations contributed to the recognition of humanistic ideals as essential to the play therapy process. Allen concentrated on the importance of providing a child with a therapeutic intervention in which the child and therapist co-construct a world that allows the child to be fully authentic.

This is the point at which Carl Rogers arrived on the scene in the world of child therapy. In fact, Rogers' first published book focused on child therapy, *The Clinical Treatment of the Problem Child* (Rogers, 1939). The title alone implies a philosophy that belies Rogers' later approach in that the reference to a person as a 'problem child' seems problematic. For anyone who has read Rogers' subsequent works, this first book may be unrecognisable in its philosophy. It concentrates on diagnosis and treatment protocols for children. However, there are inklings of his growing but nascent belief system when he addresses his work with parents as requiring a therapeutic, warm relationship. In comparing Rogers' later publications with this initial offering, it appears that Rogers may have been unfamiliar with how to apply his approach to the developmental level of children.

As Rogers (1942) clarified and strengthened his person-centred therapeutic principles, the classical approach thrived as a humanistic intervention that recognised the actualising process of the person, the need for an empathic therapist stance, and the potential for growth and change within the therapeutic relationship. Yet, there appeared to be a struggle in how to apply these principles for children. When Rogers was teaching at Ohio State University, he met Virginia Axline (1947a) who began as his student and later became his colleague at the University of Chicago. Axline had been a successful teacher of young children and was drawn to Rogers' philosophy and work. She quickly drew connections between her knowledge of children and how Rogers' philosophy could be enacted in a developmentally meaningful way. Axline was the first person to structure play therapy based on the person-centered approach by developing methods in which children were provided with an opportunity to autonomously use play as their language while remaining grounded within the primacy of the child-therapist relationship.

Axline referred to her approach as *non-directive play therapy*, yet she is widely known as the originator of CCPT. Just as Rogers exemplified his work through research and case studies, Axline provided the same methods to explore therapeutic effectiveness through research, and also presented detailed case examples of play therapy. Her most famous work is the case study of *Dibs: In search of self* (Axline, 1964), in which she gives a moving account of a relationship in play therapy with a child who suffers from intense loneliness and isolation.

Through Axline's efforts, non-directive play therapy grew in popularity and she became a key figure in teaching others this new, and now empirically-supported, form of play therapy. Clark Moustakas (1959) studied under Axline specifically to learn the non-directive play therapy approach with children. Although Moustakas may currently be more broadly known as a fundamental contributor to phenomenological qualitative research approaches, he was a primary figure in play therapy. Moustakas embraced the essential elements of the child-centred approach for play therapy, yet his existential leanings led him to conclude that Axline's structure to play therapy limited the therapist's experience and presentation of authenticity, which in turn resulted in a limited therapeutic relationship. Moustakas furthered the child-centred approach to child therapy in his thick description, research and case excerpts that demonstrated the effect of play therapy when the therapist's use of self is blended with principles of non-directivity, such as respect for the uniqueness of the child, focus on the present living experience, empathy for and unqualified acceptance of the child, and freedom of expression for the child (Ray, 2019). Moustakas originally referred to his modifications of Axline's non-directive play therapy as 'existential child therapy'. In his later years, he referred to his approach as 'relationship play therapy' (Moustakas, 1997). His contribution to current practices of CCPT include the therapist's use of self, the relational nature of limit-setting with children, and the level at which a play therapist presents authentically to child.

Haim Ginott (1959) was a teacher who immigrated to the US from Israel and studied under Axline at Columbia University. As a child psychologist, Ginott was drawn to the humanistic perspective of the power of relationships proposed in non-directive play therapy. Ginott became a popular media figure in the US in the 1960s and extended the principles of CCPT to providing parenting and teaching advice. Ginott was the first person to coin the term *child-centered play therapy*, marking a change in the nomenclature towards more outwardly aligning with Rogers' person-centred approach. Although Ginott maintained roots in psychoanalytic conceptualisations of children's problems, he contributed to the development of CCPT through his concentration on building the autonomy of the child, the importance of the child–therapist relationship, and best practices in working with parents and teachers.

CCPT, more commonly known as non-directive play therapy at the time, grew in its development and acceptance in the 1960s but quickly lost favour against the prevalence of behaviourism in schools and increasing dominance of cognitive-behavioural therapy in mental health settings. Throughout the 1970s and 1980s, play therapists continued to dedicate efforts to the expansion and examination of CCPT, with little recognition from the mental health community. Bernard and Louise Guerney (2001) created *filial therapy*, a play therapy intervention that used CCPT methods adapted for parents and teachers. The Guerneys also conducted research on the effectiveness and use of CCPT in the 1970s. Garry Landreth (2023) founded the Center for Play Therapy and produced a prolific number of process and outcome studies on CCPT throughout the 1990s and early 2000s. Landreth is credited with refining the practice of play therapy through defining the verbal and non-verbal roles of the therapist that lead to deeper relationships with children. He also organised the training of therapists in the practice of CCPT, nationally and internationally, resulting in the expansion of CCPT across communities and cultures. Landreth's (2023) seminal text, *Play Therapy: The art of the relationship*, is in its fourth edition and has been translated into numerous languages across the world.

Multiple texts define the philosophy and practice of CCPT (Cochran et al., 2022; Landreth, 2023; Ray, 2011; West, 1996; Wilson & Ryan, 2006), which is still more widely known as non-directive play therapy in Europe. Due to the evidence-based mental health movement in the US and lack of quantitative research support for CCPT, the new millennium brought increased threat to the practice of CCPT in governmental and community settings. In order to respond to evidence-based standards, I (Ray, 2011) introduced the CCPT protocol manual for use in training and research, as well as intervention fidelity methods (Ray et al., 2017). In the past two decades, play therapy researchers have increased the number of quantitative intervention effectiveness studies, improving both methodological rigour and analyses, resulting in the recognition of CCPT as an evidence-based practice among several major governmental agencies in the US.

As in the rest of Europe, in the UK, the preferred term for CCPT is 'non-directive play therapy'. However, this unspecified term leads to some confusion about the specific approach enacted in play therapy. 'Non-directive' is also used as an umbrella term for a psychoanalytic-leaning therapy, using play therapy as a means for interpretation, or sometimes a general term for play therapy in which content and process is actually decided by the therapist, undermining the principles of a classical person-centred approach. However, Wilson and Ryan (2006), play therapists based in the UK, argue that they prefer the use of the 'non-directive play therapy' term as it distinguishes the approach from other play therapy approaches in the UK that use the term 'child-centred' but are not in fact grounded in person-centred principles.

Elements and applications of child-centred play therapy

CCPT's philosophy is most closely aligned with classical person-centred therapy in its belief in the self-actualising tendency, the necessity and sufficiency of the therapeutic conditions, and the primacy of the therapist's non-directive role (see Sanders, 2012). Remaining aligned with Rogers' person-centred theory, Axline (1947a) emphasised permissiveness in play therapy, by which a child is trusted to decide the content and process of their play. The level of permissiveness in CCPT allows the therapist to provide the UPR necessary to unleash the child's potential. Axline provided few restrictions in the way of structure, yet she conceptualised CCPT in a way that provides direction for what occurs during sessions. Although Axline's (1947a) original work on play therapy is more than 80 years old, her eight principles of therapy are still currently used as the foundation for CCPT. These are:

1. The therapist develops a warm, friendly relationship with the child as soon as possible.
2. The therapist accepts the child exactly as they are, not wishing the child were different in some way.
3. The therapist establishes a feeling of permissiveness in the relationship so that the child can fully express their thoughts and feelings.
4. The therapist is attuned to the child's feelings and reflects those back to the child to help gain insight into their behaviour.
5. The therapist respects the child's ability to solve problems, leaving the responsibility to make choices to the child.
6. The therapist does not direct the child's behaviour or conversation. The therapist follows the child.
7. The therapist does not attempt to rush therapy, recognising the gradual nature of the therapeutic process.
8. The therapist sets only those limits that anchor the child to reality or make the child aware of responsibilities in the relationship. (1947a, pp.73–74)

Although all principles are essential to the application of CCPT, Axline prioritised the order by placing the building of a warm relationship as the first principle, while the eighth principle is the setting of limits. Axline emphasised the primacy of the therapeutic relationship, unconditional positive regard for the child, and empathic understanding and communication to the child. In addressing limits, Axline remarked that limits are set as part of relationship responsibilities, demonstrating that limits are seen as contributing to the relationship, not as tools for compliance.

The play therapy room and materials

Because toys serve as children's words and play as their language, the structure of the play therapy room itself serves as an environment for sending messages of unconditional positive regard and empathic understanding. The play therapy room is designed to immediately convey to the child that they belong and that their world is the most important world in this room. The recommended room size is 12 x 15 feet (3.7 x 4.6m) (Landreth, 2023), yet play therapy spaces vary in size. Some therapists conduct play therapy in small spaces within larger rooms; other therapists offer mobile play therapy and transition the spaces from session to session. As is true for any therapy, play therapy rooms/spaces require attention to confidentiality. Even when conducting play therapy in larger spaces or settings such as schools, the CCPT therapist ensures confidentiality. Play therapy room spaces typically have shelves to display the toys and materials, as well as open space for movement. Figure 12.1 shows an example of a typical play therapy room.

Toys and materials in the play therapy room are carefully selected for inclusion. Aligned with the philosophy of CCPT and person-centred theory, the materials in the play therapy room are chosen to encourage the child to explore and express themself, as well as to build

Figure 12.1: A typical play therapy room

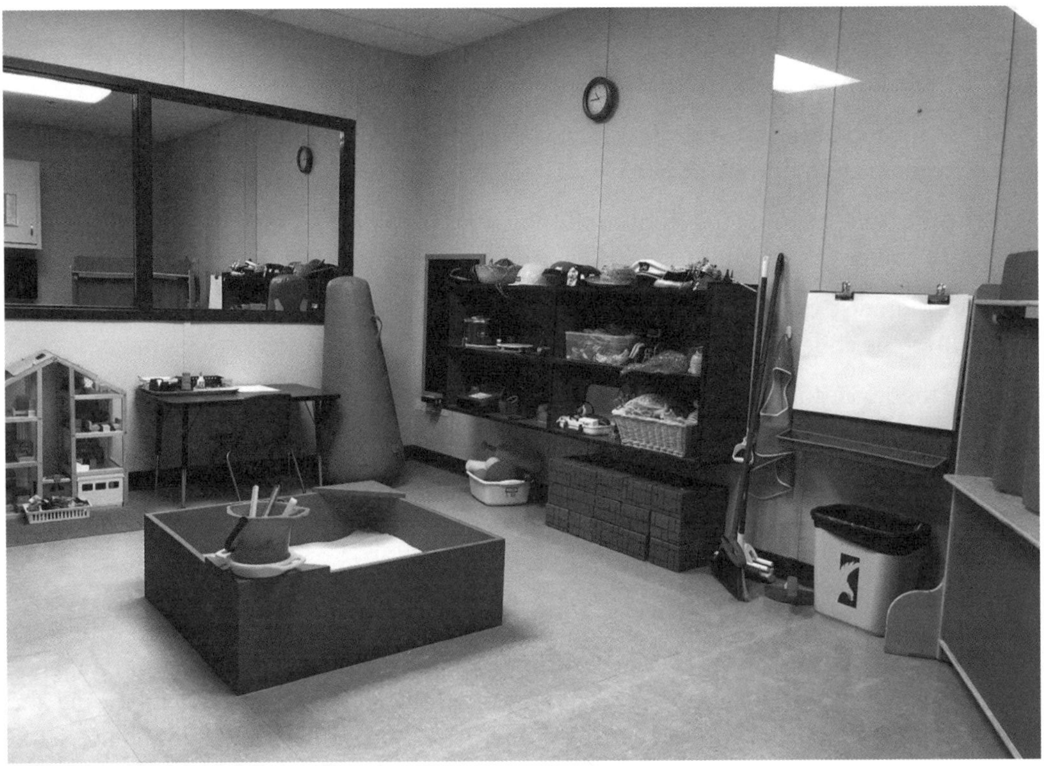

a relationship with the therapist. Hence, certain materials are deemed inappropriate for the CCPT play therapy room. Toys such as board games, technology-based materials and traditional teaching materials (i.e. books) are not used in CCPT, due to their potential to restrict relationship-building and expression. Board games and books are often used for instructional purposes, and seen by children to be used in strictly delineated ways (e.g. board games have rules, books are to be read). Technology-based materials, such as electronics and video games, although popular among children, offer limited opportunities for meaningful interaction or child expression.

Toys and materials included in the play therapy room are presented in a consistent order, in the same place each time the child enters the room. Consistency of the room structure allows the child to build a sense of safety there and with the therapist – a fundamental need for children and acknowledgement of the therapist's empathic understanding of the child's world. Although CCPT therapists vary in the specific toys they offer, most therapists adhere to including and arranging the toys according to categories. Landreth (2023) suggests three categories of toys and materials: real-life toys; acting-out aggressive-release toys, and toys for creative expression and emotional release. Real-life toys, such as dolls, puppets, cash registers and so forth, allow children to play out events in their lives. Acting-out aggressive-release toys, such as inflatable punch-bags, toy soldiers and aggressive animal figures, allow children to express feelings of anger, hostility or power. Creative expression and emotional release toys are unstructured media, such as water, sand and paints, that allow for unlimited expression.

In order to send messages of empathic understanding, CCPT therapists are deeply concerned to demonstrate cultural inclusion in the materials they offer in the play therapy room. In a recent study on expanding the CCPT play therapy room to be more culturally inclusive, our team noted that play therapists recommended the selection of materials that are (Ray et al., 2022):

> accessible, diverse, and representative of many cultures, including but not limited to materials for categories of household, kitchen, food, dolls and figures, expressive materials, costumes, and transportation, with particular attention to forms, textures and colors that are diverse and representative of many cultures. (p.290)

CCPT therapists enact the practice of empathic understanding and UPR through the provision of materials that help children feel a sense of belonging and acceptance of their whole selves, including their intersectional cultural identities. Culturally inclusive materials also allow children to explore and express their identities in a rapidly diversifying world.

In an attempt to be less prescriptive about the selection of play therapy materials and possibly more aligned with the permissive nature of person-centred therapy, I originally proposed three questions to aid therapists in intentional decision-making, and our multicultural research team has recently updated them to four (Ray, 2011; Ray et al., 2022). These questions are:

1. What therapeutic purpose will this toy/material serve for children who use this room?
2. How will this toy/material help children express themselves?
3. How will this toy/material help me build a relationship with children?
4. How does this toy/material help children feel a sense of belonging and explore their cultural identity?

If a play therapist can answer these questions with meaningful affirmative responses, the toy or material is likely to be appropriate and helpful in the play therapy room.

Therapist attitudes

Much has been said about the therapist attitudes necessary for person-centred therapy. Volumes have been dedicated to the importance and essential nature of the therapist's genuineness, UPR and empathic understanding toward the client that leads to substantive change. I hesitate to be repetitive in a book dedicated to the tribes of person-centred theory. However, the experience of these attitudes towards and with children can sometimes manifest differently and, in my estimation, they deserve attention apart from their general descriptions. I will attempt to limit my discussion to the therapist attitudinal conditions in the context of play therapy.

Genuineness and authenticity

Traditional CCPT, as explained by Axline (1947a), Landreth (2023), and others, is periodically critiqued for a lack of genuineness on the part of the therapist. Although historically CCPT promotes the importance of therapist genuineness in how the therapist presents, the therapist is typically trained to direct all their energy into non-direction of the child. This might involve not answering children's questions, lest the child becomes reliant on the therapist for direction, or not expressing the therapist's thoughts or feelings, lest the child then becomes focused on the therapist rather than themself. This approach to genuineness often leads the therapist not only to limited expression of genuineness but, more disturbingly, to limited experience of genuineness in relationship to the child.

For example, a child may direct frequent negative statements toward the therapist, such as: 'You're the stupidest person ever, I hate you;' 'You can't do anything right;' 'You'll always be stupid.' Objectively, the therapist realises that the child is sharing their world with them – the way they feel about themselves, or what they have been told by others. However, in the moment, the therapist may feel hurt, denigrated, annoyed or angry. Because adults in the wider world are taught to dismiss children's statements and therapists are taught to intellectually observe the client, play therapists may deny their genuine experiences in response to the child. Hurt feelings are suppressed under subsequent cognitions such as 'She's only six years old, she shouldn't be able to hurt my feelings;' 'I love all children so I can't be angry at this child,' or 'I'm not letting this child hurt me, they won't win this one.' These distortions of experience may suppress the therapist's awareness of congruence and subsequently lead to inauthentic interactions with the child.

When I allow therapeutic interactions into my full awareness, with attention to my self-structure and possible threats to that structure, I am freed to make intentional decisions about transparency with the client, leading to greater authenticity in the relationship. For instance, supposing in the example above I, as the therapist, have given an inaccurate reflection to the child before they call me 'stupid'. When the child says I'm stupid, I begin to question my competency. But, rather than ignore this internal process, I acknowledge that the child has just touched on something real within me, my ongoing self-doubt. In my split second of acknowledgement, I make the decision to deal with my insecurities after the session, and this decision releases me to be fully present with the child. I might respond, 'You're thinking of things to say to hurt my feelings.' If I go in the other direction and do not allow the experience into my awareness, I might move into a defensive mode: 'I'm not for calling names.' This type of response is not a damaging response to the child, but it does not derive from an authentic place based on self-awareness, and hence places limitations on the genuineness in the relationship.

Because children operate in a non-verbal world, they are especially attuned to the non-verbals of others. Any message of inauthenticity sent by the therapist, such as facial expression, eye movement or body tension, is a felt interaction to the child. A child is likely to interpret the therapist as untrustworthy or experience themselves as unacceptable, which interferes with the messages of empathic understanding and unconditional positive regard.

Unconditional positive regard

As emphasised in classical person-centred theory, CCPT is predicated on the essential nature of UPR as a condition for change. In the wider culture, UPR is rarely valued by adults in their relationships with children. In CCPT, UPR is characterised by three attitudes, including acceptance, belief in the child and prizing of the child. In her eight principles, Axline (1947a) clarified acceptance as not wishing the child were different in some way. Because adults typically refer children to therapy for the very purpose of changing something about them, CCPT therapists are pressured from intake to 'change' the child. Embracing the concept that the child does not need to be changed requires resolve on the part of the therapist to combat the greater adult culture.

Another cultural mismatch between CCPT and adult norms is the therapist's belief in a child's capability to solve their own problems and to know what they need to do in therapy. The adult world sends strong cultural messages that children are incapable and must be guided to know how to think and act. The therapist's belief in the child's activated actualising tendency is one of the most powerful messages sent to the child because it is so rarely experienced by children in the presence of adults. Finally, the therapist's feeling of prizing their time with children is especially salient for children who have experienced themselves as being unworthy or unlovable. Through UPR, the therapist sends the message to the child that they are someone who the therapist wants to be with and enjoys being with, even in the tough times. The experience and communication of UPR is a unique feature of CCPT in the world of child therapy: in CCPT, the child is considered the best arbiter of what they need and how they use therapy.

Empathic understanding

A child's experience of therapist empathic understanding sends the message to the child that the therapist values the child's world and is willing to engage with the child in that world. In CCPT, empathic understanding starts with the use of play as the child's primary form of communication, sending the message that the therapist is willing to move into the child's world rather than expecting the child to move into the adult verbal world. The therapist then seeks to listen and understand what the child communicates through play and verbalisations in order to communicate accurate empathic understanding to the child. Accurate empathic understanding is predicated on a therapist's cultural humility and their recognition that truths and experiences are deeply rooted in a person's identity, background and experiences, and are therefore myriad in their diversity, just as we are (Davis et al., 2018). Specific to children, CCPT therapists may struggle with hearing young children voice or play out their most negative self-thoughts and feelings.

In comparison with my facilitation of adult therapy, I have experienced much more of a need to rescue children in their communication of negative self-perceptions. I attribute a need to rescue children from their feelings and thoughts as rooted in the wider culture's insistence that children should be happy and that adults hold the responsibility to make children happy. When a child states, 'I'm so stupid', the natural inclination is to quickly respond with, 'No, you're not. You're really brilliant.' This type of response sends the message to the child that it is not okay to have bad feelings or thoughts or to talk about them, thereby sending messages of therapist unwillingness to engage in empathic understanding. In CCPT, I would respond with, 'You're feeling bad about yourself right now,' or 'You just don't think you can do it.' These types of responses send the message that the therapist hears and understands the child and sees the pain, and that the child and therapist can journey through the pain together. The child is not alone.

The willingness to engage in empathic understanding with children involves tremendous internal resources on the part of the therapist. I believe the essential difference in therapist engagement in empathic understanding with children versus adults is the recognition that children have very little agency over their external circumstances. For children, therapists acknowledge that much of the pain they experience is inflicted by adults or societal systems. Knowing that children are powerless to change their external circumstances is, in many cases, likely to elicit sympathy responses rather than empathy responses from therapists. The CCPT therapist is highly aware of the impact of the external and seeks to advocate for changes in wider society. However, the CCPT therapist contributes meaningfully to the child when they experience and communicate empathic understanding that activates the child's ability to change what can be changed.

Therapist skills

Although CCPT is grounded in and holds to classical person-centred principles, the approach is characterised by a considerable amount of structure to support its facilitation. The developmental level of children requires attention to physical movement and safety, means of communication and engagement with parents/caregivers. Axline's principles provided a broad understanding of the essential characteristics of CCPT, yet considerations of practical application were incomplete. Subsequently, CCPT theorists and therapists (e.g. Guerney, 2001; Landreth, 2023) pulled together decades of literature on CCPT to offer more guidelines on structure that honours person-centred theory. In their efforts to provide pragmatic guidance, one result might arguably be a movement away from classical person-centred therapy. Specifically, the addition of certain types of responses within the structure of CCPT by including 'other conditions, methods or techniques' may be interpreted as violating the sufficiency assumption of the conditions (Sanders, 2012, p.239).

Furthering this debate, in an effort to move CCPT toward evidence-based recognition in the US, I developed the CCPT research and training protocol (Ray, 2011). I trained as a classical person-centred therapist and have a high admiration for and integration of person-centred principles, so I was hesitant to move CCPT into what might be perceived as a formulaic method for conducting therapy. However, it had become evident in the US mental health community that CCPT was being rejected as a viable intervention, based on its exclusion from lists of evidence-based therapies. One of the primary reasons for excluding CCPT research findings was that the studies generally lacked the clear methods and protocols required by the authorities who decide standards of evidence-based interventions (such as the UK's National Institute for Health and Care Excellence (NICE)). The good news was that here in the US, a protocol did not require step-by-step instructions on how to conduct therapy; it simply required a clear explanation of the theory and methods. In the next section, I present the non-verbal and verbal therapist skills outlined in the CCPT protocol (Ray, 2011).

Non-verbal skills

Because children are more likely to operate in the emotional world through neuroception (Porges, 2021), the CCPT therapist conveys genuineness, UPR and empathic understanding most effectively through their presence and way of being with the child. In CCPT, we use non-verbal skills to send messages of safety and belonging in the play therapy room. The therapist sits in a designated chair in the play therapy room to send the message that the use of the room and materials is decided by the child. The therapist may move from their chair at the request of the child, but the therapist does not initiate movement within the room. The therapist does not lead the play or verbalisations but follows the child's lead through reflective responding or playing in response to the child's request. The therapist does not label toys unless the child labels the toy. Because toys serve as children's words, the child is the one who decides what each toy is in the play therapy room. An elephant can be a monster, a ball can be a bomb, or a car can be a plane. The child's use of the materials represents the child's phenomenological world, and the therapist seeks to enter that world. The therapist also sends the message that they value the child's lead by sitting in an open posture and turning their whole body to face the child if and as the child moves through the room.

Although most therapists seek to present themselves as genuine through their facial expressions and tone of voice, these factors are especially salient in working with children in play therapy. Often, children are more likely to perceive the adult's tone of voice or eye movement before their actual words. Children, especially children who have experienced

Table 12.1: CCPT verbal response categories

Response category	Description	Examples
Tracking behaviour	Therapist verbally responds to behaviour of the child by stating what is observed.	'You're picking that up.'
Reflecting content	Therapist paraphrases the verbal interaction of the child.	'You went to see the pirate movie and there was a lot of action in it.'
Reflecting feeling	Therapist verbally responds to emotions expressed by child.	'You're angry about being here and want to go home.'
Returning responsibility	Therapist verbalises statements to help the child experience their own capability and take responsibility for it.	'You decided you would be the boss and take charge.' 'That looks like something you can do.'
Facilitating creativity	Therapist verbalises statements that help the child experience a sense of freedom and creativity.	'In here, it can be whatever you want it be.'
Esteem-building	Therapist verbalises statements to help the child experience a stronger and capable sense of self.	'You did it. You tried hard and figured it out.'
Facilitating relationship	Therapist reflects statements that build the relationship between therapist and child.	'You wanted to be close to me.' 'You wanted to do something to help me.'
Reflecting deeper meaning	Therapist notices and verbalises patterns in the child's play.	'When you come into the playroom, you want to be the one in charge.'
Limit-setting	Limits are set according to a three-step procedure of reflecting the child's intention of feeling; setting a definitive limit, and providing an appropriate alternative.	'You are really angry with me but I'm not for throwing sand at. You can throw the sand in the sandbox.'

incongruent relationships with adults, are hypervigilant to adult non-verbal expressions and spend considerable energy attempting to interpret them. The CCPT therapist is careful to match their tone of voice with their words to communicate genuineness; that their non-verbal expression matches their verbal expressions reassures the child that they are an adult who can be trusted. The CCPT therapist also seeks to match the child's tone in their play and verbalisations in order to send messages of empathic understanding. If a child is angry or frustrated, the CCPT therapist responds with a lower tone, rather than succumbing to the inclination to use a lighter, happier tone to 'make' the child feel happier.

Verbal skills

Although the therapist's non-verbal way of being in the play therapy room is profound, the CCPT therapist also uses verbal responses to build the relationship. As CCPT has evolved over the decades, nine specific verbal skills have been identified as responses that contribute to its objectives (Landreth, 2023) by sending messages of trust in the child's self-direction, belief in the child's capabilities and care for the child and the child's world. Table 12.1 provides a listing of each verbal skill and examples of therapist responses for the skill. The verbal skills currently serve as the elements of the CCPT research protocol (Ray, 2011) and are used for intervention fidelity (Ray et al., 2017), as well as in training for new therapists.

Identification of CCPT verbal skills was not intended to prescribe the words or actions of the therapist. Building on the work of early CCPT therapists (i.e. Axline, Moustakas, Ginott, Guerney), Landreth (2023) began categorising the skills in order to provide structure for therapists to convey therapist attitudes in developmentally appropriate reflection responses. Over time, others have contributed to the list of categories to include responses that build the child's autonomy, develop the therapeutic relationship and, most uniquely to CCPT, place limits on problematic behaviours. The verbal categories help CCPT therapists structure responses to keep the child in the lead (i.e. tracking, reflecting content and feeling, reflecting deeper meaning), build the child's autonomy (i.e. returning responsibility, facilitating creativity, encouragement), and facilitate a meaningful therapeutic relationship (i.e. facilitating relationship). Within the CCPT structure, the therapist chooses how to respond in the context of the relationship with each individual child. Although new play therapists may concretely use the categories as prescribed responses for sessions, seasoned play therapists respond to the individual person of the child. When an experienced CCPT therapist embraces the person-centred conditions and operates more genuinely with a child, the verbal responses are a natural extension of providing attitudinal conditions and are intuitively used by the therapist to build a relationship with the child.

Here is one example that might help illustrate the use of verbal skills to meet the needs of an individual child. Jonathan, an eight-year-old boy, is building a fort with the wooden blocks. Jonathan says, 'I'm going to build the best fort ever. It's going to have really tall walls and no one is going to get in. Do you see it?' Based on Jonathan's previous actions and the therapist's experience of him, the therapist may make any of the following choices that are intended to be specific to Jonathan.

> Therapist: You're excited about the fort you're building. (*Therapist is reflecting feeling in order to communicate empathic understanding*)
>
> Therapist: It's important to you that no one can get in your fort. (*Therapist is reflecting deeper meaning in the context that Jonathan often plays in ways that keep him safe from others*)
>
> Therapist: You really want me to see how you can build the best fort. (*Therapist gives a facilitating relationship response to reciprocate Jonathan's reaching out to her*)
>
> Therapist: You're trying your hardest to make the fort just like you want. (*Therapist gives an encouragement response based on Jonathan's previous play in which he shares that he is not capable and cannot do things*)

Any of these responses are within the CCPT verbal categories, yet the therapist's accurate empathic understanding of Jonathan drives the choice of response. The therapist chooses the response that most accurately communicates what Jonathan needs in that moment, based on empathic understanding.

Limit-setting is perhaps the most distinctive therapist verbal skill that sets CCPT apart from classical person-centred therapy. Children in play therapy are likely to engage in behaviours that may be harmful to themselves, the therapist or to the materials or room. The therapist is responsible for keeping each person in the play therapy room safe, and has the practical duty to protect materials that cannot be easily replaced. This safety responsibility is juxtaposed with the premise of permissiveness, which is so greatly needed to unleash the actualising tendency of the child. CCPT therapists often struggle with balancing these elements of therapy. Landreth (2023) built on Ginott's (1965) method of limit-setting when he created the ACT model for limit-setting. In ACT, the therapist Acknowledges the child's feelings/desires (A), Communicates the limit (C), and Targets an alternative (T).

So, for example, the therapist might say: 'Sophie, you're excited about the paint (A) but the paint isn't for throwing on the walls (C), you can paint the paper (T).' In this example, the therapist prioritises the child's feelings to ensure communication of empathic understanding in the first step. In the second step, the therapist intentionally avoids directly telling the child what to do (e.g. 'You can't…'); the therapist simply states what is not for doing. Communicating the limit lets the child know the boundary but leaves the decision about following the boundary to the child, thereby respecting the child's autonomy and sending a message of trust in the child's capability to make decisions.

The AC part of ACT is somewhat unique to CCPT as a person-centred tribe, yet can still be contextualised within the philosophy of person-centred therapy. However, targeting the alternative diverges from classical person-centred therapy in that the therapist is suggesting an alternative action. Targeting the alternative can be described as a variation of therapy based on child development rather than person-centred principles. If Sophie is four years old and becomes very excited about the colour and feel of the paint, she will need time to regulate so she can access her cognitive abilities to brainstorm other ideas for the paint. During this time of emotionality, sometimes conceptualised as dysregulation,

Sophie may act immediately by dumping the paint on the floor or pouring the paint over her head. Yet, when the therapist provides an alternative, Sophie's energy is immediately re-directed to a more appropriate action. Thus, Sophie can use the alternative and then have time to regulate to make a decision about whether she wants to continue to follow the limit, find other alternatives, or break the limit. When CCPT therapists set limits with older children or with children who are regulated, they often choose to only use the AC of ACT in order to remain permissive and trusting of the child and so more consistent with the classical person-centred approach.

Developmental modifications to child-centred play therapy

Although CCPT as a protocol is designed for children from the ages of three to 10 years, its emphasis on the therapeutic relationship signifies that the structure and many of the skills used are applicable to children at younger and older ages. Play is the recognised symbolic form of communication for children aged three to 10; however, children younger than three use various forms of play to build relationships, explore their understanding of the world and develop a sense of competency. Their play is typically very concrete and focused on the immediate. Because the main goal of development for children up to three years old is to develop meaningful attachment relationships with primary caregivers, CCPT therapists will more often work with parents to develop skills within structured play times, rather than recommend individual therapy for the child. Yet, at times (e.g. parents/caretakers are inaccessible; the child has experienced trauma), CCPT individual sessions directly with the child can be effective. At the other end of the spectrum, children older than 10 are in various developmental stages where play may or may not be a primary communication tool. Children older than 10 often benefit from the therapist's use of CCPT skills in a more developmentally appropriate therapy space, such as a therapy room that offers activity materials matched to the child's developmental level – for example, cooking, construction or working with more expressive materials. The primacy of a relationship that keenly respects children's play across childhood allows for CCPT to be modified to fit the needs of children at different stages of development.

Parent/caretaker consultation

CCPT is predicated on the belief that children have the internal resources to know the content and processes that are of most significance to them. However, as Rogers so elegantly described (Wilkins, 2015), children are vulnerable to people with whom they are in relationship. Most essentially, children are in the reciprocal process of developing and being influenced by their parents or primary caretakers. Hence, CCPT is an intervention that is facilitated directly with the child, with added systemic intervention with parents/caretakers. The purpose of parent/caretaker consultation in CCPT is to help them provide a growth environment for their child that is characterised by the attitudinal conditions of genuineness, UPR and empathic understanding.

CCPT therapists typically meet with parents/caretakers after every three and five play therapy sessions (Landreth, 2023). The consultations do not follow a predetermined structure, which means there is much variation in what takes place. Typically, however, play therapists use parent/caretaker consultation sessions to listen to carer concerns, report on general progress in play therapy, and possibly teach skills such as reflective listening, limit-setting or encouragement. Some CCPT therapists hold to a classical person-centred approach by following the parent/caretaker in their listening and reflecting; other CCPT therapists engage in psychoeducation. Even if therapists are using instructional methods in CCPT parent consultations, the goal is to teach caretakers how to build relationships with their children through the attitudinal conditions.

Axline proposed that CCPT was effective without parent involvement, and current research has found this to be true. Often, parents/caretakers may be unavailable or unwilling to participate in therapy, due to myriad issues, such as their own background of trauma, custodial circumstances or disinterest. In my line of research (e.g. Ray et al., 2022; Ray et al., 2015; Ray et al., 2013), I have concentrated on demonstrating effects of CCPT when there is no therapeutic contact with parents/caretakers. Outcomes have been positive and demonstrate that children have a substantial ability to change their relational systems.

However, research has also demonstrated that the effects are stronger when parents are involved in the process (Bratton et al., 2005). Building empathic relationships with parents appears to promote the development of the child because the parent is then more likely to maintain an increase in empathic understanding and UPR outside the therapy context. The CCPT protocol recognises the autonomy and internal strengths of children but also honours the primacy of the child-parent relationship and its powerful impact on the child. Parent consultations are considered an essential feature of CCPT and integrated component of working effectively with children.

Case example: Theo

Theo, a seven-year-old boy, was referred to play therapy by his mother, who was concerned about his refusal to go to school. Theo's mother explained that Theo had been strong-willed and determined since birth. He walked and talked earlier than expected. He liked to play sports and was fiercely competitive, even at a young age. He was often perfectionistic and would destroy his own creations when he believed they were not done well. When Theo entered primary school at age five, he was excited to go, to play with friends and learn about flying. Theo's father was an airline pilot. After several months at school, Theo's teacher told his parents that Theo struggled with reading and writing and would often refuse to do assignments. Within the first year, Theo began to say he did not want to go to school. When his parents asked why, Theo only said that the other children were stupid, his teacher was stupid and school was stupid. Although Theo continued to say he did not want to go to school throughout the first two years, he reluctantly attended, with minimal resistance.

Theo's mother further reported that Theo's father had moved out of the home six months previously, and the two were seeking a divorce. Because their marriage had been contentious, with loud arguments, Theo's mother felt the home environment was calmer and healthier for Theo now that his father had moved out. However, two months before coming to therapy, Theo began to refuse to go to school. His refusal behaviours included yelling, screaming, hiding, crying and throwing items in the home. At times, Theo's mother or father physically picked him up to take him into the school. The teacher reported that Theo would frequently stand by the door, refusing to participate in activities, and that he was no longer playing with friends at recess. In the first play therapy session, the therapist introduced the room to Theo.

Therapist: Theo, in here is the playroom. You can play with the toys in lots of the ways you like.

Theo: (*Arms crossed, stands in middle of room saying nothing*)

Therapist: You're not sure what to think about this place.

Theo: What's that? (*Points to the toy plane*)

Therapist: You see something you're interested in. You're wondering what that is.

Theo: (*In a tone as if the therapist was stupid*) I know what it is. It's a plane. Don't you know that?

Therapist: You knew just what it was, and you think I should know too.

Theo: Can I play with it?

Therapist: In here, you can decide what you want to play with.

Theo: (*Picks up plane and looks at it closely*)

Therapist: You're checking it out. Seeing what you think.

Theo: It's a Boeing 747. They are the fastest.

Therapist: You knew just what that was. It sounds like you know about those.

Theo: I know all the planes. 717, 737, 777 but 747 is the best one.

Following this conversation, Theo played only with the plane for the rest of the session. He did not talk but made airplane sounds as he flew the plane through the room. The therapist tracked his play and reflected on his enjoyment in playing. As the sessions progressed, Theo began to create storylines for the plane in the sandbox. The plane would often crash into a house or car and then blow up. After the blow up, Theo would bury and leave the plane under the sand as he left the session. His verbalisations increased but remained solely on the storyline of the plane crashes. In the fourth session, Theo increased his verbalisation of the storyline.

Theo: (*Holding the plane and the house*) This time he's going to make it. Here he comes… (*Flies the plane close to the top of the house*)

Therapist: Oh, you think this time is going to be different. He's going to make it.

Theo: (*Crashes the plane into the house. In a disappointed voice*) He couldn't do it. He couldn't make it. It was just too hard. He broke the house.

Therapist: You're sad about the crash. You really thought he could do it.

Theo: Yeah, he's the best flyer and he has the best plane.

Therapist: Even though he's the best, he just couldn't make it work.

Theo: At least he didn't die this time. (*Places the plane above the sand in the corner of the box*)

Therapist: So, he survived this time. You sound hopeful.

Theo: He just needs to learn to fly better.

Therapist: If he would only learn to fly better, he wouldn't crash into the house.

Theo: He doesn't mean to break the house.

Therapist: You know he doesn't mean it. You know he wants to do better.

In the following two sessions, Theo played out similar scenes except he changed the storyline by giving the pilot resources and telling the pilot what to do in order to avoid crashing into the house. In the seventh session, Theo landed the plane beside the house with no crash. In the last five minutes of the session, Theo moved to the craft table and pulled out a piece of paper and marker. This was the first time Theo had played at the table.

Theo: Okay, we're going to have a spelling test.

Therapist: You decided it's time for a spelling test.

Theo: Yep! I call out the words and you spell them on this paper. (*Hands marker to therapist*)

Therapist: So, you want me to take the spelling test. You give the words and I spell them.

Theo: Yep! The word is 'school'.

Therapist: (*Writes out the word 'school'*)

Theo: (*Yells angrily*) Nope! That's wrong!

Therapist: You're angry that I got it wrong.

Theo: (*In angry voice*) Do it again! Spell 'airplane'.

Therapist: (*Whispers to Theo*) How should I spell it?

Theo: (*Raises voice in anger*) I don't care! Spell it right. Airplane.

Therapist: (*Writes out 'airplane'*)

Theo: (*Before therapist finishes the word, yells*) Nope! Wrong! Wrong! Wrong! You're the stupidest!

Therapist: You are angry that I can't seem to do it right.

The session ended. In the subsequent two sessions, Theo began each session by placing the plane and house carefully on the sand beside each other. Then he quickly moved to the craft table, where he proceeded to give the therapist spelling tests. The therapist failed all the spelling tests.

> Theo: Why are you so stupid?
>
> Therapist: If I can't spell right, it feels like there's something wrong with me.
>
> Theo: Yep, there is something wrong with you. You should be smarter.
>
> Therapist: You wish I was smarter.
>
> Theo: You're nice and all. I like you, but you should be smarter.
>
> Therapist: You're confused because it seems like you like me, but you don't like that I'm not smart enough.
>
> Theo: No, I like you. You can be stupid.
>
> Therapist: You can still like me even if I'm stupid.
>
> Theo: You're not really stupid.
>
> Therapist: You want me to feel better.

In the following five sessions, Theo no longer gave the therapist spelling tests but began to write sentences on the paper. Early on, when writing out a word, he asked the therapist if it was correct. The therapist replied, 'In here you decide how it's spelled.' As the sessions progressed, Theo stopped asking the therapist if the word was correct and began to verbalise his process as he was writing. In the 14th session, Theo began the session at the craft table with paper and marker.

> Therapist: It looks like you have a plan.
>
> Theo: Yep! I'm going to write a story.
>
> Therapist: You do have a plan and you know just what you want to do.
>
> Theo: So, in the first sentence, you start with an uppercase letter. See what I'm doing here. (*Theo writes 'This room…' and shows it to therapist*)
>
> Therapist: You want me to see just what you're doing.
>
> Theo: (*Continues to write 'This room is my fevrit room'*) At the end, you put a period.
>
> Therapist: You sound confident in how to write that sentence.
>
> Theo: (*Picks up paper and holds it close to his eyes. Points to the word 'fevrit'*) I don't think this is right.
>
> Therapist: You're just not sure about that one.

> Theo: It's supposed to say 'favourite' but in here I get to decide how to spell it.
>
> Therapist: Yep, in here, you know you're the one who decides how it's done.
>
> Theo: That's why this is my favourite room.

The therapist regularly met with Theo's mother outside of session. After the fifth session, his mother reported that Theo was no longer refusing to go to school. The therapist worked with the mother on planning consistent visits with Theo's father and worked with Theo's father on creating a place that was specifically for Theo in his new home. The therapist worked with both parents on reflective listening and having special playtimes with Theo where he could lead the play and his parents used reflective listening. The therapist also worked with the parents on limit-setting with Theo when he became destructive or refused tasks. By the 14th session, both parents reported that Theo now looked forward to going to school and the teacher had reported that he was participating in assignments and playing with friends.

In Theo's case, the therapist noted that Theo's developmental history indicated that he was a fairly anxious child with perfectionistic tendencies. When Theo entered school, the environment was overwhelming in the context of his need to be the best. The need to succeed in school and the messages that he was not doing so had been introjected as a sense of failure and unworthiness. Theo's coping skill of controlling his environment began to fail him once his parents separated and there was no way for him to control the instability. In play therapy, Theo's first play theme related to the separation of his parents, and his fear of losing both his parents was played out in his plane crash scene, probably because the divorce was the most immediate threat to his self-structure and hence the most immediate need for him to express in play therapy. Once he felt safe to express his confusion and felt understood and accepted by the therapist, Theo moved to a place of acceptance and hope that the plane and the house would both survive. Having taken care of these immediate and existential fears, Theo seemed to feel strong enough to work on his self-concept related to school. The spelling play allowed Theo to express his negative self-thoughts, his strong feelings, and how he had integrated a general sense of unworthiness into his self-structure. The therapist's understanding and acceptance of Theo's struggles freed Theo to explore different ways of looking at himself and integrate a new concept of self. Because Theo valued the therapeutic relationship so highly (as did the therapist), Theo seemed to know that he could care about the play therapist even if she was stupid, and maybe she was not that stupid after all. This nurturing of the therapist appeared to allow Theo to see the value in caring for and valuing himself.

Research in child-centred play therapy

CCPT has a long and rich history of research on its effectiveness. As noted, Axline followed Rogers' lead in emphasising the need to study intervention and its effects. She conducted early studies on the effects of CCPT with children with intellectual disabilities and academic challenges (Axline, 1947b; Axline, 1949), and found that children who had emotional disturbances were freed to reach their potential academically after participating in CCPT. In the almost 80 years since Axline's initial research, researchers have remained committed to exploring the effectiveness of CCPT with diverse populations and presenting issues.

Due to the robust number of individual CCPT studies, several meta-analyses have been conducted that present promising results for children who participated in CCPT. In their review of 52 randomised controlled trials, Lin and Bratton (2015) examined outcomes for studies conducted from 1995 to 2010. They found that children who participated in CCPT made statistically significant improvements over children on a waitlist or receiving alternative interventions, on measures of problem behaviours, relationship stress, self-efficacy and academic performance, with a moderate treatment effect (Cohen's $d = 0.47$). Lin and Bratton reported that children of colour who participated in CCPT improved at an even larger effect size level of 0.76. Ray and colleagues (2015) explored the results of 23 randomised controlled trials on CCPT conducted in schools in the US and found that children who participated in a mean of 12 sessions reported statistically significant improvement over peers on waitlist or in alternative interventions, with varying effect sizes. More recently, Parker and colleagues (2021) conducted a meta-analysis of 23 studies of children who were referred for disruptive behaviours. Including studies conducted between 1999 and 2018, Parker and colleagues found that children in CCPT improved at a statistically significant level, with a moderate effect size of 0.48 over peers in waitlist or alternative treatment groups. In order to capture the effects of CCPT in multiple single case-design studies, Pester and colleagues (2019) conducted a meta-analysis on 11 CCPT single case studies representing 43 children and reported moderate effect sizes of 0.43 for externalising problem behaviours and 0.51 for internalising problems, which were achieved in as few as eight sessions.

One unique characteristic of CCPT studies in comparison with other child intervention research is the young age of the participants. Lin and Bratton (2015) reported a mean age of 6.7 years while the participants in Parker and colleagues' study (2021) were a median age of 6.0 years. Ray and colleagues (2015) included children aged three to 12 years old, while Pester and colleagues (2019) researched children aged three to 10 years old. The concentration on young children sets CCPT apart from other interventions in demonstrating that classical person-centred principles are effective with even the youngest of clients. Additionally, CCPT research has shown CCPT to be effective across diverse populations (e.g. Lin & Bratton, 2015) and presenting issues (Lin & Bratton, 2015; Ray et al., 2015).

Resources

Key books

- Axline, V.M. (1947). *Play therapy.* Ballantine.
  The seminal historical document on the definition, description and practice of CCPT.
- Landreth, G. (2023). *Play therapy: The art of the relationship* (4th ed.). Routledge.
  The most widely used description of CCPT practice in current publication, including rationale, case studies, and systemic applications.
- Ray, D. (2011). *Advanced play therapy: Conditions, knowledge, and skills for child practice.* Routledge.
  The companion book to Landreth's *Art of the Relationship*, which offers depth into the connection between CCPT and the classical person-centered approach, including the research protocol for CCPT.
- Ray, D. (2016). *A therapist's guide to development: The extraordinarily normal years.* Routledge.
  A practical guide to understanding the development of young children from birth to 12 years old, including descriptive handouts of developmental markers for each year of childhood.

Websites

- Association for Play Therapy – www.A4pt.org
- British Association of Play Therapists – www.bapt.info
- Center for Play Therapy at University of North Texas – https://cpt.unt.edu/center-play-therapy

Journal

- *International Journal of Play Therapy,* published by the American Psychological Association
  www.apa.org/pubs/journals/pla

References

Allen, F. (1942/2011). *Psychotherapy with children.* Gleed Press.

Axline, V.M. (1947a). *Play therapy.* Ballantine.

Axline, V.M. (1947b). Nondirective therapy for poor readers. *Journal of Consulting Psychology, 11*(2), 61–69. https://doi.org/10.1037/h0063079

Axline, V.M. (1949). Mental deficiency – symptom or disease? *Journal of Consulting Psychology, 13*(5), 313–327. https://doi.org/10.1037/h0059597

Axline, V. (1964). *Dibs in search of self.* Ballantine.

Badenoch, B. (2008). *Being a brain-wise therapist: A practical guide to interpersonal neurobiology*. W.W. Norton.

Badenoch, B. (2018). *The heart of trauma: Healing the embodied brain in the context of relationships*. W.W. Norton.

Behr, M. (2003). Interactive resonance in work with children and adolescents: A theory-based concept of interpersonal relationship through play and the use of toys. *Person-Centered & Experiential Psychotherapies, 2*, 89–103.

Behr, M. & Cornelius-White, J. (Eds.). (2008). *Facilitating young people's development: International perspectives on person-centred theory and practice*. PCCS Books.

Bozarth, J. (1998). *Person-centered therapy: A revolutionary paradigm*. PCCS Books.

Bratton, S.C., Ray, D., Rhine, T. & Jones, L. (2005). The efficacy of play therapy with children: A meta-analytic review of treatment outcomes. *Professional Psychology: Research and Practice, 36*(4), 376–390. https://doi.org/10.1037/0735-7028.36.4.376

British Association for Counselling and Psychotherapy. (2022). *Counsellors' guide: The competences for humanistic counselling with children and young people (4–18 years)*. BACP.

Cochran, N.H., Nordling, W.J. & Cochran, J.L. (2022). *Child-centered play therapy: A practical guide to developing therapeutic relationships with children* (2nd ed.). Routledge.

Davis, D.E., DeBlaere, C., Owen, J., Hook, J.N., Rivera, D.P., Choe, E., Van Tongeren, D.R., Worthington, E.L., Jr. & Placeres, V. (2018). The multicultural orientation framework: A narrative review. *Psychotherapy, 55*(1), 89–100. doi:10.1037/pst0000160.supp

Freud, A. (1946). *The psycho-analytical treatment of children*. International Universities Press.

Freud, S. (1909/1955). *The case of 'Little Hans' and the 'Rat Man'*. Hogarth Press.

Ginott, H. (1959). The theory and practice of therapeutic intervention in child treatment. *Journal of Consulting Psychology, 23*, 160–167.

Ginott, H. (1965). *Between parent and child*. Avon.

Guerney, L. (2001). Child-centered play therapy. *International Journal of Play Therapy, 10*, 13–31.

Klein, M. (1932/1975). *The psychoanalysis of children*. Hogarth Press.

Landreth, G. (2023). *Play therapy: The art of the relationship* (4th ed.). Routledge.

Lin, Y. & Bratton, S.C. (2015). A meta-analytic review of child-centered play therapy approaches. *Journal of Counseling and Development, 93*(1), 45–58. https://doi.org/10.1002/j.1556-6676.2015.00180.x

Moustakas, C. (1959). *Psychotherapy with children: The living relationship*. Harper & Row.

Moustakas, C. (1997). *Relationship play therapy*. Jason Aronson.

Parker, M.M., Hunnicutt Hollenbaugh, K.M. & Kelly, C.T. (2021). Exploring the impact of child-centered play therapy for children exhibiting behavioral problems: A meta-analysis. *International Journal of Play Therapy, 30*(4), 259–271. https://doi.org/10.1037/pla0000128

Pester, D., Lenz, A.S. & Dell'Aquila, J. (2019). Meta-analysis of single-case evaluations of child-centered play therapy for treating mental health symptoms. *International Journal of Play Therapy, 28*(3), 144–156. https://doi.org/10.1037/pla0000098

Porges, S. (2021). *Polyvagal safety: Attachment, communication, self-regulation*. W.W. Norton.

Ray, D.C. (2011). *Advanced play therapy: Essential conditions, knowledge, and skills for child practice*. Routledge.

Ray, D.C. (Ed.). (2016). *A therapist's guide to child development: The extraordinarily normal years*. Routledge.

Ray, D.C. (2019). The child and the counselor: Relational humanism in the playroom and beyond. *Journal of Humanistic Counseling, 58*(1), 68–82. https://doi.org/10.1002/johc.12090

Ray, D.C. (2023). *Playful education: Using play therapy strategies to elevate your classroom*. Routledge.

Ray, D.C., Armstrong, S.A., Balkin, R.S. & Jayne, K.M. (2015). Child-centered play therapy in the schools: Review and meta-analysis. *Psychology in the Schools, 52*(2), 107–123. https://doi.org/10.1002/pits.21798

Ray, D.C., Chung, R.K., Turner, K.K. & Aguilar, E.V. (2022). The multicultural playroom. In D. C. Ray, Y. Ogawa, & Y. Cheng (Eds.), *Multicultural play therapy: Making the most of cultural opportunities with children* (pp.29–43). Routledge.

Ray, D.C., Ogawa, Y. & Cheng, Y. (2022). *Multicultural play therapy: Making the most of cultural opportunities*. Routledge.

Ray, D.C., Purswell, K., Haas, S. & Aldrete, C. (2017). Child-centered play therapy-research integrity checklist: Development, reliability, and use. *International Journal of Play Therapy, 26*(4), 207–217. https://doi.org/10.1037/pla0000046

Ray, D.C., Stulmaker, H.L., Lee, K.R. & Silverman, W.K. (2013). Child-centered play therapy and impairment: Exploring relationships and constructs. *International Journal of Play Therapy, 22*(1), 13–27. https://doi.org/10.1037/a0030403

Rogers, C. (1939). *The clinical treatment of the problem child*. Houghton Mifflin.

Rogers, C. (1942). *Counseling and psychotherapy*. Houghton Mifflin.

Rogers, C. (1951). *Client-centered therapy: Its current practice, implications and theory*. Houghton-Mifflin.

Rogers, C. (1957). The necessary and sufficient conditions of therapeutic personality change. *Journal of Consulting Psychology, 21*, 95–103.

Russ, S., Fiorelli, J. & Spannagel, S. (2011). Cognitive and affective processes in play. In S. Russ & L. Niec (Eds.), *Play in clinical practice: Evidence-based approaches* (pp.3–22). Guilford.

Sanders, P. (2012). Mapping person-centred approaches to counselling and psychotherapy. In P. Sanders (Ed.), *The tribes of the person-centred nation: An introduction to the schools of therapy related to the person-centered approach* (2nd ed.) (pp.233–246). PCCS Books.

Vygotsky, L. (1966). Play and its role in the mental development of the child. *Voprosy Psikhologii, 12*, 6–18.

West, J. (1996). *Child centred play therapy* (2nd ed.). Arnold.

Wilkins, P. (2015). *Person-centred therapy: 100 key points* (2nd ed.). Routledge.

Wilson, K. & Ryan, V. (2006). *Play therapy: A non-directive approach for children and adolescents* (2nd ed.). Bailliere Tindall.

Conclusion

Mick Cooper

If you started this book thinking person-centred therapy was one thing, we hope by now you'll have a much richer, more complex and more nuanced sense of the whole. The person-centred tribes form a dynamic, vibrant kaleidoscope of approaches, suited to a wide range of mental wellbeing needs in the 21st century. There are approaches to helping children, people who lose the ability to sustain relational contact, people with substance use problems, reflective approaches for clients wanting space and time in therapy, structured practices for those wanting more guidance, and creative arts interventions. Far from the stereotype of the 'nodding dog' therapist – repeating the last sentence that the client said and nodding sagely – person-centred therapy emerges as a sophisticated and multifaceted set of contemporary practices that has stood the test of time.

Dimensions and differences across the person-centred tribes

In making sense of this whole, it may be useful to identify some of the key dimensions along which person-centred approaches tend to differ – although, of course, there are always also variations by practitioner, by client, and even by the particular session and point in time. Probably the most fundamental dimension, from Gendlin's focusing (see Chapter 4) onwards, is between those tribes in which the therapist directs the therapeutic process in some way versus those in which the client is wholly encouraged to take the lead: 'sitting forward' and 'sitting back' stances, respectively. In the latter camp is the classical person-centred approach (Chapter 2) as well as child-centred play therapy (Chapter 12). At the other end of the spectrum tends to be emotion-focused therapy (Chapter 5) and motivational interviewing (Chapter 7). The other tribes lie somewhere in between.

Those tribes at the client-led end of this spectrum tend to see Rogers' six conditions as necessary and sufficient (see Chapter 1) and consider this the basis for practice. Those at the process-directive end, on the other hand, tend to see clients as sometimes needing 'something more' in order to heal. What this 'more' is, however, is dependent on the particular tribe and their model of human being. For focusing (Chapter 4), the 'more' is helping clients connect with, and carry forward their felt senses; for EFT (Chapter 5), it is primarily helping clients to access and process emotions and 'emotion scheme'. Motivational interviewing (Chapter 7) focuses on reinforcing and eliciting clients' 'change talk', while in existentially informed person-centred therapy (Chapter 8), the 'help' involves supporting clients to face the existential givens of life. There is more. For the creative arts approaches (Chapter 10), it is the client's creativity that is the focus of the therapist's efforts; in pluralistic person-centred therapy (Chapter 9), a wide range of tools and techniques can be used, depending on the client's particular needs, goals and wishes at a particular point in time (and the therapist's training).

Conceptually, we can also say that the client-led tribes have a fundamental faith in a human tendency to actualise, while the process-directive approaches hold a more ambivalent view, seeing a potential both for growthful and ungrowthful ways of being. In EFT (Chapter 5), for instance, the client's 'primary emotions' are generally seen as constructive, but there is also a belief that our natural and basic emotional responses can lead us at times in unhelpful directions. Similarly, existentially informed approaches (Chapter 8) hold that, to some extent, our natural human tendency is to 'bury our heads in the sand' and not face the reality of our existential condition. Understandings of human being such as these lead naturally, then, to more process-directive approaches. If clients are organismically constructive, as the classical person-centred approaches hold, then the role of the therapist is to get out of the way and let the client's own healing process unfurl. But if clients can naturally, organismically, also get things wrong, the therapist may need to take a more active role in guiding the client towards what is helpful.

Another dimension of person-centred practice, closely aligned to the process-directive-client-led one, is between those approaches that are more integrative – drawing on theories and practices from across the therapy palette of choices – and those that are more purely 'Rogerian'. Again, at one end, we have the classical person-centred approach (Chapter 2), with a view of the six conditions as necessary and sufficient, and at the other end of this spectrum, we have tribes like pluralistic person-centred therapy (Chapter 9), EFT (Chapter 5), and motivational interviewing (Chapter 7), which draw on ideas and practices from such sources as Gestalt therapy, behavioural psychology and attachment theory.

There is also something of a difference between those approaches that see human beings in two-person, relational terms (the relational approach, Chapter 3; and to some extent pluralistic person-centred therapy, Chapter 9), and those that tend to adopt a more individual-oriented perspective (such as the classical approach, see Chapter 2). This is a subtle difference, particularly in practice, but while the former approaches are more likely to emphasise dialogue and the co-creation of the therapeutic relationship, the latter are more likely to conceptualise the therapist's role in terms of being a 'crucible', 'container', or 'tool' for the client's internal process of change. In the former approaches, there may also be a greater tendency for therapists to bring themselves into the therapeutic work: more self-disclosure, more here-and-now immediacy, more 'meta-therapeutic communication' about the nature of the therapeutic work. In these two-person approaches, healing is conceptualised as taking place in the space 'between' therapist and client. In the more individual-oriented tribes, the healing is within the client's own psyche.

A concept of 'the unconscious' in person-centred creative arts (Chapter 10) can also be contrasted against the phenomenological approach adopted by most other tribes (i.e. they stay with the client's experiences, as implicitly or explicitly expressed). Again, this is not an 'either/or' polarity but a gradated spectrum, with varying beliefs about the extent to which human beings may suppress – and/or be unaware of – their own material. For the person-centred creative arts approaches, which use the term 'unconscious' liberally (and, indeed, 'collective unconscious'), there are things that human beings cannot see in their own minds. What follows on from this is more interpretative-like questions to the client – for instance, 'What does red mean?' or 'Why is the giraffe sad?' – to try to elicit those hidden aspects of the psyche. As de la Prida makes clear in her chapter (Chapter 10), however, these are still interpretations emanating from the client, rather than the therapist's beliefs or hypotheses about what these things mean.

More practically, what also differs across the person-centred tribes is the particular client groups to which they are oriented. Most person-centred tribes have been developed for adult clients, but child-centred play therapy (Chapter 12), as the name suggests, was specifically developed for children. Similarly, while most person-centred tribes were developed for working with a wide range of client issues, motivational interviewing (Chapter 7) emerged specifically for clients with alcohol use problems – although it is now used across a range of health and wellbeing contexts, including, as in this case example, smoking cessation. Pre-therapy (Chapter 11) was developed for clients who have a severe lack, or loss, of psychological contact. Initially, this tended to be clients experiencing psychosis, although it has now been applied to such groups as clients with dementia and learning disabilities, and those on the autistic spectrum. Pre-therapy, like focusing-oriented therapy (Chapter 4), were also both, initially, developed as precursors to therapy – something to prepare clients for 'actual' therapeutic work – though both are now considered therapies in their own right.

Our commonalities

While we should recognise, celebrate and debate our differences, as Margaret Warner (2000) says (see Introduction), we should also remember that we are under a common person-centred umbrella, and that our commonalities outweigh that which divides us. What are those commonalities? Across the different tribes, we see a fundamental commitment to engaging with clients in deeply valuing and respectful ways and prioritising the quality of the relationship over any particular methods or techniques. Closely related to that, we see a desire to empower clients: to help them draw on, and bring out, their own strengths and abilities. Across the person-centred therapies, there is a desire to relate to clients – all clients – in non-pathologising, non-objectifying ways. Clients, from all person-centred standpoints, are people like us – striving to make the best of their lives in the best ways they know how. Closely related to that is a commitment across the tribes to therapist reflexivity: to recognising that we, too, are beings in the process of growth and actualisation, and that there is always more we can learn.

What we also see, across the tribes, is a desire to work with clients in terms of their subjective experiencing: to help them focus on their emotions, feelings, perceptions, needs and desires. This contrasts with approaches that focus primarily on cognitions, behaviours, external 'truths' or hypothetical 'unconscious' processes. To a great extent this emerges, as above, from the person-centred value base: that the client is not an object to us but a subjectively experiencing being – someone we stand alongside so that we can empathically enter into their lived worlds, not someone we are trying to 'do to'.

What also unites the person-centred tribes is a willingness to value diversity and difference. Each client is understood as a unique being, with experiences and qualities that can never be fully known in advance. When we meet a client, then, it is with an openness of heart, and with a deep respect for the particular culture or tradition that they come from, recognising that there may be much there that we are unfamiliar with and need to learn. Paradoxically, then, what may also unite the tribes is a willingness to value and respect our own internal diversities, recognising that there are many different ways of being person-centred, and that each of the tribes has much to contribute to the rich kaleidoscope of person-centred theories and practices.

The future

What does the future hold for the person-centred tribes? Here are a few personal reflections.

First, for me, is the question of whether we will see more division and differentiation across the tribes, or whether we will see more integration and re-uniting. From the standpoint of person-centred theories of growth (Rogers, 1961), one could see it both ways. On the one hand, the actualising process is a movement towards greater specialisation, greater differentiation, more uniqueness and development of each individual part – like the spreading branches of a tree. On the other hand, actualisation means a greater relating between the parts: a coming-together-into-a-whole. Perhaps, ideally, both processes would take place: growth and development of each individual tribe, but also a greater degree of inter-relating and a sharing of ideas and practices. Like a great work of art, different colours need to have some distinctiveness – a big mushy brownness is not particularly compelling – yet 'the art' lies in their relationships as a complex whole. And, indeed, my personal sense is that we are moving in that direction: towards both greater differentiation and greater integration (helped, I would like to think, by the publication of this book). In recent years, we have seen advocates of different approaches engaging more across boundaries, while at the same time developing their own, unique ideas and practices. Hopefully, the days of near-stand-up fights at person-centred conferences are long gone.

What about the evolution of new tribes – new branches of the tree and new flowerings? That would certainly be my hope, that we add to the richness, colour and breadth of this person-centred nation. One source of such developments might be the increased recognition of particular psychological issues and/or ways of being in contemporary society. This, inevitably, leads to questions such as what might a person-centred therapy for clients on the autistic spectrum look like, or for trans clients, or for isolated older adults? Developing tailored person-centred therapies for such client groups, drawing extensively from an understanding of that group's unique experiences and needs, as well as from collaborative research endeavours, would almost certainly generate person-centred therapies with particular flavours, if not fully-fledged tribes.

Another principal source for new developments may be particular cultural traditions. Multicultural approaches to therapy have evolved rapidly in recent years (see, for instance, Ratts et al., 2016), with the recognition that no one type of therapy is suitable across all cultures. What works for a white, middle-aged, British man may not also work for a young, disabled woman of the global majority. Recognising such differences has not always been at the forefront of the person-centred movement (with its universally-applicable 'necessary and sufficient' conditions), but it is fundamentally consistent with its deeper values (see 'Our Commonalities', above). We may see, then, person-centred approaches emerging for particular cultural groups: as, for instance, Ioane and Tudor's (2023) proposal for a 'family-centred therapy', drawing on Pacific spirituality. More than that, we may see person-centred approaches emerging from particular cultural groups that may then disseminate out into the wider field. My hope would be that the days when person-centred tribes – at least in the English-speaking world – emerged almost exclusively from English-speaking, white males (including, I recognise, me), are hopefully also gone.

Finally, my view is that research evidence will, almost inevitably, play a part in the development, generation and, indeed, survival of tribes. Today, in order to be funded and commissioned to deliver any kind of public service, it is rarely enough to say, 'I know this works, trust me.' Service providers, and, indeed, service users, want evidence; they want to know, from some quasi-independent source, that something works. So, if an approach to person-centred therapy can show robust positive benefits – as, for instance, EFT (Chapter 5) has done so brilliantly over the past few decades – it is likely to thrive, while those approaches that fail to generate evidence may be increasingly limited to the realm of private practice.

But research can be about so much more than just trying to prove one's worth. It can be a means of developing and evolving one's approach, of finding new, and more helpful, forms of practice. And, of course, research does not just mean highly experimental, controlled trials. There is qualitative research: for instance, asking service users what they found helpful and unhelpful in a particular approach, or descriptions of pieces of client work, written ideally in collaboration with their subject, that can serve to evaluate and develop particular theories. Even with quantitative research, there is an increasing number of measures that can be used to assess outcomes and processes in a person-centred way, such as the Authenticity Scale (Moerken & Cooper, 2023) and the Person-Centred and Experiential Psychotherapy Scale (Freire et al., 2014).

Summary

In this conclusion, I have drawn together some of the key differences across the person-centred tribes. The most fundamental of these is the process-directive vs client-led dimension, with the latter placing greater faith in the necessity and sufficiency of Rogers' conditions and the human tendency to actualise. Other dimensions are the degree of integration versus purism, two-person versus one-person models of human being, and a belief in unconscious processes versus a more strictly phenomenological approach. For those approaches that are more process-directive, we also see differences in how they try to support the client, and there are also differences where tribes have been developed for particular groups of clients. Such differences, however, should not mask the commonalities within the person-centred umbrella: a deep respect for clients, their experiencing, and their differences from us, the therapists. For the future, the tribes may move towards both greater differentiation and greater integration, will flower across multicultural lines, and will need to attend more fully to the research agenda. But, of course, things may evolve in entirely different ways. What do you think? And where do you stand in this great, evolving person-centred nation?

References

Freire, E., Elliott, R. & Westwell, G. (2014). Person-Centred and Experiential Psychotherapy Scale: Development and reliability of an adherence/competence measure for person-centred and experiential psychotherapies. *Counselling and Psychotherapy Research, 14*(3), 220–226. https://doi.org/10.1080/14733145.2013.808682

Ioane, J. & Tudor, K. (2023). Family-centered therapy: Implications of Pacific spirituality for person-centered theory and practice. *Person-Centered & Experiential Psychotherapies, 22*(1), 58–76. https://doi.org/10.1080/14779757.2022.2100812

Moerken, D. & Cooper, M. (2023). The Authenticity Scale as an outcome measure for psychotherapy: A psychometric evaluation. *Journal of Humanistic Psychology*; Online First. https://doi.org/10.1177/00221678231159152

Ratts, M.J., Singh, A.A., Nassar-McMillan, S., Butler, S.K. & McCullough, J.R. (2016). Multicultural and social justice counseling competencies: Guidelines for the counseling profession. *Journal of Multicultural Counseling and Development, 44*(1), 28–48. https://doi.org/10.1002/jmcd.12035

Rogers, C.R. (1961). *On becoming a person: A therapist's view of therapy*. Constable.

Warner, M.S. (2000). Person-centered psychotherapy: One nation, many tribes. *Person-Centered Journal, 7*(1), 28–39.

Contributors

Nicola Blunden

During my initial training as a person-centred therapist in the late 1990s, I was also employed as a youth worker, based in a council estate in the multiply deprived South Wales valleys. My first job was to design an alternative curriculum for teens who had stopped attending school. The poverty in the area was crippling, with high levels of unemployment and early mortality, and low levels of hope. To my truant teens, there seemed little point in going to school. As a passionate person-centred therapist in training, it appeared entirely obvious to me how to engage them. I believed wholeheartedly – and still do – in the potency of people being more in touch with what they think, feel and want, and less in touch with the exterior urgings of conformity. I invited the teens to write their own curriculum, and we all knuckled down to make it happen. They went on to achieve near-perfect attendance, and the project was regarded as a flagship model of best practice in the alternative curriculum movement.

What I saw as a 'person-centred approach to youth work' relied on something that I later learned to call 'coproduction'. Coproduction is about involving people from the first moment in co-creating services that affect them. It is not about 'doing *to* people' (imposing a service) or even 'doing *for* people' (deciding on their behalf). It is about 'doing *with* people'. It's a radical commitment to collaboration.

That has been my approach to therapy too, for 25 years. The revolutionary possibilities that emerge in person-centred therapy do so because the client is alive to themselves, when society would prefer that they are silent. For me, that always means inviting a person to 'design their own curriculum'.

The person-centred world has not always agreed with me. On my first day as course leader of the person-centred counselling programme at Metanoia Institute, I shocked many students by beginning a therapy demonstration with the words, 'What would you like to come from this short session?' I had broken their first rule of person-centred counselling in the first 10 seconds, by asking the client a direct question. I'm very happy to be a radical in this way. Being person-centred is more about possibility than it is about limits and more about discovery than it is about rules. It's about liberation. I am honoured to be part of this book and to contribute something that emerged from my work with those teens 25 years ago. They taught me how to let go of what is already established to make space for what is needed.

Mick Cooper

My first counselling course was a person-centred certificate, but I subsequently trained for four years in existential psychotherapy. I loved the values of the person-centred approach but got unbearably frustrated with the lack of direction on my certificate, where it felt like we would spend interminable hours deciding whether to have our lunch breaks at 12.30 or 12.45! In my existential training, I think I also came to experience a deeper acceptance of the intense feelings of anxiety, panic and mournfulness that I had experienced from childhood, and continue to experience (see Chapter 8). Here, these feelings were deeply accepted as expressions of a very meaningful and valid perception of the reality of my, and human, existence. On completing my existential training, however, I returned to the person-centred fold for many years (the Counselling Unit at the University of Strathclyde), and much of the reason for this was the feelings of community, warmth and 'relational depth' that I experienced within this world.

However, working on *Politicizing the Person-Centred Approach* (Proctor et al., 2006), I came to recognise that what I really cared about was not any one particular therapeutic orientation, but a set of political and ethical values: a deep valuing and respect for our clients. So, in recent years, I have moved towards a perspective that John McLeod, I and others have termed 'pluralistic'. For me, this perspective is an articulation of the very essence of a person-centred approach: a commitment to prizing our individual clients over and above any theories that we might hold about them. More than that, it's a way of celebrating the value, richness and diversity of the person-centred tribes, without holding that one is superior to another. This is exactly what this book is about, and why I was deeply honoured to take over its stewardship.

In recent years, my concern with ethical, social and environmental issues has taken me further in the direction of exploring the interface between therapy and politics. My most recent authored book is *Psychology at the Heart of Social Change: Towards a progressive vision of society* (Policy Press, 2023), and I have also been involved in the establishment of a Therapy and Social Change (TaSC) network.

- Cooper, M. (2023). *Psychology at the Heart of Social Change: Towards a progressive vision of society.* Policy Press.
- Proctor, G., Cooper, M., Sanders, P. & Malcolm, B. (2006). *Politicizing the Person-Centred Approach.* PCCS Books.

Steve Cox

I became a person-centred therapist in the early 1990s. My initial interest in talking therapy came from a personal reaction towards psychiatry. During my late teens and early 20s, I was hospitalised many times in psychiatric institutions. It was an experience that was prolonged because I would not accept the treatment model and actively fought against it. Even at my most distressed, I realised that diagnosis and the subsequent use of psychotropic drugs couldn't provide the healing that I required; indeed, it made things worse.

In my 30s I sought my own answers to my wellbeing, and it was during this time that I started to learn about the many different kinds of therapy and self-help methods, and counselling became a particular interest. As my interest in counselling grew, I applied and was accepted onto a person-centred counselling training course. I did not specifically seek out Carl Rogers or person-centred therapy. However, as I studied Rogers, his understanding and meaning of life deeply resonated with me. Rogers wasn't teaching me anything I didn't already know, but he affirmed and awoke meaning and understandings that were rooted in me. He provided language and structure that clarified hitherto unvoiced sensing. Rogers' conviction regarding self-determination, personal connection, development and integration, and interconnection has provided me with a guiding light with which to explore my being and living. It has also meant that I found a way to make a living that I can give my heart to.

From the outset of my 30-year career as a therapist, I have always understood that connection, and therefore relationship, is key to person-centred practice. Over time I have a deepening experience of people-centredness in which a relational breadth is experienced, encompassing person, people and place. Over the years I have held various practitioner positions under the umbrella of person-centred: therapist, supervisor and trainer. I have worked for mental health charities, drug and alcohol agencies, hospices, colleges, universities and psychiatric hospitals. To practise authentically and uphold person-centred values, I have had to challenge the authority of all of the organisations that I have worked for, particularly concerning my clients' and my own agency. Over the past few years, I feel very comfortable as an independent practitioner working from my cabin at the bottom of my garden.

Ani de la Prida

I have a diverse heritage with family dotted around the world, many of whom don't speak the same languages. I learned to use creative, non-verbal ways to communicate as I listened to their stories of trauma, survival and loss. This sowed the seeds of my interest in creative expression and psychological healing. I took courses in dance movement therapy, play therapy, expressive arts and child psychology, and did a placement in a school in East London with children with behavioural difficulties. My own experience of art therapy was important, but it was my experience of person-centred counselling that I found most valuable.

When I discovered Liesl Silverstone's Person-Centred Art Therapy (PCAT) in 1999, which combined art and person-centred therapy, I felt I had found my tribe. I then trained as a person-centred counsellor at Havering College. I saw the person-centred approach as simple and yet profound, able to work with and beyond mental health issues.

My first job in 2003 was running a person-centred art therapy group with offenders on a drug treatment programme in East London. The group was intense and raw, and I saw how art could access places that words cannot reach. Since then, I've worked in a wide range of settings with children and adults, and in private practice since 2005. Both my training courses were deeply person-centred; we negotiated, planned and shaped the curriculum in a challenging and empowering experience of transformational learning.

I started teaching the PCAT approach in 2005 and met Liesl the same year when I joined her tutor supervision group. Liesl was brilliant, rigorous and an inspirational mentor. I started teaching at Havering College on the BA in person-centred counselling in 2007, became a course leader at Renew in 2011, and moved on to teach on the pluralistic BSc at the University of East London from 2020.

Over the years, the person-centred creative approach has stagnated. Its validity was questioned, with some seeing its innate pluralistic integration of a range of theories and methods as directive. Little new material was published, there was a lack of development and very few trained practitioners. I became deeply concerned that this approach might disappear, and so in 2020 I founded the Association of Person-Centred Creative Arts (APCCA) to promote its development and visibility.

My chapter is an opportunity to develop a clear theoretical basis for the approach as a valid tribe of the person-centred nation, with a contemporary perspective relevant to our new digital context. I hope it helps to illustrate the approach, and that it will encourage practitioners to bring more creativity into training and practice.

Gina di Malta

My fascination with the person-centred approach stems from the influence of Carl Rogers – an influence that has not only shaped my career but also touched my own experiences in profound ways. The acknowledgment and fostering of an individual's innate potential for personal growth and healing, in particular, have always resonated with me.

My own journey as a researcher and psychologist has been marked by an exploration of how some of these principles can be harnessed to create an impactful therapeutic experience. One concept that's become a central focus of my work is relational depth, a notion that has been significantly developed by Mick Cooper.

It was my first experience of relational depth with one of my early clients that was pivotal in making me see the transformative powers of therapy. This moment changed our therapeutic relationship to become a haven and new realm of therapeutic possibilities. After that, the work of psychologists also took on a new spiritual meaning for me. I later found the words to explain this early experience when I started my doctorate in counselling psychology at the University of Roehampton and came across the book *Working at Relational Depth in Counselling and Psychotherapy*, then in its first edition (Mearns & Cooper, 2005/2018).

Relational depth goes beyond the conventional therapeutic relationship. It's about forging an environment where clients feel not only safe but also profoundly valued and wholly unjudged. It's in these moments that clients can delve into the depths of their most inner senses. Through my academic pursuits, I've sought to unravel the intricacies of relational depth with the view to support more authentic connections with others, ultimately cultivating a space where growth and healing are not just possible but likely.

In our chapter for this present book, we aspired to bridge a deep-seated appreciation of person-centred therapy and draw on research and our experiences of deep moments of connection to begin defining what might be a relational approach to person-centred therapy. We hope our chapter will inspire therapists and practitioners to cultivate richer and more meaningful connections in their practice of person-centred therapy, enhancing the therapeutic journey for individuals seeking support and healing.

- Mearns, D. & Cooper, M. (2005/2018). *Working at relational depth in counselling and psychotherapy.* Sage.

Richard Doyle

My interest in the person-centred experiential approach stems from a long-held and deep curiosity about people and communities, as well as about the wider world. From a young age, I had a fascination for atoms and molecules as much as personalities and personal growth.

While I undertook my teenage work experience at a university psychology department, I went on to study science, completing a doctorate in chemical physics and working in some fascinating research environments. Looking back, I feel my logical and analytical skills became well developed over these years, and yet I was searching for something more.

My interest was sparked following some personal therapy in my 30s, and I took an introductory evening course in counselling skills at the Norwich Centre, followed by a certificate-level qualification. It was not long before I developed a strong affinity with this way of being, and a growing awareness of its power as a force for change and growth in myself and others.

Eventually I made the leap, choosing to retrain as a person-centred therapist and initiating a major career change. I gained experience as a counsellor in a voluntary organisation, a student counselling service and private practice. I engaged with further training in person-centred relationship counselling, emotion-focused therapy, focusing and person-centred experiential counselling for depression. Further, I began research into various counselling scales and measurements and got involved in course facilitation as a tutor on a person-centred diploma.

All of this experience I found demanding, while also immensely rewarding and real. In late 2021, I joined the School of Education at the University of Nottingham as an assistant professor. As well as undertaking my own research, I am a facilitator on the MA in person-centred experiential counselling and psychotherapy and on a course in person-centred experiential counselling for depression (PCE-CfD). I feel I have found my direction and look forward to what comes next.

Robert Elliott

My interest in person-centred-experiential therapy grows out of a deep curiosity about other people's experience. My first psychotherapy training (in the 1970s) was in client-centred therapy from Jerry Goodman, a student of Carl Rogers. Goodman also encouraged my interest in therapy process research, and I began a 50-year exploration of clients' experiences of therapy. In spite of these interests, however, much of my professional training was psychodynamic, and I also received training in family therapy and early forms of cognitive therapy.

In 1977, I heard Laura Rice and Les Greenberg present their research at a conference. I immediately began incorporating experiential tasks into my work as a therapist. Thus, by the time I completed my PhD, I was an eclectic therapist who conceptualised clients in psychodynamic terms and preferred a combination of psychodynamic interpretation and experiential therapy tasks. In 1985, while on sabbatical in England, I decided to return to my humanistic therapy roots. I began working with Laura and Les to develop what became emotion-focused therapy. They brought the theory and the therapeutic experience, while

I was doing research testing out the new therapy with depressed clients, was an expert on clients' in-session experiences, and was good at organising ideas.

In 2006, I left American clinical psychology and moved to Scotland to teach counsellors. There I found myself for the first time in a solidly humanistic training environment and entered into a stimulating and fruitful dialogue with my more classically person-centred colleagues. After a stimulating and exciting 16 years teaching person-centred/experiential counselling, I retired in 2022, and subsequently moved permanently back to California.

Today, I maintain an active practice as an EFT supervisor and trainer. I continue to learn from my clients (who have always been my main teachers), and also from the discipline of trying to teach EFT in a clear, appealing manner. The things I enjoy most about EFT are the opportunities it provides for getting inside others' experiences, the combination of relational and task-focused elements, and the excitement of helping to develop something new.

Sheila Haugh

I am one of those people who, on reading Carl Rogers for the first time, found someone who was articulating 'stuff' I had been vaguely thinking and feeling but had not been able to put into words. To be honest, first off, his theories of personality development didn't really interest me much. I was completely taken by his ideas on how to be with people in a way that helped; how it might be okay to care about people (including clients and service users) and not be pathologised as the 'wounded healer' or 'over-involved'. After studying psychodynamic theory and practice for 18 months, I knew I had to find a different way to work with people.

Around that time Carl Rogers came to London speak at an event for youth workers. I wasn't able to go to that event, but through trying to join it, I came into contact with the facilitators from the Person-Centred Approach Institute (INT) and, to cut a longish story short, started my three-year, part-time, residential training with them. This programme involved visiting facilitators from the US, including Peggy Natiello, Nat Raskin, Jerold Bozarth and Valerie Henderson. Along with Irene Fairhurst and Chuck Devonshire, these people showed me a person-centred way of being that was unique to each of them. From Chuck Devonshire in particular, I found an excitement with theory as well as practice, each deeply informing the other. Having buried myself in person-centred theory and practice, I decided I also wanted (and needed) a bit more knowledge about other theories and approaches and undertook a master's in (integrative/existential) psychotherapy and counselling. The master's brought home to me how there are grains of truth in all approaches to therapy. For me, simply put, the grains of truth in person-centred theory and practice are the biggest.

I work as a person-centred therapist and facilitator and am currently Director of Studies for the Dip/MSc in contemporary person-centred psychotherapy and application at the Metanoia Institute, London. I have had the privilege to work across Central Eastern Europe on different trainings for person-centred therapists and to facilitate international encounter groups. The philosophy and values of the person-centred approach have always sat very easily with me – in theory – if not always without challenges in the practice of life.

Rosanne Knox

My interest in relational depth was initially sparked by my own experiences with clients and, indeed, with my therapist when a client myself. My interest deepened further while undertaking a research study on a separate topic; I found myself frequently being led back to the same thing – profound moments of deep connection – and I wanted to know more. It was Pete Sanders who guided me towards Glasgow, where I discovered that Dave Mearns and Mick Cooper were in the finishing stages of the first edition of *Working at Relational Depth in Counselling and Psychotherapy* (2005). It was, for me, one of those magical 'right place at the right time' moments, and soon I was embarking on research into clients' experiences of relational depth. I have encountered so many incredible people on my journey, with so many deeply moving and powerful stories to tell. At the core of them all has been the power of the therapeutic relationship, serving only to draw me deeper into my conviction that relational depth, as the articulation of a deep encounter between client and therapist, is a powerful element of the person-centred approach.

I have been working as a person-centred counsellor for about 20 years and have been training counsellors in the approach for 10 years.

I feel honoured to have been given the opportunity to contribute to the new edition of this important book, partly because it feels like a validation of all those years of research, but mostly because I feel that, for many clients, the power and depth of the relationship is an integral part of the therapeutic process. I am delighted that the mini-chapter in the previous edition has now been developed into a full chapter for the new edition, and I feel privileged to be in the company of fellow authors Gina, Mick and Steve.

- Mearns, D. & Cooper, M. (2005/2018). *Working at relational depth in counselling and psychotherapy.* Sage.

Tony Merry (1948–2004)

I was first introduced to Carl Rogers' work in the mid-1970s, and I subsequently trained in client-centred therapy from 1981 to 1984. I also had some contact with other therapeutic methods, including Gestalt and transactional analysis, and I had some quite extensive experience of various forms of group encounter, some of which I found helpful, some entertaining and some downright offensive. Meeting and working with Rogers towards the end of his life were very affirming experiences. It seemed to me that the close, empathic attention that Rogers both espoused and 'lived' was the most gently powerful factor in creating opportunities for positive change in both myself and in others. I became a follower of Rogers' approach, and later an advocate for it. However, I have never viewed person-centred therapy with anything other than a critical eye. I am, by nature, a sceptical person with a questioning outlook on life generally. I have a great desire to understand and to create my own 'sense' and meaning from what I read and experience, and I am not easily persuaded of any particular 'truth'. One of the most enduring things I learned from my undergraduate biological science training (which in most other respects was old-fashioned and alienating) was to question the nature of 'evidence' and to remain open-minded to the existence of other explanations and models.

In this sense, I don't regard my position as a 'classical' person-centred therapist as the correct position, and other positions as wrong. It is simply that, in my experience, understanding and individual meaning-making, this classical position is most consistent with what I observe in myself and others about how human relationships can most reliably become constructive and creative. In the 'classical' position, I see all the elements required to make psychotherapy effective. I see in it a deep respect for and trust in the positive potentials present within human persons, even though these potentials may have become so damaged that their recovery and expression are threatened sometimes, it seems, beyond endurance.

I see the classical position as attending to the whole person – with equal respect for content and process, feeling and thinking, and being and becoming. While I have certainly been influenced by the other models and approaches described in this book, I see much of what they say as being already present within the classical approach, either implicitly or explicitly. There are, of course, some divisions between us, some more obvious than others, but I don't see this book as representing a competition between the various approaches described here. How these divisions can be resolved, if indeed some of them can be, is a matter for each reader.

William R. Miller

I was trained in a behaviourally-oriented clinical programme that required a nine-month course in psychotherapy skills before learning and practising behaviour therapies. In our year, none of the clinical psychology faculty were available to teach the course, so they looked across campus to hire a counselling psychology faculty member to mentor us. She had been a student of Leona Tyler, and thus was an academic grandchild of Carl Rogers. The person-centred approach to which she introduced us fit me very well, as I was more naturally humanist than behaviourist. Over the course of pre-doctoral training, I developed a humanistic style for practising and teaching cognitive-behaviour therapies (CBT). Subsequently, at the University of New Mexico, I trained my own pre-doctoral clinical students in both person-centred and CBT approaches.

In an early randomised clinical trial treating people with alcohol use disorders, we observed the nine therapists for adherence to manual-guided CBT procedures and also for skilfulness in accurate empathy, as measured by the Truax and Carkhuff scale. The varieties of CBT methods that we studied made little difference in outcomes, whereas the therapist skill of accurate empathy accounted for two-thirds of clients' subsequent alcohol use. Clients treated by high-empathy counsellors drank significantly less, whereas clients of low-empathy therapists drank more than those in a self-help control condition. This mirrors the broader finding in treatment research that client outcomes are substantially more impacted by therapist skills than by specific treatment techniques or schools of psychotherapy.

My behavioural training also served me well. Therapeutic skills such as accurate empathy vary significantly and are not common to all therapists. These skills are specifiable, measurable and learnable, and predict client outcomes. Carl Rogers laid foundations for clinical science in psychology, documenting therapist skills that predict client outcomes. The same close observation of practice led to the development of motivational interviewing as a person-centred approach that is now being used in helping professions around the world, having been evaluated in more than 2,000 controlled clinical trials. Like person-centred therapies more generally, motivational interviewing began not with a pre-conceived theory but with careful observation of clinical practice and client outcomes.

- Miller, W.R. & Moyers, T.B. (2017). Motivational interviewing and the clinical science of Carl Rogers. *Journal of Consulting and Clinical Psychology, 85*(8), 757–766.
- Miller, W.R. (in press). The evolution of motivational interviewing. *Behavioural and Cognitive Psychotherapy.*

David Murphy

How did I come to be involved in person-centred counselling? Having left school in the mid-1980s at age 16, I became a roof slater. I had one O level in English and a CSE grade 1 in woodwork. I suppose I could say that I learnt about Rogers' theory of education and human development through experiences that were the antithesis of his approach. On the upside, that made it very easy to understand the theory when I finally read it! His description of the development of personality resonated so strongly, I could feel the words written on the page in my body. The theory fitted with my experiencing.

I became familiar with humanistic psychology and person-centred counselling in a more formal sense in 1993–96, when studying psychology. I had returned to education after nearly a decade in the building trade. After getting a degree in psychology, I completed four years of training in person-centred counselling, starting in 1999 at the University of Nottingham. I never left the university. What I valued most and oriented me towards the person-centred approach are the philosophical foundations: an absolute trust in the capacity of a person for self-direction, our capacity for knowing ourselves, our socially constructive nature and our innate tendency towards relationship as social beings. These ideas continue to resonate for me and act as guiding principles.

I have developed many interests in our field. I have a concern with understanding the relationship conditions for growth – something I still believe we know very little about. I am interested in how the person-centred approach applies across disciplinary fields. I am concerned that progress in the person-centred paradigm is limited by our collusion with the medical model and its role within the neoliberal regime. We are where we are because of what we do.

It is therefore an ironic twist that I am co-authoring a chapter on person-centred counselling as it is applied for people experiencing depression, in a healthcare setting, using a manualised form of therapy. All three of these things contrast with my position as a person-centred counsellor. However, it is through this work that I have come to the conclusion that person-centred counselling is a pedagogical rather than a healthcare practice: I see the counselling process as facilitating the reconstruction of experience, and I see the reconstruction of experience as a process of experiential learning.

Campbell Purton

I first learned about focusing around 1985, on my initial person-centred training course. I found it interesting but did not follow it up. Then, in 1994, at a person-centred and experiential psychotherapy conference in Gmunden, Austria, I was fascinated by a presentation about the work of the Japanese therapist Fujio Tomoda. Tomoda's work is little known in the West, but someone told me that there were similarities with focusing. I went along to some of the focusing presentations at the conference and knew that I had to learn more about this. I then did a focusing training course with Barbara McGavin and began to read Gendlin's work.

My original training, like Gendlin's, was in philosophy, and reading his work threw a whole new light on person-centred theory for me. I introduced more focusing-oriented material into our postgraduate counselling diploma course at the University of East Anglia and, with much help and support from Judy Moore, set up a diploma and MA course in focusing and experiential psychotherapy. Later I taught focusing-oriented therapy to students in China, where, as in Japan, there is considerable interest in the approach.

Since then, I have come to think in a new way about some of the basic focusing concepts. Some of this new thinking is included in the revised edition of my chapter in this book. I have tried to explain how it has come about that focusing-oriented therapy has often been seen as something different from person-centred therapy, although for Gendlin it was simply a continuation of Rogers' original 'client-centred therapy'. Looking back after nearly 40 years, I think now that it may have been a mistake to re-name client-centred therapy as 'person-centred therapy'. The original name catches precisely what was central to Rogers' approach, whereas 'person-centred' can mean different things to different people, as testified indeed by the present book. More importantly, I think it was a mistake to insist that therapists need to give up their own preferred modes of therapy if they are to be 'person-centred'. What both Rogers and Gendlin held was that being 'person-centred' is not a matter of the kind of procedures a therapist uses, but whether they use those procedures in a 'client-centred' way.

Focusing, in spite of being so simple, can be curiously difficult to learn, but as it becomes better appreciated, and people are helped by it (as I have been), I think that there will be an increasing interest in it. I hope my chapter can make some small contribution to this development within the person-centred approach.

Dee C. Ray

My road to person-centred work was twisty and unclear, mostly due to the need to work on my own unconditional positive self-regard. From my first course in counselling, I was attracted to the work of Carl Rogers, his view of human nature and his approach to counselling. Yet, something within me could not accept that humans could be trusted to know what they needed and how to work toward the betterment of self and others. In hindsight, this reluctance to embrace person-centred therapy was a reluctance to accept myself. I have spent many years deconstructing my early versions of self and learning to attune to my own organismic valuing process. I continue to do this work as an essential component of being a person-centred therapist.

Following years of study, practice and my own therapy, I re-read Rogers and it all started to make more sense. I had become disillusioned with the cognitive behavioural approaches, feeling that they were missing the essence and complexity of the ability to heal through relationship. As I embraced humanistic tenets and ways of working with adolescents and adults in my early career, I was taught that such less directive methods would never work with children because children needed more guidance and behavioural reinforcements. Stumbling upon child-centred play therapy in my doctoral programme brought clarity to my professional path. I say stumbled because it was never my intention to work with children. I had resigned myself to the conclusion that I would not be able to work with children because I was not a believer in behaviourism.

My introduction to child-centred play therapy was life-changing. In the study and practice of child-centred play therapy, I experienced the tenets of person-centred come to life. In working with children, I saw Rogers' 19 propositions come to life in real time. And I saw how the therapeutic relationship could provide the antidote to the conditions of worth being internalised at the very moments of development. I continue to see child-centred play therapy make a difference in children's lives on a daily basis as they engage in therapeutic relationships that provide strength toward a belief in their own worth and capabilities.

Siebrecht Vanhooren

I clearly remember my first encounter with the broad field of the person-centred approach in 1993. As young graduate students in the clinical psychology programme at Ghent University (Belgium), we had been introduced to many psychological theories and psychotherapies. All theories made a kind of sense, but I could not imagine working in such a fashion with clients. It all felt very distant and paternalising in one way or another. In the third year of the programme, we were introduced to experiential psychotherapy. I can recall that very first lecture, where Professor Dr Willemaers introduced us to the work of Carl Rogers. Something deeply resonated for me with this approach to therapy. Reading a chapter of *On Becoming a Person*, I recognised what I had been missing in the other approaches: a warmth, a humanity, and the sense that we are all just humans trying to make sense of our existence. It felt immediately as a kind of home-coming. I felt the same click with the work of Gendlin and focusing. This also felt very natural.

After graduating, I started working in mental health centres that were focused on working with victims of violence, and later I worked in forensic settings, while having a small private practice. In the midst of it, I took on a postgraduate training in 2001 in person-centred and experiential psychotherapy at the training centre Faculteit voor Mens en Samenleving (Belgium), led by Claude Missiaen at that time. Just as during my clinical psychology training and following the Belgian person-centred tradition, person-centred therapy was taught in a very integrative way, meaning that all person-centred 'tribes' were integrated in the training. I enjoyed learning about focusing-oriented, emotion-focused and existential therapy as well.

Following my path in life, and having been confronted with death anxiety from a young age and being sensitive to felt sensing and the spiritual, I continued my training in existential therapy with Mick Cooper (2006) and focusing-oriented therapy. I became involved in the International Focusing Institute from 2010, and more recently the Gendlin Center for Research in Experiential Philosophy and Psychology. My continuous search to integrate person-centred, focusing-oriented and experiential practices led to my current position as a professor at the university in Leuven (KU Leuven, Belgium) and co-authoring the chapter on existentially informed person-centred therapy in this book.

Dion Van Werde

I was 16 years old when I wrote down the word 'empathy' on my calendar at my small desk at home. I had run into that word, was intrigued by it, and was curious to understand what it exactly meant. This interest never went away…

I did a master's in psychology at the University of Leuven (Belgium), followed by a postgraduate specialisation in person-centred/experiential psychotherapy.

To get a feel of the person-centred world out there, I participated in a cross-cultural conference with Carl Rogers in Szeged, Hungary, in 1986, and later visited the Center for Studies of the Person in La Jolla, USA.

Participating in Garry Prouty's second European workshop in 1987 resonated so much with me that I decided to go study pre-therapy in Chicago. I became a pre-therapy staff fellow of the Chicago Counseling and Psychotherapy Center and was later designated a certified pre-therapy trainer.

During my stays in Chicago and during the numerous workshops Prouty did all over Europe, my initial understanding of person-centred therapy deepened. I witnessed Garry radically practise what I became to understand as the essence of Carl Rogers' work.

In 1989, Garry introduced me to Eugene Gendlin. In a workshop on focusing and dreams, Gendlin worked with a dream of mine – which we published in a joint article afterwards. The dreamwork further enhanced my understanding of the person-centred/experiential approach.

From 1985 on, I worked for 32 years in residential psychiatric care for people suffering psychotic experiencing. Translating Prouty's work into a multidisciplinary treatment milieu was my contribution to my mentor's legacy.

In 1995, Jill and Garry Prouty founded the Pre-Therapy International Network, which I have coordinated by myself ever since.

In 2018, I moved to Germany and worked for five years in the field of occupational rehabilitation. I worked with long-time unemployed people, often socially isolated and marginalised due to multiple problems. Visiting these people at home, and trying to connect and support them, deeply touched me. Again, as in pre-therapy, the focus of my endeavour was how to make contact with someone locked up in his/her idiosyncratic world.

I am now retired and work as an independent supervisor for individuals, small groups and teams, besides still being passionately involved in spreading the word about pre-therapy through workshops, lectures and publications and by coordinating the Pre-Therapy International Network.

Name index

Subject index

C

D